M

HIV/AIDS in U.S. Communities of Color

Valerie Stone • Bisola Ojikutu
M. Keith Rawlings • Kimberly Y. Simth
Editors

HIV/AIDS in U.S.
Communities of Color

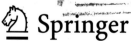 Springer

Editors

Valerie Stone
Harvard Medical School
Massachusetts General Hospital
Divisions of Infectious Diseases
and General Medicine
55 Fruit St., Boston MA 02114
Bulfinch 130, USA

Bisola Ojikutu
Harvard Medical School
Massachusetts General Hospital
Division of Infectious Diseases
Gray-Jackson 504
55 Fruit Street
Boston MA 02114
USA

M. Keith Rawlings
AIDS Arms Inc.,
Peabody Health Center
1906 Peabody St.
Dallas TX 75215
USA

Kimberly Y. Smith
Rush-Presbyterian-St. Luke's
Medical Center
Section of Infectious Diseases
600 S. Paulina St.
Chicago IL 60612, USA

ISBN 978-0-387-98151-2   e-ISBN 978-0-387-98152-9
DOI 10.1007/978-0-387-98152-9
Springer Dordrecht Heidelberg London New York

Library of Congress Control Number: 2009921801

Printed on acid-free paper

Springer is part of Springer Science + Business Media (www.springer.com)

Preface

From the onset of the HIV/AIDS epidemic, communities of color have been disproportionately affected. Yet with the passage of time, the face of HIV/AIDS in the U.S. has increasingly become that of a racial/ethnic minority. While most chronic diseases disproportionately impact racial/ethnic minorities in the U.S., HIV/AIDS leads the way. The disparities in incidence, prevalence, and death rates in blacks and Latinos are 3–10 times higher than those seen in the U.S. majority population, dwarfing the substantial disparities seen in cancer, cardiac disease, and even diabetes mellitus. Indeed, minorities now contribute to the majority of the HIV/AIDS epidemic in the U.S. in terms of numbers of persons living with HIV/AIDS, new diagnoses, and deaths due to HIV/AIDS.

Much has been written about HIV/AIDS, but what has been written about this disease in U.S. minorities has either been focused on only one area such as epidemiology or research challenges, or has been comprehensive but brief. The goal of this book is to provide a comprehensive guide to the HIV/AIDS epidemic among U.S. racial/minorities, including prevention strategies and clinical management of those living with HIV/AIDS. We hope to provide expert perspectives on how to approach the care of diverse minority populations with HIV/AIDS, many of whom may have other life challenges and often several other clinical conditions – ranging from Hepatitis C to depression or pregnancy. The intended audience for this text is broad, including clinical providers of all types, medical trainees, and mental health providers. In addition, we expect that many chapters will be useful to public health professionals and community health leaders and advocates. We hope that this resource will lead to better understanding of the needs of racial/ethnic minorities with HIV/AIDS and ultimately improved HIV care and outcomes in U.S. communities of color.

Boston, MA   Valerie E. Stone
Boston, MA   Bisola O. Ojikutu
Dallas, TX   M. Keith Rawlings
Chicago, IL   Kimberly Y. Smith

Contents

List of Contributors

Oluwatoyin Adeyemi, MD
Section of Infectious Disease, Rush University Medical Center, Chicago, IL

Arlene Bardequez, MD, MPH
University of Medicine and Dentistry of New Jersey, Newark, NJ

Loida Bonney, MD, MPH
Division of General Medicine, Emory University School of Medicine, Atlanta, GA

Christina Camp, PhD
Rollins School of Public Health (Emory), Atlanta, GA

Rafael Campo, MD
Division of Infectious Diseases, Adult HIV Service of Jackson Memorial Hospital, University of Miami School of Medicine, Miami, FL

Victoria Cargill, MD, MSc
Office of AIDS Research, National Institutes of Health, Bethesda, MD

Hannah Cooper, ScD
Rollins School of Public Health (Emory), Atlanta, GA

Carlos del Rio, MD
Emory University School of Medicine, Atlanta, GA

Ralph J. DiClemente, PhD
Rollins School of Public Health (Emory), Atlanta, GA

Jodie Dionne-Odom, MD
Infectious Disease Fellow, Emory University Medical School, Atlanta, GA

Kristin Dunkle, PhD
Rollins School of Public Health (Emory), Atlanta, GA

Kevin A. Fenton, MD, PhD
National Center for HIV/AIDS, Viral Hepatitis, STD, and TB Prevention,
Centers for Disease Control and Prevention, Atlanta, GA

Jamal Harris, MD
Center for AIDS Prevention Studies, University of California,
San Francisco, San Francisco, CA

Dionne Jones, PhD
Services Research Branch, Division of Epidemiology, Services & Prevention
Research, National Institute on Drug Abuse, Bethesda, MD

William King, MD, JD
Department of Psychiatry/Family Medicine UCLA, Los Angeles, CA

Claudia Martorell, MD, MPH, FACP
The Research Institute, Springfield, MA

Bisola O. Ojikutu, MD, MPH
Massachusetts General Hospital, Office of International Programs, Division of
AIDS, Harvard Medical School, Boston, MA

Deborah Parham, PhD, MSPH, RN
Health and Human Services Administration, Rockville, MD

M. Keith Rawlings, MD
Peabody Health Center, AIDS Arms Inc., Dallas, TX

George W. Roberts, PhD
Division of Partnerships and Strategic Alliances, Centers for Disease Control
and Prevention, Atlanta, GA

Kimberly Y. Smith, MD, MPH
Section of Infectious Diseases, Rush University Medical Center, Chicago, IL

Valerie E. Stone, MD, MPH
Harvard Medical School, Divisions of Infectious Diseases and General Internal
Medicine, Massachusetts General Hospital, Harvard Medical School, Boston, MA

Dina Strachan, MD, PC
Private Practice, New York, NY

Leo Wilton, PhD
Department of Human Development, College of Community and Public Affairs,
State University of New York at Binghamton, Binghamton, NY

Gina Wingood, ScD, MPH
Department of Behavioral Sciences and Health Education, Rollins School of Public
Health (Emory), Atlanta, GA

The Epidemiology, Prevention, and Control of HIV/AIDS Among African Americans

Victoria Cargill and Kevin A. Fenton

Introduction

Twenty-six years after five cases of *Pneumocystis carinii* pneumonia were reported in white gay men, the U.S. faces a mature AIDS epidemic.[1] An infectious disorder with profound morbidity and mortality, this epidemic rivals virtually every other infectious disease outbreak in human history – from its impact upon communities, social structures, and health care systems to the disruption of the fabric of daily life. While many gains have been made in the HIV/AIDS epidemic, from testing modalities to the diagnosis, care, and management of the HIV infection and its complications, these gains have not been realized uniformly. Disparities exist across race, gender, and socioeconomic status, and these disparities not only continue to drive the epidemic, but also the profound economic and human costs associated with it.

With the introduction of newer therapies, specifically protease inhibitors in 1995, and other classes of drugs, there has been a significant improvement in the quality of life and quantity of life. As a result, simply counting the number of AIDS cases in a region or municipality would not provide sufficient information about the trajectory of the epidemic, given the lag between HIV infection and progression to AIDS (as long as 10 years or more). Tracking the number of cases of HIV infection provides a more complete picture of the epidemic, yielding additional data about HIV-infected populations at all stages of HIV disease. Such data not only enhance local, state, and regional efforts to prevent HIV transmission, but also facilitate allocation of important resources for treatment services, and further assessment of the impact of a number of public health interventions.[2]

In 1994, the CDC implemented a uniform system for national, integrated HIV and AIDS surveillance. Initially, 25 states began submitting confidential name-based

V. Cargill (✉)
Office of AIDS Research, National Institutes of Health, 5635 Fishers Lane, Suite 4000, Bethesda, MD 20892, U.S.
E-mail: vc52x@nih.gov

V. Stone et al. (eds.), *HIV/AIDS in U.S. Communities of Color*.
DOI: 10.1007/978-0-387-98152-9_1, © Springer Science + Business Media, LLC 2009

derived data, and since 2001, data have been available from 33 states, which now include U.S.-dependent territories.[3] As of January 2008, 33 states and four U.S.-dependent territories utilize this national integrated HIV and AIDS surveillance system. From these data, a time-elapsed snapshot of the HIV/AIDS epidemic in the black community emerges. It is a picture of disparity, differential risk, unequal access to care, late presentation for care, and differential survival. In this chapter, we will present an overview of the HIV epidemic in African Americans, with specific attention to subgroups within the African American community exhibiting accelerating rates of HIV transmission. As will become apparent, there are significant differences in the rates of HIV transmission between whites and blacks – differences that will be highlighted and potential causes for these differences suggested. This picture of HIV infection over the 25-year history of the AIDS epidemic raises very important questions about the critical next steps to decrease transmission in African American communities.

Overview of the Epidemic in African Americans

Although the first cases of *Pneumocystic carinii* pneumonia were reported in white, homosexual men, HIV/AIDS has never been an exclusive disease of white gay males. From the earliest beginnings of the epidemic, HIV infection had occurred in black men, women, and children. In 1982, African Americans comprised 23% of the new AIDS cases reported, and yet constituted only 12% of the U.S. population.[4] During this time period, HIV/AIDS cases were on the rise at rates that were virtually logarithmic; the incidence of AIDS essentially doubled every 6 months between 1980 and 1982, with an average of five to six new AIDS case reports received by CDC each day.[5] This accelerating epidemic with its disproportionate impact of HIV/AIDS upon African Americans continued unabated, despite the introduction of protease inhibitors at the end of 1995.

The introduction of protease inhibitors, and thus potent combination antiretroviral therapy, to the HIV treatment armamentarium had early and significant effects; however, these effects did not quickly translate into increased survival with HIV infection or decreased transmission for blacks. In 2000, black non-Hispanic adolescents and adults of age 13–34 years accounted for the largest number of persons living with AIDS.[6] At the end of 2000, 3,22,796 persons were living with AIDS, nearly twice the number of those at the end of 1994. As the epidemic matured, so did the treatment regimens and options to manage HIV infection. The number of prevention interventions increased and the push for increased entry into care continued. Nevertheless, the epidemiology of HIV/AIDS continued to demonstrate that prevention and care interventions were not stemming the epidemic in blacks. The impact of the epidemic was widening as non-Hispanic blacks were an increasing proportion of the AIDS cases.

Between 1985 and 2004, blacks accounted for a steadily increasing proportion of the AIDS cases reported, increasing from 25% in 1985 to 49% in 2004 (Fig. 1).

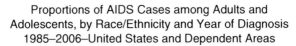

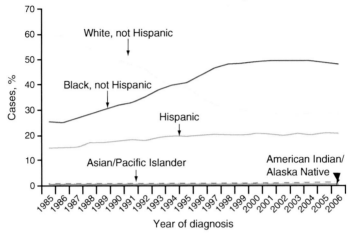

Fig. 1 Proportion of AIDS cases among adults and adolescents, by race and ethnicity – year of diagnosis: 1985–2006 in U.S. and dependent areas

During this same time period, blacks accounted for 12% of the U.S. population in 1985 and 13% of the U.S. population in 2004, confirming the significant over-representation in the reported AIDS cases. McQuillan et al. conducted an analysis of national household survey data from 1999 to 2002 demonstrating that 2.2% of African Americans in the U.S. tested positive for HIV infection, which is higher than any other population group. African Americans were also the only group for which the HIV prevalence had increased significantly over time.[7] As a result of this increased HIV prevalence among blacks, the 2004 AIDS case rate among black adults and adolescents per 1,00,000 population was over 10 times that among whites. The mortality of AIDS was greater in blacks, accounting for 55% of the 2002 AIDS deaths (Fig. 2). HIV became the third leading cause of death in African Americans of age 25–34 in 2002.[8] The surveillance data also revealed another interesting aspect of the epidemic among blacks, namely, that it was concentrated in specific geographic areas: the Northeast, the South, the Mid-Atlantic, and the West coast.

From 2001 to 2005, the estimated number of AIDS cases increased among all racial and ethnic groups including blacks. The number of people living with AIDS increased for both whites and blacks: an increase of 31% for blacks compared with that of 20% for whites. The number of AIDS deaths decreased for both whites and African Americans. Despite this decline in AIDS deaths, over one-third of persons diagnosed with HIV in the 33 states with confidential name-based reporting developed AIDS less than 12 months after the HIV diagnosis. This finding suggests late testing, which represents missed opportunities for prevention, management, and care interventions.

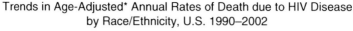

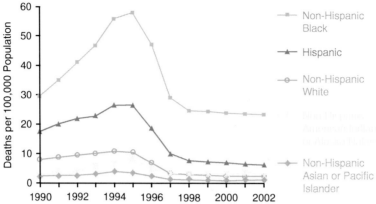

Fig. 2 Trends in age-adjusted annual rates of death due to HIV disease by race and ethnicity, U.S., 1990–2002

Dramatic increase in the numbers of a specific population infected with a management-intensive disease such as HIV infection has ramifications for the health care and other systems that support these individuals. Several studies during this time period demonstrated inequalities by race in access to care, quality of care, and delays in accessing care. The HIV Costs and Services Utilization Study (HCSUS) demonstrated that, despite the large increase in HIV/AIDS case numbers, African Americans had less access to care and lower quality care when compared with whites. While these differences waned as the epidemic continued, they did not completely abate.[9] Delays in accessing care that were attributable to race were well demonstrated by Turner et al.,[10] and differential receipt of antiretroviral therapy based on race has also been demonstrated.[11]

These differences in care and treatment have implications for the ensuing HIV epidemic among African Americans. Treatment with an appropriate antiretroviral therapy has the potential to decrease genital viral shedding, and hence reduce an individual's likelihood of transmitting HIV.[12, 13] Entry into comprehensive HIV health care provides opportunities for repeated exposure to important health messages for those living with HIV infection, including a review of safer drug and sexual practices to prevent further HIV transmission. Thus, if a heavily impacted population group is disproportionately delayed or unable to access health care services, and thus fails to receive effective antiretroviral treatment, then ongoing transmission of infection within that population group can be anticipated.

To fully appreciate the impact of HIV infection among African Americans, it is important to look closely at specific subpopulations, including women, men who have sex with men (MSM), and adolescents. While the epidemiology of HIV infection among African Americans presents a compelling story of disparities in disease impact and transmission, without examination of these subpopulations the picture is incomplete.

The Epidemic in Specific Subpopulations

HIV Infection Among Black Women

The disproportionate impact of HIV infection among black women has been long-standing. The number of reported AIDS cases among women in 1990 was 34% higher than that reported in 1989, and black women accounted for the majority of the AIDS cases among women. Of the HIV tests that returned positive in federally funded voluntary counseling and testing facilities during 1989 and 1990, the majority of the positive test results were among black and Hispanic women.[14] In 1999, women accounted for 18% of the AIDS cases, an increase of 11.3% from 1986. More of these cases were in the South, among black women and with an increasing number lacking an identified or reported risk.[15] Trends in HIV seroprevalence among women of childbearing potential continued to show a disproportionate burden of HIV infection among women of color, especially African American and Hispanic women. The highest rates were along the Atlantic coast, with the greatest proportion from the Northeast. However, the seroprevalence rates in the South eventually surpassed the rates in the Northeast, with African American women being disproportionately represented.[16]

This disparity in HIV infection among women was not limited to simply those living with HIV infection. In 2002, AIDS was the leading cause of death for African American women of age 25–34.[17] Between 1999 and 2004, more cases of HIV were reported for black women than for Hispanic or white women. HIV cases in black women exceeded by more than twofold the number of cases in their white counterparts.[18] Black women accounted for 13% of the U.S. population of women, but 64% of the *new* AIDS cases – almost five times greater than their representation in the population. Of all the AIDS cases among blacks in 2004, black women were 36% of the cases.[19] In 2004, death from HIV infection among black women of age 25–44 was 20 times higher than that among white women, and was the third leading cause of death in this age group in that time period.[18] Black women continue to account for the majority of new AIDS cases among women (Fig. 3).

HIV Infection Among Black MSM

HIV infection has disproportionately impacted black MSM since the early days of the AIDS epidemic. Too often MSM have been considered as a single category, when there are critical cultural, economic, and social differences between white and black MSM. From 1990 to 1999, the proportion of black MSM with AIDS almost doubled from 19% to 34% of the total MSM AIDS cases. However, these males were not exclusively sexually active with males, as 35% reported having a sexual contact with a female partner.[20]

With the introduction of highly active antiretroviral therapy (HAART), AIDS incidence declined among all MSM between 1996 and 1998 including black MSM. The AIDS incidence rates declined the least in black MSM, and remained the

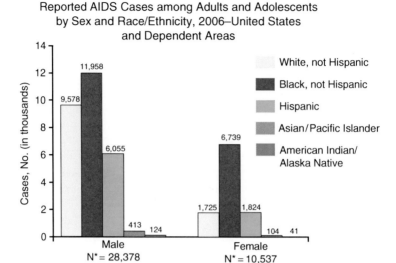

Fig. 3 Reported AIDS cases, by sex, race/ethnicity – 2006 in U.S. and dependent areas

highest for black MSM. Similarly, AIDS deaths declined for all MSM from 1996 to 1998, but the lowest rate of decline was among black MSM. For each year between 1996 and 1998, rates were higher for black MSM than for all other MSM despite these declines.[20]

HAART has decreased the morbidity and mortality of HIV infection; however, those gains can be offset by increases in high-risk behavior, or a significant increase in the number of HIV-infected persons. Between 2001 and 2004, among all age groups, HIV diagnosis rates were higher for black MSM than for white MSM. In 2004 alone, the HIV diagnosis rate per 1,00,000 for black MSM was five times higher than for white MSM, and these differences become even more pronounced when compared by age category. For black MSM of age 13–19 years, the HIV diagnosis rate was 19 times higher than that for white MSM of the same age (Fig. 4).[21]

Disease progression in the HAART era also shows a clear disparity between white and black MSM. Progression from HIV to AIDS within 3 years was more likely among black MSM than among white MSM. Similarly, death from AIDS was greater in black MSM than in whites. That is, black MSM were less likely to be living 3 years after an AIDS diagnosis compared with their white counterparts.[21] Disease progression, however, can be confounded by a number of characteristics of a population. These characteristics include advanced stage at the time of diagnosis, higher rates of other comorbid conditions associated with disease progression, late testing, and delayed presentation for care as well as decreased access to care. A recent study analyzed the data from five of 17 cities that participated in the National HIV Behavioral Surveillance (NHBS) system. Of the 1,767 men tested for HIV infection, 450 (25%) were found to be HIV infected, 64% of whom were blacks.

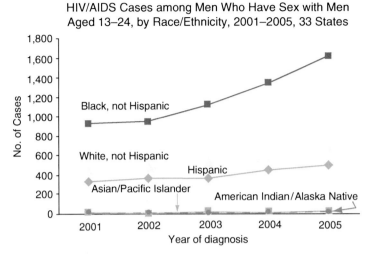

Fig. 4 HIV/AIDS cases among men who have sex with men aged 13–24, 2001–2005, 33 states

Of the 450 who tested positive, 217 (or 48%) were unaware of their HIV-positive status,[22] suggesting that lack of awareness of serostatus may also contribute to the disparity in disease progression between white and black MSM. Ironically, 92% had a prior HIV test, but most had not been tested in the prior year.

HIV Infection Among Black Adolescents

As noted with the other subpopulations, adolescents have consistently exhibited a disproportionate burden of HIV infection. This burden carries the toll of significant disease and early death to adolescents, especially black adolescents. Despite declines in risk behavior in general in the U.S., data continue to demonstrate high-risk behavior among adolescents and young adults of age 13–24, especially those who are racial and ethnic minority. In 2002, HIV/AIDS was a major cause of death for black males and females aged 15–24, ranking among the top ten causes of mortality in this age group.[23] On balance, between 1991 and 2001, the Youth Risk Behavior Survey demonstrated a decline in sexual debut rates, and a trend away from multiple sexual partners.[24] However, during this same time period, HIV infection rates among black adolescents continued to be high, in part driven by the high HIV prevalence rates among MSM and the impact of HIV upon heterosexual males and females in the South.[25,26]

At the end of 2003, almost one-third of the U.S. adolescents and young adults living with AIDS were between 13 and 19 years. Half of the cases occurred in males, and the predominant mode of exposure was perinatal. However, new AIDS diagnoses in 2003 demonstrated that ongoing HIV transmission was robust in black communities with the highest AIDS rates occurring in blacks for each of the age groups between 13 and 24 years (13–15, 15–19, and 19–24). These rates were highest in the South, followed by the Northeast.[23] HIV diagnoses from the 33 reporting surveillance areas revealed a slightly different picture; among those aged 13–15 years, the highest proportion of infections was among females, and the majority of these were black females. The majority of all HIV diagnoses in this age group were in blacks (78%). By age 15–19, the proportion of HIV diagnoses was nearly identical between males and females, with the highest proportion of the diagnoses again occurring in black individuals (71%).[23]

These statistics have broader ramifications. HIV and pregnancy have a great deal of overlap in black communities. While HIV infection disproportionately impacts black females, pregnancy disproportionately impacts black female teens as well. While black teens represent 16% of the U.S. population of teens in 2005, they were 69% of the new AIDS cases reported in teens in 2005.[27] Approximately 20% of non-Hispanic blacks give birth before the age of 20 years compared with 8% of non-Hispanic whites.[28] These findings underscore the extent of unprotected sexual activity, further supported by the high sexually transmitted infection rates in this population.

Disparities in HIV Infection Rates Between Whites and Blacks: Possible Causes

There are a number of reasons that HIV infection within African American communities is a serious health disparity. Exploring these reasons may provide clues for future interventions to control and dramatically reduce HIV transmission, as well as sexually transmitted infections in general. The root causes for these differences between HIV and STD transmission rates among whites and blacks stem from very basic and longstanding inequities between the two communities.

Poverty is a major driver of the many health disparities between whites and blacks, including HIV infection. Nowhere is this association clearer than in the southern U.S. where HIV infection rates have increased dramatically. HIV infection is increasing the fastest in the South, as demonstrated by having the highest number of (1) new AIDS cases, (2) new AIDS diagnoses, and (3) AIDS fatalities. The Deep South (historically defined as those Southern states that actively promoted slavery and whose agricultural and economic base was in cotton) has over one-third of the U.S. African American population, and all six of the states constituting the Deep South are included among the 15 states with the highest AIDS death rates. The Deep South also has the lowest rates of educational attainment and health insurance coverage, as well as higher rates of poverty and unemployment.[29]

Lack of educational attainment, unemployment and underemployment, incarceration, and limited or no health insurance all are products of poverty – the final common pathway that links socioeconomic status and HIV risk. Limited educational attainment also includes limited health education and health literacy, a factor infrequently considered as a contributor to the disparity between whites and blacks with respect to HIV infection and its outcomes.[30] Therefore, poverty commonly results in decreased access to prevention services, and delayed health care access. A direct relationship between poverty and rates of HIV infection has been well documented.[31,32] Level of educational attainment has even been found to correlate with the level of HIV risk behavior in African American injection drug users.[33]

Health insurance status is also a reflection of socioeconomic status, which in turn affects the ability to access quality health care, as well as when individuals enter care. Blacks with HIV/AIDS are more likely to have Medicaid or be uninsured compared with their white counterparts.[8] For example, in the Deep South, blacks are 1.5 times more likely to be without health insurance compared with whites, with about half of the blacks living at 200% below the poverty line.[29] Given this degree of poverty it is easy to envision competing subsistence demands, with the need for food, clothing, and housing leading to a postponement of care and ultimately lower access to care.[15]

Delayed entrance into care and limited access to care also have significant health related and associated economic consequences. Those who present for care with advanced HIV disease have poorer health status, as well as a greater risk of experiencing HIV treatment side effects, and a number of comorbid conditions that reflect advanced immunodeficiency. Patient analysis from the Canadian health system controlling for barriers to access and treatment clearly demonstrated that delayed presentation renders HIV care more costly.[34] Similar findings have been noted in the U.S.[35] Therefore, the economic burden of HIV is borne more heavily by racial and ethnic minorities. The productivity losses associated with HIV mortality were higher for blacks than for whites.[36]

Access to quality health care and treatment are not the only casualties of poverty. The ability to seek and obtain stable housing is negatively impacted by poverty, and the availability of quality stable housing is directly proportional to the income of the individual. Competing demands for food, housing, clothing, and other basic needs further complicate limited housing options, increasing the risk for unstable housing, marginal housing, and homelessness. Homelessness is associated with increased risk for HIV infection. Housing is clearly related to social and racial class, with racial and ethnic minorities disproportionately represented at the bottom of the income scales. Homelessness significantly impacts African Americans, as demonstrated in the 2004 survey of 27 cities by the U.S. Conference of Mayors; the homeless in that sample were 49% African Americans, 35% Caucasians, 13% Hispanics, 2% Native Americans, and 1% Asians.[37]

In Los Angeles, black and Hispanic low-income homeless women had two to five times the risk of their low-income housed counterparts of having multiple sexual partners in the past 6 months, increasing their risk of HIV infection.[38] Being homeless or marginally housed facilitates more pervasive risk behavior. Competing needs and limited financial resources place the individual in a web of escalating risks from survival sex (exchanging sex for shelter, food, money, and/or drugs), to drug use for self-medication, and introduction into social and sexual networks with a high prevalence of HIV infection.[39,40] This effect extends to those already engaged in high-risk behavior.

Salazar et al. have reported that homeless black men who inject drugs are more than twice as likely to engage in a number of high-risk behaviors, including needle sharing, unprotected sexual contact, and multiple sexual partners compared with their counterparts in stable housing.[41] Homelessness and unstable housing are also markers of other HIV-associated risks. Prevalence rates of childhood sexual abuse, intimate partner violence, physical abuse, and sexual abuse are all higher among homeless individuals. Such experiences are not only strongly associated with a risk of subsequent abuse and homelessness, but are also correlated with depressive symptoms and subsequent substance abuse.[42]

The impact of homelessness cannot be underestimated, as housing needs are a significant barrier to consistent HIV care. Lack of stable housing jeopardizes not only receipt of medical care but also adherence to therapeutic regimens,[42] thereby adversely affecting virtually any effort to prevent and/or manage HIV infection.[43] Given the comorbidities associated with unstable housing, including mental health disorders, substance abuse, prior physical, sexual, and/or emotional abuse, unstable housing is a marker for a complex interplay of conditions that fuel HIV transmission in African American communities.

Substance abuse is also related to homelessness, poverty, and race, and clearly elevates the risk of HIV infection and transmission for black men and women. Substance abuse increases HIV risk in a number of ways, including but not limited to (1) increasing risk behavior (unprotected sexual encounters, needle sharing), (2) disinhibition that accompanies an intoxicated state, thereby decreasing safer practices such as condom use, (3) exchanging sex for money and/or drugs, and (4) negatively impacting the immune system and/or enhancing viral replication.

Therefore, substance abuse contributes significantly to the heterosexual transmission of HIV infection among black men. Focus groups with low-income black men confirm that substance abuse affects risk behavior, and that prioritization of scarce resources may place procurement of drugs ahead of purchasing condoms.[44] Similarly in black women, substance abuse, especially crack cocaine was associated with high-risk sexual behavior. Early in the epidemic, crack cocaine was associated not only with HIV transmission, but also with other STIs such as syphilis.[45] This risk arises from both the impact of crack cocaine on high-risk behavior, especially unprotected sexual contact with multiple sexual partners, as well as an independent effect upon viral replication in peripheral mononuclear cells.[46] Furthermore, severe crack cocaine addiction was associated with unstable housing, depression, and profoundly limited economic resources. Substance abuse and the intersection of poverty and homelessness serve as powerful drivers of the HIV epidemic in African American communities.

Depression, conduct disorders, and substance abuse are associated with increased risk of HIV infection in adolescent girls.[47] In addition to an earlier sexual debut, sexually transmitted infections, unintended pregnancy, and multiple sexual partners are prevalent among black adolescent females.[47] While injection drug use may not be as prevalent, alcohol, marijuana, and crack cocaine are commonly used substances among adolescents, and all are associated with more sexual partners, more STIs, and less frequent condom use.[48] Predictors of high-risk sexual activity in urban low-income black female adolescents included older age and substance use (alcohol, marijuana, and cocaine). Black adolescents have less illicit drug use compared with their white counterparts, but higher risk when engaging in normative sexual behaviors compared with their white counterparts.[49,50]

In the last two decades, there has been a pronounced increase in the number of individuals incarcerated with a gross disproportion of these incarcerations occurring among black men, such that one out of three black males has been incarcerated. Between 1980 and 1995, drug offenders accounted for half of the growth in state prison populations and over 80% of the growth in federal prison populations. The number of white inmates incarcerated for drug offenses increased by over 300% between 1985 and 1995, but the number of black inmates incarcerated for drug offenses increased by over 700% in the same time period.[51] Furthermore, between 1980 and 1990, the female incarcerated population has tripled, and these rates have increased more rapidly among black women than among white women.[51] Prisons represent amplification centers in the HIV epidemic for the African American community. Although prison reporting is unreliable and many men will not report what occurs inside, incarceration represents exposure to increased HIV risk through drug use and sexual behaviors. Given the clandestine nature of the activities, and the often scarce resources to decrease the risk of the proscribed behavior, jails and prisons facilitate HIV transmission among inmates and back to the wider community upon release of HIV-infected inmates.

With such high rates of incarceration in the African American community, the ramifications for a community can be, and are profound. Several studies have suggested a direct association between high incarceration rates and other evidence of social disruption within a community – increased rates of STIs, teen pregnancy, and poverty.[52,53] The impact of incarceration upon communities is further effected through social networks and sexual bridging. Increasingly social networks are becoming appreciated as an avenue for exploring and deciphering the drivers of the HIV disparity between blacks and whites. A recent examination of the sexual and drug patterns of whites and non-Hispanic blacks using data from the National Longitudinal Study of Adolescent Health demonstrated that even when black young adults were engaging in normative behavior, their risk was high for acquiring HIV or other STIs.[50] Moreover, the density of sexual networks with sexual bridging to the general population plays a critical role in increasing heterosexual HIV infection among blacks.[54] This social network structure facilitates HIV infection by serving as a mediator of the many factors reviewed earlier: poverty, racial discrimination, and high rates of incarceration.[54]

Where to Go from Here?

From the beginning of the epidemic, strengthening HIV/AIDS prevention has been a key strategy for reducing the impact of this infection on the lives of Americans. The mission of the Centers for Disease Control and Prevention (CDC) has been to prevent HIV infection and reduce HIV-related illness and death. The agency funds programs that (1) help people learn their HIV status, (2) help high-risk HIV-negative persons avoid infection, (3) support prevention services for persons living with HIV infection and their partners, (4) link persons living with HIV infection to appropriate care and treatment services to reduce risk behaviors, prevent further transmission of new HIV infections, and decrease mother-to-child HIV transmission, and (5) help track the course of the epidemic and identify new and enhanced interventions. The CDC currently addresses HIV/AIDS prevention through a range of public health activities including monitoring disease impact, facilitating and supporting partnerships, implementing prevention programs, conducting intervention research and program evaluation, delivering technical assistance to build the capacity of organizations to offer prevention services, and developing policy and communications to support HIV prevention. These activities are conducted with a wide range of public- and private-sector partners, including state and local health departments, community-based organizations, and other nongovernmental organizations, universities, businesses, and the media.

A national HIV Prevention Strategic Plan was first developed by CDC in 2001 to guide the agency's efforts to more effectively address HIV infection and AIDS. The central focus of the plan was to reduce racial and ethnic disparities in HIV/AIDS.[55] The plan was updated further in 2007 to serve as CDC's strategic guide for HIV prevention through 2010, and includes a short-term goal of reducing new HIV infections by 5% per year, or at least by 10% by the end of 2010. To achieve this goal, the Extended Plan includes an expanded set of objectives and performance indicators that make priorities more explicit and ensure that key issues are effectively addressed. Specifically, new objectives were added and others modified to make more explicit the focus on African American and MSM communities, as well as to address advances in knowledge about the important role of acute HIV infection. Additional areas of emphasis included the role of incarceration in the HIV epidemic, technical advances in HIV rapid testing, and the priority of increasing HIV screening in medical care settings – all reflecting the recent data about racial disparities in knowledge of individual HIV serostatus, especially among MSM.

CDC's commitment to providing national leadership in reducing HIV/AIDS among African Americans culminated in the March 2007 launch of the Heightened National Response to HIV/AIDS initiative.[56] The Agency reiterated the severity of the HIV/AIDS crisis within the African American community and articulated the need for urgent, sustained, coordinated, intensified progress to be made in four areas: (1) intensifying efforts to make sure that prevention services reach those most in need, (2) promoting early diagnosis and treatment of HIV/AIDS, (3) ensuring effective risk-reduction interventions for African American populations, and (4) mobilizing African American communities to become more aware of HIV prevention strategies to preserve their health.

In addition to the CDC, other national organizations have created "call to action" documents that focus on the need for new activities, expanded resources, and increased action at local, state, and national levels. The National Alliance of State and Territorial AIDS Directors (NASTAD) released its report, "A turning point: Confronting HIV/AIDS in African American communities," in November 2005.[57]

The document provides recommendations in the areas of (1) strategic prioritization/resource allocation, (2) policy education, (3) research, (4) strategic collaboration, and (5) coalition and partnership building. The Black AIDS Institute (BAI) released its call to action, "AIDS in blackface: 25 Years of an epidemic," in June 2006.[58] This report focuses on developing a comprehensive and coordinated effort to address the epidemic among African Americans. Its recommendations encompass the issues of stigma, need for evidence-based programs, and efforts to educate and hold policy makers and other leaders accountable. In addition, the National Minority AIDS Council (NMAC) published its report, "African Americans, health disparities and HIV/AIDS," in November 2006.[59] The document stresses the importance of addressing underlying factors (previously discussed in this chapter) such as lack of housing, incarceration, and poverty that are associated with the HIV/AIDS epidemic among blacks.[64] Many of the recommendations contained in these reports are consistent with a socioecological model of the epidemic, reflecting the overarching strategies and specific activities of CDC's Heightened National Response action plan.

Expanding the Reach of Prevention Services

Looking ahead, it is imperative that greater coverage and penetration of effective HIV prevention services into communities of color is achieved. After nearly three decades, there remain substantial areas where greater coverage and scale-up of these interventions are needed and subpopulations that require intensification of prevention interventions. Expanding the reach of prevention services will require partnering with other organizations that provide related social and health services to African Americans (such as employment services, mental health, and housing) to increase the availability of HIV prevention information and services. Strategies aimed at facilitating and strengthening collaborative efforts among health departments, AIDS service organizations, local businesses, media outlets, and faith-based organizations to disseminate appropriate HIV prevention information and resource materials to African Americans must be prioritized. Similarly, sharing of technical assistance resources to build the capacities of AIDS service organizations to develop sound infrastructures that support effective program services for African Americans is essential. Finally, it will be important to ensure that HIV prevention programs serving African Americans are more effective at delivering culturally and contextually appropriate interventions and services to reduce the risks of transmitting or acquiring HIV.

Increasing Opportunities for Diagnosing and Treating HIV

HIV testing remains a major and important gateway for individuals to know their HIV status, receive appropriate care, and take steps to protect themselves and their partners from acquiring HIV. Although African Americans report higher rates of

HIV testing than other communities in the U.S., the high background prevalence within the community, coupled with bridging between risk groups, is likely to drive higher disease incidence. Consequently, more frequent and earlier testing may be required to get ahead of the curve. One strategy for improving access to HIV testing for all Americans is ensuring that HIV testing is made more routine, as recommended in CDC's 2006 revised recommendations on HIV testing.[60] Key opportunities for increasing HIV testing among African Americans will require increasing communication and health marketing efforts to spread the message that HIV testing and knowledge of one's HIV serostatus are important prevention interventions – interventions that individuals and communities are able to utilize. It will also be important to ensure that HIV testing is a regular part of health evaluations and screenings for all African Americans, in accordance with CDC's expanded testing initiative. Efforts should be made to increase access to HIV testing and treatment services by either offering these services or partnering with community organizations that offer these services to African Americans. Such places would include, but are not be limited to, emergency rooms, primary care practices, urgent care settings, and walk-in clinics. Finally, federal and state agencies must continue to work with community organizations to make HIV testing services available to African Americans in all settings that are appropriate.

Developing New, Effective Prevention Interventions

It is crucial that efforts are made to increase the range and cultural relevance of available prevention interventions for African Americans. CDC encourages all HIV prevention partners, including health departments and community-based organizations, to move toward better evidence-based practice. Identifying and selecting evidence-based HIV behavioral interventions for programmatic implementation are necessary, as well as guiding agencies delivering locally developed interventions on how to build their evidence for their local program (see later). Although substantial progress has been made to increase the number of proven effective interventions targeting African Americans, it remains a sad reality that relatively few were specifically developed for African Americans, and fewer still are available to meet the needs of African Americans at highest risk (e.g., MSM, MSM/IDUs, youth, and heterosexual men).[61]

Increasing the pool and involvement of African American investigators will be essential in developing HIV prevention interventions for African Americans. There also needs to be greater involvement of African American community stakeholders in developing and implementing research designs that address a range of issues related to accessing HIV prevention, treatment, and care. Finally, work with prisons, jails, and detention centers should be prioritized to develop behavioral-, social-, and system-level interventions to address the HIV prevention needs of incarcerated persons.

Mobilizing Broader Community Action

Mobilization efforts should ideally be geared toward ending the silence about AIDS, while increasing awareness of HIV/AIDS within and across all sectors of the African American community. Partnerships will need to be developed and strengthened with African American leaders with the explicit objectives of changing community perceptions and norms regarding HIV/AIDS, challenging the stigma associated with HIV/AIDS, motivating people to seek early HIV diagnosis and treatment, and encouraging healthy behaviors that prevent the spread of HIV. There remains a critical need for broader communication about HIV/AIDS in places where African Americans socialize, combined with partnering with civil society serving African Americans to assist them in linking their customers and clients to relevant prevention programs and HIV testing services. Other key needs and strategies might involve using mobilization to create community change by connecting HIV/AIDS prevention with efforts against the macrostructural forces that underlie the HIV crisis in African Americans: racism, homophobia, joblessness, sexual violence, homelessness, substance use, mental illness, and poverty. Finally, it will be essential to identify credible messengers, including health and other professionals, to conduct culturally appropriate presentations on epidemiologic data and preventive action strategies to raise awareness of HIV/AIDS and to encourage coalitions of local health departments, African American health providers, and community organizations to mobilize against HIV/AIDS.

Tackling Social Determinants of HIV/AIDS

The CDC's Heightened National Response Initiative focuses largely on strategies for influencing individual- and community-level determinants of HIV transmission. Behavioral change and targeted efforts are vitally important for managing the epidemic, and an expansion of such efforts will be required if the U.S. is to prevent the spread of the personal consequences of HIV/AIDS among African Americans as well as provide appropriate treatment and care to those living with HIV/AIDS. CDC recognizes that focusing upon only behavioral change may inadvertently reinforce the belief that HIV transmission is solely the result of personal shortcomings and group dynamics. A salient lesson from tobacco control or efforts to improve seatbelt use is that people do not change their behavior on the basis of an intellectual awareness of placing themselves at risk. This is particularly true for those most vulnerable to HIV infection. Individual-level interventions focused on behavioral modification, while essential in the short term, are not a long-term solution.

There are abundant data that HIV/AIDS in the U.S. is also a social justice issue, which will require a conceptualization of our society in which justice is achieved in all sectors of our society, rather than only in the administration of laws and statutes, or expanded access to medical services. A key aspect of this shift in focus will be understanding and tackling the social determinants of HIV/AIDS. These social determinants include the economic and social conditions in which people live and which subsequently affect their health. HIV/AIDS, like many other major diseases, is primarily determined by specific exposures to these conditions, and these conditions are a result of social, economic, and political forces. Without action on these social determinants of disease, communities in greatest need will continue to bear the brunt of this epidemic. Relying too heavily upon the health care system for strictly medical solutions for the HIV/AIDS epidemic in African Americans could diminish the overall population health by consuming resources that could otherwise be committed to efforts that will make a lasting difference. For many, addressing these upstream determinants of health may seem daunting, and clearly it will not fall within the purview of any single agency. Consequently, meaningful success will only be achieved by closer interagency collaboration in conjunction with a concerted effort in three main areas: (1) national leadership, (2) research and education, and (3) coordination and collaboration.

National Leadership

Committed, nonpartisan leadership at the highest levels in the African American community and in governments across the country is required to combat this devastating epidemic. This leadership must continue to be embedded within a public health approach to prevent and control HIV/AIDS in the U.S. and incorporate concepts of social justice. These efforts would include strategies to reduce the income and other inequalities evident in the U.S. (e.g., through taxation or employment initiatives), reduction of the high and disparate rates of incarceration, improved income security, enhanced access to health care, expanded access to comprehensive sexual health and relationship education in schools, special efforts to retain youth in the school system, and an increased public commitment to social housing. Societal efforts to address stigma and discrimination will be crucial – in particular, a commitment to ensure that discrimination is mitigated among those who are socially isolated or marginalized, especially due to illnesses, disability, sexual orientation, race, culture, or gender. Cooperation and coordination, research and education, and applying the lessons of population health must all be among these action steps as detailed later.

Research and Evidence Base

Building leadership, commitment, and a public consensus will require efforts that place HIV/AIDS epidemiology and prevention research for African Americans more clearly within a social determinants and social justice framework. Research is needed to provide robust evidence regarding the association between social determinants with HIV/AIDS outcomes for African Americans, to identify opportunities for promoting population health for African Americans within the different public sectors that can contribute to the improving social determinants, and to articulate the potential cost savings and public health benefits associated with a socioecological approach. National research institutions should be encouraged to commit to funding research in this arena and to ensure that the evidence base is continually reviewed, collated, and critiqued. Efforts will be required to help African American communities understand how a focus on tackling the social determinants of health can be transformed from a theoretical model into a practical reality. A best practices inventory of community initiatives that have incorporated this perspective into their daily activities may be a good beginning. Furthermore, the federal agencies, especially the CDC and National Institutes of Health (NIH) could jointly support investigators and research entities to enhance their ability to share their knowledge with a broader and more general audience. Much of the population health and epidemiologic evidence available today is not available to the communities from which the data were collected and whose support was and is required for pursuing a population health model.

Interagency Coordination and Collaboration

Partnerships must be built across all levels of government and between institutions, departments, and sectors if resources for health are to be harnessed and health impact accelerated. There currently exists a strong foundation for cooperation and coordination across agencies and jurisdictions. The CDC's 2010 HIV Prevention Strategy calls for greater collaboration and coordination across health and human service federal agencies.[62] Groups such as the President's Advisory Commission on HIV/AIDS (PACHA) have called for enhanced efforts across government departments within the context of a national planning framework.[63] Strategic partnerships such as these can be used to broaden the understanding of the public and population health approaches to HIV prevention and build a consensus around the need for tackling the social determinants of HIV/AIDS transmission. In building this commitment and consensus, it will be important to reach out to those departments and nongovernmental agencies that are not traditionally involved in developing social policy, for example, Treasury or Interior Departments and to include business coalitions and leaders. As we shift our focus to the social determinants of this epidemic, we can no longer regard HIV/AIDS among African Americans as a health issue alone, or as a moral issue, but as a legal, human rights, and health equity issue. Doing so will require leadership, commitment, and sustained effort to build social cohesion by addressing poverty, unemployment, illiteracy, inadequate housing, social isolation, violence, abuse, and racial discrimination. Without efforts to fundamentally improve community health and well-being through interagency collaboration and coordination, African Americans will continue to struggle with the manifestations rather than the root causes of the HIV/AIDS epidemic.

Summary

The HIV epidemic in African American communities is a reflection of a confluence of biomedical, economic, social, and historical factors. African American communities are disproportionately impacted by poverty and all of its attendant complications, including limited education, low health literacy, substance abuse, incarceration, sexually transmitted infections, unstable housing, and limited medical access and care. To decrease and ultimately stop the robust transmission of HIV in this community will require a multilevel, multidisciplinary approach that accounts for the social as well as the behavioral determinants of risk.

Given the disproportionate impact of HIV infection upon specific subpopulations within the African American community, especially women and MSM, potential biologic susceptibility must be explored, in addition to culturally and contextually appropriate prevention interventions. Most importantly, African American communities must recognize the profound threat that HIV infection poses and be prepared to respond to this crisis with partnerships that include community organizations, community leaders, policy makers, investigators, city and state health departments, and federal health agencies. Silence is the accelerant of the HIV brushfire, as ignorance and discrimination are the kindling.

The way forward will not be found in short-term interventions, but in a sustained commitment to address not only the superficial issues that HIV infection raises (HIV testing, access to quality HIV care, and modifying high-risk sexual/drug behavior), but also the root causes such as decades of economic, social, and political disenfranchisement that has blinded many to the full toll of this unchecked epidemic. HIV infection in African American communities has been a tale of deprivation, disparity, and denial. However, this need not become the status quo. An honest assessment of the response is needed, and the steps to meet this challenge can be the engine that drives the change that will make real inroads into the disparities that exist in many health outcomes for African Americans. HIV infection may be the prism through which a number of social injustices and inequities can be highlighted; however, the devastating impact of this infection upon the African American community requires that we move beyond observation to action at all levels and within all sectors. Effective community, academic, and federal partnerships are needed to limit and ultimately halt the ongoing transmission of HIV infection.

References

1. Gottlieb MS, Schanker HM, Fan PT, Saxon A, Weisman JD et al. Pneumocystis pneumonia – Los Angeles. MMWR Morb Mortal Wkly Rep 1981; 30: 250–2.
2. Centers for Disease Control and Prevention. Guidelines for national human immunodeficiency virus case surveillance, including monitoring for human immunodeficiency virus infection and acquired immunodeficiency syndrome. MMWR Recomm Rep 1999; 48(RR-13): 1–27, 29–31.
3. CDC. HIV/AIDS Surveillance Report 2005, Vol 17, Rev. ed. Atlanta: United States Department of Health and Human Services, CDC, 2007: 5.
4. CDC. Update on Kaposi's sarcoma and opportunistic infections in previously healthy persons – United States. MMWR Morb Mortal Wkly Rep 1982; 31(22): 294, 300–1.
5. Dowdle WR. The Epidemiology of AIDS. Public Health Rep 1983; 98(4): 308–12.
6. CDC. AIDS cases in adolescents and adults by age – United States, 1994–2000. HIV/AIDS Surveill Suppl Rep 2003; 9(1): 5–6.

7. McQuillan G et al. The Prevalence of HIV in the United States Household Population: The National Health and Nutrition Examination Surveys, 1988 to 2002, Abstract 166. 12th Conference on Retroviruses and Opportunistic Infections, Boston, MA, February 2005.
8. Kaiser Family Foundation. HIV Policy Fact Sheet: HIV and Black Americans. July 2007. Available at: http://www.kff.org/hivaids/upload/6089-04.pdf. Last accessed January 30, 2008.
9. Shapiro MF et al. Variations in the care of HIV-infected adults in the United States. JAMA 1999; 281(24): 2305–15.
10. Turner BJ, Cunningham WE, Duan N et al. Delayed medical care after diagnosis in a U.S. national probability sample of persons infected with HIV. Arch Int Med 2000; 160: 2614–22.
11. King WD, Wong MD, Shapiro MF et al. Does racial concordance between HIV-positive patients and their physicians affect the time to receipt of protease inhibitors? J Gen Intern Med 2004; 19(11): 1146–53.
12. Zhang H, Dornadula G, Beumont M, Livornese L Jr, Van Uitert B, Henning K, Pomerantz RJ. Human immunodeficiency virus type 1 in the semen of men receiving highly active antiretroviral therapy. N Engl J Med 1998; 339(25): 1803–9.
13. Graham SM, Holteb SE, Peshuf NM, Richardson BA, Panteleeff DD. Initiation of antiretroviral therapy leads to a rapid decline in cervical and vaginal HIV-1 shedding. AIDS 2007; 21: 501–7.
14. CDC. Current trends characteristics of, and HIV infection among, women served by publicly funded HIV counseling and testing services – United States, 1989–1990. MMWR Morb Mortal Wkly Rep 1991; 40(12): 195–6, 203–4.
15. Hader SL, Smith DK, Moore JS, Holmberg SD. HIV Infection in women in the United States: Status at the millennium. JAMA 2001; 285: 1186–92.
16. Davis SF, Rosen DH, Steinberg S, Wortley PM, Karon JM, Gwinn M. Trends in HIV prevalence among childbearing women in the United States, 1989–1994. J Acquir Immune Defic Syndr Hum Retrovirol 1998; 19(2): 158–64.
17. Anderson RN, Smith BL. Deaths: Leading causes for 2002. Natl Vital Stat Rep 2005; 53(17): 1–89.
18. McDavid K, Li J, Lee LM. Racial and ethnic disparities in HIV diagnoses for women in the United States. J Acquir Immune Defic Syndr 2006; 42(1): 101–7.
19. CDC. HIV/AIDS Surveillance Report, Vol. 16. Atlanta: United States Department of Health and Human Services, CDC, 2005.
20. Blair JM, Fleming PL, Karon JM. Trends in AIDS incidence and survival among racial/ethnic minority men who have sex with men, United States, 1990–1999. J Acquir Immune Defic Syndr 2002; 31(3): 339–47.
21. Hall HI, Byers RH, Ling Q, Espinoza L. Racial/ethnic and age disparities in HIV prevalence and disease progression among men who have sex with men in the United States. Am J Public Health 2007; 97(6): 1060–6.
22. CDC. HIV prevalence, unrecognized infection, and HIV testing among men who have sex with men – Five U.S. cities. MMWR Morb Mortal Wkly Rep 2005; 54: 597–601.
23. Rangel MC, Gavin L, Reed C, Fowler MG, Lee LM. Epidemiology of HIV and AIDS among adolescents and young adults in the United States. J Adolesc Health 2006; 39(2): 156–63.
24. CDC. Trends in sexual risk behaviors among high school students, United States, 1991–2001. MWWR Morb Mortal Wkly Rep 2002; 51(38): 856–9.
25. CDC. Cluster of HIV-infected adolescents and young adults – Mississippi, 1999. MMWR Morb Mortal Wkly Rep 1999; 49: 861–4.
26. CDC. HIV transmission among black college student and non-student men who have sex with men – North Carolina, 2003. MMWR Morb Mortal Wkly Rep 2004; 53: 731–4.
27. CDC. Slide set: HIV/AIDS surveillance in adolescents and young adults (through 2005). Available at: http://www.cdc.gov/hiv/topics/surveillance/resources/slides/adolescents/index.htm. Last accessed January 6, 2008.
28. Abma JC, Martinez GM, Mosher WD, Dawson BS. Teenagers in the United States: Sexual activity, contraceptive use, and childbearing, 2002. National Center for Health Statistics. Vital Health Stat 2004; 23: 1–48.

29. Reif S, Geonnotti BS, Whetten K. HIV infection and AIDS in the Deep South. Am J Public Health 2006; 96: 970–3.
30. Osborn CY, Paasche-Orlow M, David TC, Wolf MS. Health literacy – An overlooked factor in understanding HIV health disparities. Am J Prev Med 2007; 33(5): 374–8.
31. Diaz T, Chu S, Buehler J et al. Socioeconomic differences among people with AIDS: Results from a multistate surveillance project. Am J Prev Med 1994; 10: 217–22.
32. Karon JM, Fleming PL, Steketee RW, De Cock KM. HIV in the United States at the turn of the century: An epidemic in transition. Am J Public Health 2001; 91(7): 1060–8.
33. Hasnain M, Levy A, Mensah EK, Sinacore JM. Association of educational attainment with HIV risk in African American active injection drug users. AIDS Care 2007; 19(1): 87–91.
34. Krentz HB, Auld MC, Gill MJ. The high cost of medical care for patients who present late with HIV infection. HIV Med 2004; 5: 93–8.
35. Fleishman JA, Gebo KA, Reilly ED, Conviser R, Mathews WC, Korthuis PT. Hospital and outpatient health services utilization among HIV-infected adults in care 2000–2002. Med Care 2005; 43(9 Suppl): III-40–52.
36. Hutchinson AB, Farnham PG, Dean HD, Donatus U, del Rio C et al. The economic burden of HIV in the United States in the era of highly active antiretroviral therapy. J Acquir Immune Defic Syndr 2006; 43: 451–7.
37. National Coalition for the Homeless. Who is homeless: Fact sheet. August 2007. Available at: http://www.nationalhomeless.org. Last accessed June 23, 2008.
38. Wenzel SL, Tucker JS, Elliott MN, Hambarsoomians K. Sexual risk among impoverished women – Understanding the role of housing status. AIDS Behav 2007; 11(6 Suppl): 9–20.
39. Aidala AA, Sumartojo E. Why housing? AIDS Behav 2007; 11: S1–6.
40. Adimora A, Schoenbach VJ. Social context, sexual networks, and racial disparities in rates of sexually transmitted infections. J Infect Dis 2005; 191: S115–22.
41. Salazar LF, Crosby RA, Holtgrave DR, Head S, Hadsock B et al. Homelessness and HIV-associated risk behavior among African American men who inject drugs and reside in the urban south of the United States. AIDS Behav 2007; 11(6 Suppl): 70–7.
42. Henny KD, Kidder DP, Stall R, Wolistski RJ. Physical and sexual abuse among homeless and unstably housed adults living with HIV: Prevalence and associated risks. AIDS Behav 2007; 11: 842–53.
43. Aidala A, Lee G, Abramson DM, Messeri P, Siegler A. Housing need, housing assistance, and connection to HIV medical care. AIDS Behav 2007; 11: S101–15.
44. Essien EJ, Meshack AF, Peters RJ, Ogungbade GO, Osemene NI. Strategies to prevent HIV transmission among heterosexual African American men. BMC Public Health 2005; 5: 1–10.
45. Chirgwin K, DeHovitz JA, Dillon S, McCormack WM. HIV infection, genital ulcer disease and crack cocaine use among patients attending a clinic for sexually transmitted diseases. Am J Public Health 1991; 81: 1576–9.
46. Bagasra O, Pomerantz R. Human immunodeficiency virus type 1 replication in peripheral blood mononuclear cells in the presence of cocaine. J Infect Dis 1993; 168: 1157–64.
47. Bachanas PJ, Morris MK, Lewis-Gess JK, Sarett-Cuasay EJ, Flores AL et al. Psychological adjustment, substance use, HIV knowledge and risky sexual behavior in at-risk minority females. J Pediatr Psychol 2002; 27(4): 373–84.
48. Bachanas PJ, Morris MK, Lewis-Gess JK, Sarett-Cuasay EJ, Sirl K et al. Predictors of risky sexual behavior in African American adolescent girls: Implications for prevention interventions. J Pediatr Psychol 2002; 27(6): 519–30.
49. Golub A, Johnson BD. Variation in youthful risks of progression from alcohol and tobacco to marijuana and to hard drugs across generations. Am J Public Health 2001; 91(2): 225–32.
50. Hallfors D, Iritani BJ, Miller WC, Bauer DJ. Sexual and drug behavior patterns and HIV/STD racial disparities: The need for new directions. Am J Public Health 2007; 97: 125–32.
51. Blankenship KM, Smoyer AS, Bray SJ, Mattocks K. Black–white disparities in HIV/AIDS: The role of drug policy and the corrections system. J Health Care Poor Underserved 2005; 16(4 Suppl B): 140–56.
52. Thomas JC, Torrone E. Incarceration as forced migration: Effects on selected community health outcomes. Am J Public Health 2006; 96(10): 1762–5.

53. Thomas JC, Sampton I. Incarceration as a social force affecting STD rates. Rev Infect Dis 2005; 191: S55–60.

54. Adimora A, Schoenbach VJ, Doherty IA. HIV and African Americans in the southern United States: Sexual networks and social context. Sex Transm Dis 2006; 33(7): S39–S45.

55. CDC. The HIV prevention strategic plan: Extended through 2010 (extended plan). Available at: http://www.cdc.gov/hiv/resources/reports/psp/pdf/psp.pdf. Last accessed February 15, 2008.

56. Centers for Disease Control and Prevention. A heightened national response to the HIV/AIDS crisis among African Americans. Atlanta: U.S. Department of Health and Human Services, Centers for Disease Control and Prevention. March 2007. Available at: http://www.cdc.gov/hiv/topics/aa/resources/reports/pdf/heightenedresponse.pdf. Last accessed February 15, 2008.

57. National Alliance of State and Territorial AIDS Directors. A turning point: Confronting HIV/AIDS in African American communities. Available at: http://www.nastad.org/Docs/highlight/2006113_AA_Call2Action_120905_final.pdf. Last accessed February 15, 2008.

58. Black AIDS Institute. AIDS in blackface: 25 Years of an epidemic. Available at: http://www.blackaids.org/image_uploads/article202/.pdf. Last accessed February 15, 2008.

59. National Minority AIDS Council. African Americans, health disparities and HIV/AIDS: Recommendations for confronting the epidemic in black America. Available at: http://www.nmac.org. Last accessed February 15, 2008.

60. Branson BM, Handsfield HH, Lampe MA, Janssen RS, Taylor AW, Lyss SB, Clark JE, Centers for Disease Control and Prevention (CDC). Revised recommendations for HIV testing of adults, adolescents, and pregnant women in health-care settings. MMWR Recomm Rep 2006; 55(RR-14): 1–17.

61. See CDC. Updated compendium of evidence-based interventions. Available at: http://www.cdc.gov/hiv/topics/research/prs/evidence-based-interventions.htm. Last accessed February 15, 2008.

62. CDC. The HIV prevention strategic plan: Extended through 2010 (extended plan). Available at: http://www.cdc.gov/hiv/resources/reports/psp/pdf/psp.pdf. Last accessed February 15, 2008.

63. PACHA. Achieving and HIV/AIDS-free generation. Recommendations for a new American HIV strategy. Available at: http://www.pacha.gov/pdf/PACHArev113005.pdf. Last accessed February 15, 2008.

64. Wolitski RJ, Kidder DP, Fenton KA. HIV, homelessness, and public health: Critical issues and a call for increased action. AIDS Behav 2007; 11: S167–71.

HIV/AIDS and the Latino Populations in the U.S.: Epidemiology, Prevention, and Barriers to Care and Treatment

Claudia Martorell

Introduction

Latinos living in the U.S. are disproportionately affected by HIV/AIDS. Differences in immigration experiences, history, and cultural norms and expressions are common throughout Latino subpopulations and are definitive factors in shaping HIV-related knowledge and risk. In addition, socioeconomic and environmental factors have an impact on Latinos at risk for, or infected with, HIV/AIDS. By becoming aware of these factors and responding to them, providers can decrease current health care disparities.

This chapter will discuss the epidemiology, prevention, and barriers to HIV care and treatment found among diverse Latino populations in the U.S.

Diversity Among Latinos in the U.S.

Latinos are a group with varied and distinct ethnic characteristics, acculturation levels, migration patterns, and generational status. Occupational, demographic, and language profiles are also diverse amongst Latinos. These differences in historical, socioeconomic, and political factors may have direct health care status and delivery implications.

The Latino population is now the largest minority population in the U.S.[1] The most conservative estimates recognize that Latinos now comprise 13.2% of the U.S. population. The Latino population is primarily made up of those of Mexican descent (66.1%), followed by Central and South Americans (14.5%), Puerto Ricans (9%),

C. Martorell
The Research Institute, 780 Chestnut St, Suite 30, Springfield, MA 01107, U.S.
E-mail: ctmartorell@idresearchinstitute.com

V. Stone et al. (eds.), *HIV/AIDS in U.S. Communities of Color*.
DOI: 10.1007/978-0-387-98152-9_2, © Springer Science + Business Media, LLC 2009

Cubans (4%), and other Latinos (6.4%). Central and South Americans (Salvadorans, Guatemalans, and Colombians) are the fastest growing subpopulations.[1]

Latino ethnicity compromises a diverse background of indigenous, African, Anglo, European, Asian, and Middle Eastern descent. "Hispanic" is the official descriptive term adopted by the U.S. government in the 1970s. However, many Latinos believe that "Hispanic" does not credit the indigenous roots of Latin America, and hence do not feel accurately identified by the term. Additionally, several groups of non-Spanish-speaking indigenous groups from Latin America do not identify themselves as Latino or Hispanic (e.g., Brazilian immigrants who speak Portuguese).

Epidemiology of HIV/AIDS in Latino Populations

Overall, the number of AIDS cases diagnosed in the U.S. increased each year from 1986 to 1994. During the 1990s, medical advances led to a decline in the number of AIDS cases and death. However, AIDS cases among Latinos increased by 130% between 1993 and 2001, while whites experienced a 68% increase.[2]

The rate of new HIV infections amongst Latinos in the U.S. is rising faster than that amongst any other group.[3] From 1999 to 2002, rates of new infection among Latinos increased by 26.2%. In 2001, 19% of AIDS cases were among Latinos, who represented 13.2% of the population. Latinos also account for 19% of the new HIV infections that occur in U.S. each year.[4]

HIV/AIDS poses a serious threat to the Latino community. In 2005, HIV/AIDS was the fourth leading cause of death among Latino men and women aged 35–44.[5] Seventy percent of AIDS cases in 2005 were diagnosed in either black or Latino populations, according to the Center for Disease Control and Prevention (CDC). Of persons for whom AIDS was diagnosed during 2005, 49% were black (non-Latino), 28% were white (non-Latino), 21% were Hispanic, 1% were Asian/Pacific Islander, and less than 1% were American Indian/Alaska Native. The proportional distribution of AIDS diagnoses by races/ethnicities has changed since the beginning of the epidemic. The proportion of AIDS diagnoses among whites (non-Latino) has decreased; the proportion among non-Hispanic blacks and Latino has increased. The proportion of AIDS diagnoses among Asians/Pacific Islanders and American Indians/Alaska Natives has remained relatively constant, at approximately 1% of all diagnoses.[5] By the end of 2006, an estimated 80,690 Hispanics/Latinos with AIDS in the 50 states and the District of Columbia had died from AIDS-related complications.[5]

Latinos account for a disproportionate share of AIDS cases. As mentioned, Latinos comprise 13.2% of the U.S. population; yet, from 1981 through 2005, they accounted for 19% of the total number of AIDS cases reported to CDC. From 1981 through 2005, 19% of the women and 23% of the children reported as having AIDS were Hispanics.[5]

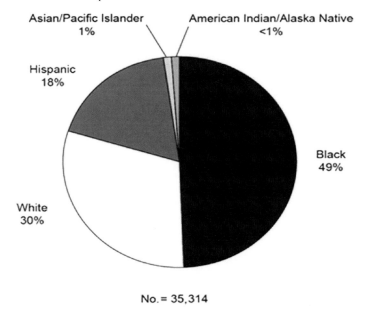

Asian/Pacific Islander 1%

American Indian/Alaska Native <1%

Hispanic 18%

White 30%

Black 49%

No. = 35,314

Fig. 1 Race/ethnicity of persons (including children) with HIV/AIDS diagnosed during 2006

In 2006, Latinos accounted for 18% of the 35,314 *new* HIV/AIDS diagnoses in 33 states (including children) (Fig. 1). Latinos accounted for 17% of the 491,727 persons (including children) living with HIV/AIDS in the 33 states.[5]

For Latino men living with HIV/AIDS, the most common methods of HIV transmission are (1) sexual contact with other men, (2) injection drug use (IDU), and (3) high-risk heterosexual contact. For Latina women living with HIV/AIDS, the most common methods of transmission were high-risk heterosexual contact and IDU.[5] Of the rates of AIDS diagnoses for adults and adolescents in all racial and ethnic groups, the second highest (after the rate for blacks) was the rate for Latinos.[5] Although Latinos made up only about 13.2% of the population of the U.S., they accounted for 16% of the estimated 9,82,498 AIDS cases diagnosed in the 50 states and the District of Columbia since the beginning of the epidemic (Table 1).[5]

Latinos with AIDS tend to be tested and diagnosed later and die more quickly (within 1 year of diagnosis) than whites.[3] AIDS cases among Latinos vary by place of birth. Latinos born in the U.S. accounted for 43% of AIDS cases reported among Latinos, followed by Latinos born in Puerto Rico (22%), and those born in Mexico (14%). Age-adjusted death rates per 1,00,000 population are 32.5 among mainland Puerto Ricans, 20 among the Commonwealth of Puerto Rico, 8 among Cubans, 4 among Mexicans, and 6 among other Latino groups.[2] AIDS case rates per 1,00,000 among Latinos are highest in the eastern part of the U.S., particularly in the northeast. Estimated AIDS prevalence among Latinos is clustered in a few states, with nine states and Puerto Rico accounting for 90% of Latinos estimated to be living with AIDS (New York, California, Florida, Texas, New Jersey, Pennsylvania, Massachusetts, Connecticut, and Illinois).[2]

Table 1 Estimated numbers of persons living with HIV/AIDS at the end of 2006, by race/ethnicity, sex, and transmission category – 33 states with confidential name-based HIV infection reporting

Transmission category	Hispanic %	Black, not Hispanic %	White, not Hispanic %
Male adult or adolescent			
Male-to-male sexual contact	57	49	77
Injection drug use	23	22	9
Male-to-male sexual contact and injection drug use	6	7	8
High-risk heterosexual contact[a]	14	22	5
Other[b]	1	1	1
Female adult or adolescent			
Injection drug use	28	23	33
High-risk heterosexual contact	71	75	65
Other[b]	2	2	2
Child (<13 years at diagnosis)			
Perinatal	92	93	84
Other[c]	8	7	16

[a] Heterosexual contact with a person known to have or to be at high risk for HIV infection
[b] Includes hemophilia, blood transfusion, perinatal exposure, and risk factor not reported or not identified
[c] Includes hemophilia, blood transfusion, and risk factor not reported or not identified

Risk Factors, Barriers to Care, and Prevention Challenges

Behavioral risk factors for HIV infection in Latinos differ by country of birth. Sexual contact with other men is the primary cause of HIV infection among Latino men born in Central or South America, Cuba, Mexico, and the U.S.[2] Latina women are also most likely to be infected with HIV as a result of sex with men.[2]

IDU continues to be a major HIV risk factor for Latinos.[2] Data suggest that Latinos born in Puerto Rico are more likely than other Latinos to contract HIV as a result of IDU or through high-risk heterosexual contact. Puerto Ricans were impacted early in the HIV epidemic secondary to high rates of IDU. Young Latinos are being introduced to IDU earlier in their lives throughout the U.S. and its territories. Both casual and chronic substance users are more likely to engage in risky sexual behaviors, such as unprotected sex, when they are under the influence of drugs or alcohol. Sharing needles when injecting drugs is a source of HIV risk for all ethnic groups. However, Latinos who inject drugs are at least one and a half times more likely than white injection drug users to be infected with HIV.[6] Data collected between 1996 and 1998 suggest that Latinos who inject drugs may be as much as four times as likely as whites to progress to AIDS, with the number of Latinos living with drug-related AIDS more than doubling between 1995 and 2000.[7]

Rates of sexually transmitted diseases, which can increase the chance of contracting HIV, are higher in Latinos. In 2006, the rate of chlamydia infection in

Latinos was about three times the rate in non-Hispanic whites, and the rate of both gonorrhea infection and syphilis for Latinos was about twice the rate noted among whites.[3]

Certain cultural beliefs may affect one's risk for HIV infection and one's choices regarding health care if infected. Clinicians who care for Latino patients must be aware of the fact that patients may be impacted by beliefs dissimilar to their own. Cultural and language barriers may impact the willingness of Latino patients to accept changes in their antiretroviral therapy regimen. According to an analysis of 289 participants in a multicenter observational trial, non-Latinos were almost three times as likely as Latino participants to be accepting their provider's recommendation to change antiretroviral therapy for such reasons as an increase in viral load, adverse drug effects, drug resistance, and declining CD4 values.[8]

Cultural beliefs, traditional gender roles, and sexual norms may become barriers to care for Latino patients infected with HIV. Deeply rooted religious beliefs and values have heavily shaped most Latino cultures. The traditional Latino family constellation is that of a heterosexual couple with children. Diversions from this lifestyle are perceived by some as a rejection of religious and cultural values. Individuals may delay or refuse treatment because of the advice and opinions of family members, thus demonstrating the importance of *familismo* (family) to the Latino patient. In some cases, a family member's advice and suggestions can be deemed more valuable to the patient than the advice and recommendations made by the heath care provider. It is common for Latinos to feel uncomfortable when asked to speak openly about sexual practices and condom use. Latino men and women have demonstrated negative attitudes toward the use of condoms due to their association with illness, sex work, and emotional distance.[9] Latinos are reported to have negative attitude about condoms and are less likely than other ethnic groups to believe than condoms protect against HIV.[10] Reasons that have been cited for refusal to use condoms among Latino males include decreased pleasure, loss of erection, time and discomfort related to their use, needing to use condoms only with promiscuous women, decreased *confianza* (trust), less intimacy, alcohol and drug use, and decreased spontaneity.

Gender differences may also play a role in the ability of Latinos to access health services and HIV prevention education. For women, embarrassment about discussing sexual matters may delay or prevent access to HIV preventive services. Childcare and responsibilities toward other family members may cause Latinas to deprioritize their own health. Latinas who attempt to convince their partners of safe sexual practices may fear suspicion of unfaithfulness. Latinas may also fear confrontation that could result in domestic violence.

For Latino men, issues such as *machismo* (virility, sexual prowess, bravery, independence, decision-making power) regarding self-sufficiency and distrust of medical treatment may delay access to preventive or treatment services.[11] Because of a sense of *machismo*, Latino males may perceive themselves as invulnerable to HIV infection and refuse to use protection, consent to HIV testing, and present for treatment. For example, among men, *machismo*, proving masculinity through power and dominance, can lead both straight and gay Hispanic/Latino men to engage in risky sexual behavior.

A commonly held belief among Latinos is that events are meant to happen to them because of fate, luck, or powers beyond their control. A sense of *fatalismo* (fatalism) may convince some Latinos that it is in their destiny to be afflicted with HIV/AIDS. Latinos are more likely than their white counterparts to think that chronic disease is determined by God, and therefore must be accepted and endured as a divine punishment for personal sins.[12]

Gender roles are well defined in the Latino population. *Marianismo*, a cultural concept in women, encompasses the qualities of chastity, virginity, abnegation, and sacredness; devotion to home and family; and self-sacrifice in the interests of the family. For some Latinas, admitting that their husbands may have infected them through infidelity could possibly be interpreted as domestic failure in their role as a wife.[13]

Latino men who have sex with men (MSM) are less likely than their white counterparts to disclose either their sexual orientation or HIV status to significant others, especially family members.[14] Homosexuality among Latinos has historically been viewed as negative and shameful. Latino men who are the inserting partner in homosexual anal intercourse may not identify this as a homosexual activity and may not self-identify as homosexual. Latino men who have sex with both women and men may identify themselves as heterosexual.[15]

Immigrated populations may not access screening, prevention, and/or treatment services for fear of deportation. The migration patterns, social structure, language barriers, and lack of regular health care among transient Latino immigrants can affect awareness and hinder access to HIV/AIDS prevention and care.

Other factors that contribute to delays in the presentation for HIV care for Latinos include poverty, unemployment, and limited access to healthcare coverage. More than 1 in 5 (21.9%) Latinos live in poverty.[4] Problems associated with poverty, including unemployment, a lack of formal education, inadequate health insurance, and limited access to high-quality health care, can increase the risk for HIV infection. Thirty percent of Latinos reported having no regular source of health care and identify inability to pay for care as a major obstacle.[16] Lack of formal education (43% of Latinos in U.S. over 25 years of age have not graduated from high school) and language (approximately one-third of Latinos in U.S. are monolingual Spanish-speaking) also limits health care access. These issues can increase the risk for HIV infection. Studies of Latinos have shown that many have inadequate health literacy, even in Spanish. For example, a four-city study of 3,260 new Medicare enrollees aged 65 or older found that 53.9% of Spanish-speaking respondents had inadequate or marginal health literacy in comparison to 33.9% of English-speaking respondents.[17] Nationwide, approximately 56% of Latinos are classified as functionally illiterate.[18] In a study of HIV-positive men and women, a significant correlation was found between years of education and health literacy, and between literacy and adherence.[19]

Research has suggested that a lack of accurate knowledge concerning HIV/AIDS may exist among Latinos.[20] Latinos seem more likely to believe myths about HIV transmission by casual contact, and less acculturated Latinos are more likely to have these beliefs.[21] Acculturation, or the level of familiarity with and incorporation of the American culture (e.g., one aspect of acculturation is English language preference), has been positively related to AIDS knowledge.[22] Many of these social, economic, and cultural barriers to care may lead to advanced disease at diagnosis and delayed presentation, which is common among Latino patients.[23] Delayed presentation results in disproportionately high numbers of AIDS cases amongst Latinos,[24] high baseline viral load, impaired immune status,[25] increased morbidity, hospitalization for opportunistic infections, and mortality.

It is important to note that the quality of the patient–provider relationship has been associated with treatment adherence in HIV-positive Latinos.[26] Racial disparities in access to effective antiretroviral therapy, including protease inhibitors or nonnucleoside reverse transcriptase inhibitors, were noted almost as soon as those agents became available. Blacks, Latinos, women, the uninsured, and patients receiving Medicaid all had less desirable patterns of care. While more recent data suggest that this disparity in access is beginning to wane, differences in access to care and willingness of prescribers to utilize particular antiretroviral drugs in certain populations are still unresolved issues.[27]

Prevention

It is important that greater coverage and penetration of effective HIV prevention services is achieved, particularly among disproportionately affected populations. HIV testing remains a major and important gateway for individuals to know their HIV status, receive appropriate care, and take steps to protect themselves and their partners from acquiring HIV. One strategy for improving access to HIV testing for all Americans is ensuring that HIV testing is made routine. In pursuit of this goal, CDC released *Revised Recommendations for HIV Testing of Adults, Adolescents, and Pregnant Women in Health-Care Settings in 2006*. These new recommendations advise routine HIV screening for adults, adolescents, and pregnant women in health care settings in the U.S. The CDC also conducts epidemiologic and behavioral research focused on Latinos, supports efforts to reduce the health disparities experienced in the communities at high risk for HIV infection, provides effective, scientifically based interventions to organizations serving Latinos and is tailoring other effective behavioral interventions to address the needs of Latinos who are at high risk for HIV infection. For these initiatives to be effective, partnerships will need to be developed and strengthened with Latino advocacy organizations and with Latino leadership with the explicit objectives of changing community perceptions and norms regarding HIV/AIDS, challenging the stigma associated with HIV/AIDS, motivating people to seek early HIV diagnosis and treatment, and encouraging healthy behaviors that prevent the spread of HIV.

Conclusion

According to the U.S. Census Bureau, by the year 2050, Latinos will represent over 25% of the U.S. population. The HIV/AIDS epidemic continues to be a major problem in the Latino community. It is essential for providers to recognize that Latinos present with a unique HIV risk profile. As the Latino population continues to experience an increase in HIV infection rates, immediate attention and resources must be allocated and targeted to better address the management of HIV/AIDS. Effective risk reduction efforts appear to be local, skill-based, and led by same race/ethnicity as the target population. Access to care and utilization of antiretroviral therapy must be improved. Adherence and patient trust are major issues for providers to overcome.

Effectively treating the Latino HIV/AIDS patient requires a commitment to culturally and linguistically competent care. Culturally and linguistically competent care will aid in the elimination of current health disparities and increase positive patient outcomes. While it is good to learn specifics about the Latino culture, providers should remember that the Latino population is very diverse. Providers must be cautious of stereotyping Latino patients. It is those providers who have embraced this diverse population who will best be known for their ability to affect the overall health of the U.S.

References

1. U.S. Census Bureau. Current Population Survey, PGR-4. 2001
2. U.S. Centers for Disease Control and Prevention (CDC). HIV/AIDS surveillance report. 2001; 13: 2, 1–44
3. U.S. Centers for Disease Control and Prevention (CDC). HIV/AIDS surveillance supplemental report. 2003; 9: 2
4. U.S. Centers for Disease Control and Prevention (CDC). HIV/AIDS update: a glance at the epidemic. 2002
5. U.S. Centers for Disease Control and Prevention (CDC). HIV/AIDS surveillance. Available at http://www.cdc.gov/hiv/topics/surveillance/resources/slides/index.htm. Accessed May 7, 2008
6. Centers for Disease Control and Prevention. National HIV serosurveillance summary results. 1992; 3: 19
7. Day D. The spread of drug-related AIDS and Hepatitis C among African Americans and Latinos. Princeton, NJ: The Dogwood Center. 2003
8. Campo RE, Narayanan S, Clay PG, Dehovitz J, Johnson D, Jordan W, Squires KE, Sajjan SG, and Markson LE. Factors influencing the acceptance of changes in antiretroviral therapy among HIV-1-infected patients. AIDS Patient Care STDS. 2007; 21: 329–338
9. Gomez CA and Marin BV. Gender, culture, and power. Barriers to HIV prevention strategies for women. J Sex Res 1996; 33: 355–362
10. Marin G and Gamba RJ. A new measurement of acculturation for Hispanics: the Bidimensional Acculturation Scale for Hispanics (BAS). Hisp J Behav Sci 1996; 18: 297–316
11. Morales S and Bigby JA (Eds.). Care for Latinos in cross-cultural medicine. Cross-cultural medicine. Philadelphia: American College of Physicians. 2003, pp. 61–95

12. Banquet CR and Hunter CP. Patterns in minorities and special populations. In: Greenwald P, Kramer B, and Weed DL (Eds.), Cancer Prevention and Control. New York: Marcel Decker, Inc. 1995, pp. 23–26

13. Shedlin M. An ethnographic approach to understanding HIV high-risk behaviors: Prostitution and drug abuse. In: Leukefeld CG and Battjes RJ (Eds.), AIDS and Intravenous Drug Use: Future Directions for Community-Based Prevention Research. Rockville, MD: National Institute on Drug Abuse. 1990, pp. 134–149

14. Mason RC, Marks G, Simoni JM, Ruiz MS, and Richardson JL. Culturally sanctioned secrets? Latino men's nondisclosure of HIV infection to family, friends, and lovers. Health Psychology 1995, 14:1, 6–12

15. Bigby J. Cross-Cultural Medicine. Philadelphia: American College of Physicians. 2002

16. Morales LS et al. Sociodemographic differences in access to care among Hispanic patients who are HIV infected in the United States. Am J Public Health 2004; 91: 7

17. Gazmararian JA, Baker DW, Williams MV, Parker RM, Scott TL, Green DC, et al. Health literacy among medicare enrollees in a managed care organization. JAMA 1999; 281: 545–551

18. Kirsh IS, Jungeblut A, Jenkins L, and Kilstad A. Adult literacy in America. A first look at the results of the National Adult Literacy Survey. U.S. Department of Education. Executive Summary. Publication No 065–000–005883. Washington DC. 1993

19. Kalichman SC, Ramachandran B, and Catz S. Adherence to combinations antiretrovirals therapies in HIV patients of low health literacy. J Gen Intern Med 1999; 14: 267–273

20. Scott SA, Jorgensen CM, and Suarez L. Concerns and dilemmas of Hispanics AIDDS information seekers: Spanish-speaking callers to CDC National AIDS hotline. Health Educ Behav 1998; 25: 501–516

21. Marin BV and Marin G. Effects of acculturation on knowledge of AIDS and HIV among Latinos. Hisp J Behav Sci 1990; 12: 110–121

22. London AS and Driscoll AK. Correlates of HIV/AIDS knowledge among U.S.-born and foreign-born Latinos in the United States. J Immigr Health 1999; 1: 195–205

23. Supplemental HIV Surveillance Study Project. Los Angeles County, Department of Health Services, January 2000

24. Turner et al. Delayed medical care after diagnosis of persons infected with HIV. Arch Intern Med 2000; 160: 2614–2622

25. Swindells S, Cobos DG, Lee N, Lien EA, Fitzgerald AP, Pauls JS, et al. Racial/ethnic differences in CD4 T cells count and viral load presentation for medical care and in follow-up after HIV-1 infection. AIDS 2002; 16: 1832–1834

26. Van Servellen G and Lombardi E. Supportive relationships and medication adherence in HIV-positive low-income Latino. West J Nurs Res 2005; 27: 1023–1039

27. Shapiro MF, Morton SC, McCaffrey DF, et al. Variations in the care of HIV-infected adults in the United States: results from the HIV cost and services utilization study. JAMA 1999; 281: 2305–2315

Antiretroviral Therapy and Communities of Color

Kimberly Smith and Rafael Campo

Introduction

The current HIV treatment guidelines from both the DHHS and IAS indicate that the best choices for first-line therapy include either efavirenz (EFV) or a ritonavir-boosted protease inhibitor combined with a fixed dose combination nucleoside backbone (Table 1).[1,2] These recommendations have evolved from a long list of clinical trials, which have shown these regimens to be very effective in suppressing HIV replication and allowing immune preservation/restoration in both the short and long term. There is little in the published literature to suggest that the treatment of choice for treatment-naïve patients should be determined by the patient's race or ethnic background. Several studies have examined the effect of race on treatment outcome with mixed results. Some studies have demonstrated that blacks (and in some cases Hispanics) have lower treatment response rates than whites while others have suggested comparable outcomes given comparable treatment access. This chapter will discuss the recommendations for initial therapy in HIV-infected individuals, review the literature on disparities in treatment response to HIV therapies, and discuss possible contributing factors that drive these disparities.

Recommended Initial Therapy for HIV-Infected Individuals

The current DHHS guidelines recommend initial antiretroviral therapy consist of a boosted protease inhibitor or efavirenz, each combined with a fixed-dose dual nucleoside analogue backbone.[1] The decision of which of these options to choose for an individual patient is dependent on multiple factors. In addition to understanding the

K. Smith (✉)
Section of Infectious Diseases, Rush University Medical Center, Chicago, IL
E-mail: ksmith2@rush.edu

V. Stone et al. (eds.), *HIV/AIDS in U.S. Communities of Color*.
DOI: 10.1007/978-0-387-98152-9_3, © Springer Science + Business Media, LLC 2009

Table 1 Recommended initial regimens for ARV-naïve patients, 2008

DHHS Guidelines "Preferred," Nov 2008[1]			
NNRTI-based regimen	EFV*		
PI-based regimen	ATV/r QD FPV/r BID LPVr BID LPV/r QD DRV/r QD	+	TDF/FTC
IAS-U.S. Guidelines "recommended," July 2008[2]			
NNRTI-based regimen	EFV		
PI-based regimen	LPV/r ATV/r FPV/r SQV/r DRV/r	+	TDF/FTC‡ ABC/3TC

*Except during first trimester of pregnancy or in women with high-pregnancy potential
**HLA B5701 negative
†Avoid in women with CD4+ cell count >250 cells/mm³
‡Or lamivudine
§Or emtricitabine
1. DHHS Guidelines. Available at: http://AIDSinfo.nih.gov
2. Hammer SM, et al. JAMA. 2008;300:555–570

characteristics of the various drugs and drug combinations, clinicians must consider many individual characteristics such as the patient's lifestyle (work schedule, housing and financial situation), co-morbid conditions and medications, reproductive plans and considerations (particularly for female patients) and patient preference when making the important decision about which drug combination best fits a particular patient.

Review of Preferred Options

Efavienz

EFV-based regimens are the most popular choice for treatment-naïve patients as a result of a plethora of studies that have shown these regimens to be both effective and durable. Moreover, while some regimens have demonstrated equivalence to EFV-based regimens, no other regimen has shown itself to be superior to an EFV-based regimen in any clinical trial to date. EFV has a long half-life, which allows for once-daily dosing, and it is a component of the first single pill fixed-dose combination regimen for HIV treatment.[3,4] This one pill per day regimen offers excellent convenience and simplicity, which enhances adherence, one of the most critical factors in HIV treatment success. Finally, the popularity of EFV-based regimens stems from their favorable tolerability in comparison to some of the boosted PI regimens that have often been associated with significant GI side effects, which can be an impediment to consistent adherence. Despite these attributes, EFV-based regimens may not be the best choice for all treatment-naïve patients. The long half-life of

EFV is an advantage that allows for once-daily dosing but it can pose a problem when EFV is combined with shorter half-life agents and missed doses occur. Following a missed dose, EFV can maintain therapeutic levels for extended periods (up to 21 days) while blood levels of other antiretroviral agents may quickly become subtherapeutic, thus leading to unintended EFV monotherapy.[5] Resistance to EFV can occur in the presence of only one mutation on the reverse transcriptase enzyme, thus it has a fairly low threshold to resistance.[3] As a consequence, individuals with poor adherence are at risk for selection of EFV-resistant virus strains, which can lead to failure of EFV-based regimens. Another factor that limits the use of EFV is tolerability. Although EFV is tolerated well by many patients, the most common side effect is CNS toxicity (dizziness, insomnia, vivid dreams), which can be observed in as many as 53% of patients in the first weeks to months of EFV treatment.[3] While this side effect typically resolves over time, it can be debilitating to some individuals. Further, the severity and frequency of the side effects may be higher in particular racial groups, as is discussed in greater detail later in this chapter.[6] Transmitted resistance to antiretroviral agents has been well documented over the past few years, and resistance to NNRTIs appears to be the most commonly observed type in a number of studies.[7,8] The presence of transmitted resistance to NNRTIs has been associated with significantly reduced response to NNRTI-based regimens, thus the DHHS guidelines recommend that baseline resistance testing be performed in all treatment-naïve patients prior to initiation of therapy.[1,9] In treatment settings where access to baseline resistance tests is limited, the effectiveness of NNRTI-based regimens may be compromised if a significant amount of transmitted NNRTI resistance is present in the population. Historically, transmitted resistance has been seen with less frequency in African American (AA) patients than in Caucasian patients.[10] This may reflect less treatment exposure in some AA communities early in the HAART era. However, as treatment access has become widespread it should be expected that transmitted resistance may also become more evenly distributed, thus the recommendation for baseline resistance testing should be followed in all treatment settings where possible. Finally, EFV has significant reproductive risk potential and is labeled pregnancy category D (avoid in pregnancy due to known risk in humans).[3] Neural tube malformations have been observed in monkeys and fetuses exposed to EFV during pregnancy.[3,11] The risk is greatest if exposure occurs during the first trimester of pregnancy. This limits the use of EFV not only in pregnant women but also in women of childbearing age who are sexually active and not using birth control and in women who desire to become pregnant in the near future. Clinicians must discuss this issue with women of childbearing age before starting therapy with EFV. In addition, women of childbearing potential who are on EFV should regularly be reminded of this reproductive risk in case their reproductive choices change. A review of the pro and cons of EFV-based therapy is summarized in Table 2.

Nevirapine is another NNRTI approved for use in treatment-naïve patients. It is listed as an alternative to EFV in the DHHS guidelines. The lower ranking of nevirapine results from several important factors. First, a large clinical trial comparing nevirapine to EFV in treatment-naïve patients found that significantly more subjects experienced treatment-limiting toxicity or virologic failure on nevirapine than on

Table 2 Efavirenz advantages and disadvantages

Efavirenz advantages
Low pill burden
Demonstrated potency in multiple clinical trials
Few metabolic effects
No known long-term side effects
Efavirenz disadvantages
Low resistance barrier
Cross-class resistance
Increasing frequency of transmitted resistance
Issues in pregnancy and women of childbearing age
CNS side effects
Rash

EFV.[12] Second, treatment with nevirapine has been associated with potentially life-threatening hypersensitivity and hepatotoxicity. The risk of this toxicity is associated with higher CD4 cell count at the start of therapy. Thus, nevirapine is contraindicated in women with pretreatment CD4 cell counts of 250 cells/mm^3 or higher and in men with pretreatment CD4 cell counts 400 cells/mm^3 or higher.[13] Nevirapine remains a reasonable option for individuals who meet these CD4 count criteria and who have contraindications or intolerance to the preferred agents for first-line therapy.

Boosted Protease Inhibitors

A "boosted" protease inhibitor (PI) is a protease inhibitor that is dosed in combination with ritonavir, a potent inhibitor of the cytochrome p-450 cyp3A4 enzyme.[14] Inhibition of the cytochrome p450 cyp3a4 enzyme allows the primary PI to be metabolized more slowly, allowing less frequent dosing and lower pill burden. Boosted PIs have been shown to be more effective and to have a higher threshold for development of resistance than unboosted PIs in multiple clinical trials, thus boosted PIs are preferred over unboosted PIs for initial therapy and therapy in treatment-experienced patients.[15–17] There are several strong arguments for using a boosted protease inhibitor as first-line therapy. Many clinical trials have demonstrated that boosted PI regimens are effective and durable and, in contrast to some of the early protease inhibitors, newer PIs are better tolerated, have once-daily dosing options and lower pill burden. Boosted PIs generally have a higher threshold to resistance since multiple mutations in the PI gene are necessary for high-level PI resistance.[18] Further, numerous trials have shown that most patients who experience virologic failure on boosted PI-based regimens have little or no primary PI resistance at the time of failure.[15, 17] As a result, boosted PI-based regimens may be more forgiving of imperfect adherence and less vulnerable in the presence of transmitted resistance. Clinicians have several options for boosted PIs from which to choose. Recent clinical trials have shown that various boosted PIs have comparable efficacy, therefore the decision of which boosted PI is best for an individual patient is often guided by the unique characteristics of that patient and the specific factors such as dosing interval, drug interactions, and side-effect profile of each agent.

Until recently, boosted lopinavir (LVP/r) was the only preferred boosted PI in the DHHS guidelines.[1] This agent has stood out due to its long history of efficacy and durability and its unique coformulation.[19] This is the only protease inhibitor in which ritonavir and a primary PI are coformulated into a single pill. All other boosted PIs require a prescription for the primary PI and a second prescription for ritonavir. This makes LPV/r regimens somewhat less complex and less vulnerable to selective nonadherence in which patients avoid the ritonavir portion of the regimen in an effort to avoid ritonavir-associated side effects.

A recent clinical trial, AACTG 5142, compared preferred agents for initial therapy LPV/r and EFV, both in combination with two nucleoside reverse transcriptase inhibitors in treatment-naïve patients. A third arm of that study examined LPV/r plus EFV without NRTIs. All the three arms performed well; however, the EFV-containing regimen was associated with a statistically greater proportion of patients achieving undetectable viral load (less than 50 copies/ml) compared with the LPV/r regimens.[16] The NNRTI-sparing (LPV/r + EFV) regimen performed similarly to the EFV-based regimen but was associated with more adverse events. LPV/r regimens were associated with statistically greater CD4 cell increases over the 96-week study, and subjects who failed with LPV/r regimens developed fewer resistance mutations than subjects who failed with EFV-based regimens.[20]

The current guidelines have added other boosted protease inhibitors as preferred initial therapy in addition to LPV/r or EFV. Atazanavir (boosted with ritonavir, ATV/r) was the first once daily boosted PI to be listed in the preferred boosted PI list.[1] This agent has become a popular choice due to its excellent tolerability profile and the convenience of once-daily dosing. The most common side effect associated with ATV/r is increased bilirubin, which results from interference with the conversion from indirect to direct bilirubin.[21] Most patients tolerate this laboratory abnormality without symptoms although a fraction (less than 5%) will experience jaundice or scleral icterus.[21] Importantly, atazanavir requires an acidic environment for adequate absorption, thus acid-reducing agents should be avoided or used with caution in patients on atazanavir.[21] A recent clinical trial compared ATV/r to LPV/r both in combination with tenofovir/emtricitabine in treatment-naïve patients.[22] The study arms were comparable statistically with 78% and 76% of subjects achieving HIV-1 viral load less than 50 copies/ml at week 48 on ATV/r and LPV/r, respectively. Subjects treated with ATV/r had statistically less triglyceride and total cholesterol elevations than LPV/r-treated subjects. CD4 count increases were similar between the two treatment groups.[22]

Fos-amprenavir (boosted with ritonavir, FPV/r) can be dosed once daily or twice daily in treatment-naïve patients; however, the twice-daily dosage is preferred in the DHHS guidelines.[1,23] Recent studies have shown the twice-daily dose of FPV/r to be comparable in efficacy and tolerability to LPV/r and the once-daily dose of FPV/r to be comparable to ATV/r.[24,25]

Table 3 Boosted protease inhibitor advantages and disadvantages

PI advantages
Demonstrated long-term efficacy
Potential immune benefit beyond antiviral effect
High barrier to resistance (boosted)
PI disadvantages
High pill burden
Lipid and metabolic abnormalities
Short-term side effects (GI)
Drug interactions

Another protease inhibitor, darunavir was approved by the FDA for treatment naïve HIV- infected patients in 2008.[26] This agent previously had proven quite effective for treatment experienced patients with resistence to other protease inhibitors.[27] Recent studies have shown it to be at least as effective as other boosted PIs in treatment naïve patients and it was recently added to the list of preferred boosted PIs in both the IAS-U.S. and DHHS treatment guidelines.[1,2,28] This agent is dosed once daily in treatment naïve patients and twice daily in treatment experienced patients. Overall it has been shown to be well tolerated with mild to moderate GI side effects as the most commonly associated side effect.[26]

Choosing a Nucleoside/Nucleotide Analogue Backbone

The recent update of the IAS-U.S. guidelines lists tenofovir plus emtricitabine fixed combination or abacavir plus lamivudine fixed dose combination as the preferred NRTI backbones for initial therapy.[2] The most recent update of the DHHS guidelines list tenofovir plus emtricitabine as the preferred NRTI backbone, with abacavir plus lamuvudine or zidovudine plus lamivudine as alternatives.[1] The decision of which of these agents is best suited for any given patient depends upon individual characteristics of that patient as well as tolerability and toxicities related to various agents. These preferred nucleoside backbone fixed dose combinations have been given preferred status due to their long history of solid efficacy and good tolerability in numerous clinical trials. The most common toxicity associated with tenofovir is nephrotoxicity and the most common abacavir associated toxicity is a hypersensitivity syndrome.[28,29]

Tenofovir and Nephrotoxicity

African American individuals are at high risk of developing chronic kidney disease in association with HIV infection; in fact, HIV-associated nephropathy (HIVAN) is the most common cause of chronic kidney disease in HIV-infected African-

Americans.[30] The incidence of chronic kidney disease severe enough to require renal transplantation is 1% per year, a figure ten times higher than it is for an age-matched African-American population.[30,31] Importantly, HIV-infected individuals with renal disease are at 2.5-fold higher risk of mortality than HIV-infected individuals with normal renal function.[32] Fortunately, the incidence of end stage renal disease due to HIV has declined in the HAART era, and numerous epidemiological surveys and case reports have shown that HAART reduces the incidence of disease progression to end stage renal disease in patients with HIVAN.[33] However, in addition to the beneficial effects of HAART, potential nephrotoxic effects of individual antiretroviral agents are well described. As mentioned earlier, tenofovir has nephrotoxicity among its potential side effects.[28] Several prospective clinical trials have reported a low incidence of renal disease associated with tenofovir; however, a number of case reports and cohort studies have described an association between the use of tenofovir and instances of renal toxicity.[34–36] In some cases African Americans have been shown to be at a greater risk for tenofovir-associated nephrotoxicity; however, this may result from the fact that African Americans are more likely than other racial groups to have pre-ART renal compromise related to HIV or other causes.[37] Baseline renal insufficiency, specifically creatinine clearance of less than 90, appears to be the greatest risk factor for tenofovir-associated declines in renal function.[36,37] Thus, while tenofovir is a preferred agent for many patients including African Americans, clinicians should be aware of the higher frequency of renal disease in AA and carefully evaluate patients for signs of subclinical renal disease (GFR <90, proteinuria, glucosuria) before initiating therapy. Tenofovir may be a reasonable option for some patients with renal disease; however, these patients may require dose adjustments and should be monitored closely.

Abacavir Hypersensitivity Reaction

Over the past few years the association of severe and sometimes fatal hypersensitivity reactions (HSR) with the use of abacavir has become well recognized. Early studies of this agent revealed that the incidence of HSR ranged from 5 to 9% in the overall patient population, but it was noted that African Americans experienced HSR at a lower rate.[29,38] One study examined a total of 5,332 patients exposed to abacavir in which 197 cases of hypersensitivity reaction were reported (3.7%). The multivariate model using all demographic data available indicated that the risk of hypersensitivity reaction among black patients (3% hypersensitivity reaction) was lower (OR = 0.59; 95% CI, 0.38–0.91) than that among other ethnic groups.[38] It has also become clear that there is a strong association between these reactions and the presence of the HLA-B*5701 major histocompatibility antigen.[39] HLA-B*5701 is most prevalent in Caucasian populations and quite rare in African-American or Hispanic populations, and this might be the explanation regarding why it is possible that suspected or confirmed abacavir HSR have been so rare among members of these two minority populations.[39] In fact, recent studies that have explored the usefulness of prospective HLA-B*5701 screening in order to prevent abacavir HSR have had logistical difficulties with African American and Hispanic patients due to the low prevalence of these reactions and the low carriage frequency of HLA-B*5701 in these populations.[40,41]

A recent study compared abacavir + lamivudine to tenofovir + emtricitabine both in combination with LPV/r dosed once daily.[42] The study found no significant difference in virologic efficacy between the treatment arms and both combinations were generally well tolerated. The incidence of abacavir HSR was low (<4%), and the incidence of tenofovir-associated renal toxicity was low (<1%). A recent ACTG study, A5202, compared tenofovir + emtricitabine to abacavir + lamivudine, each in combination with either ATV/r or EFV. Preliminary data from that study suggest a higher rate of virologic failure in abacavir-treated subjects with baseline viral loads higher than 100,000 copies/ml. Final results of this study will be available in 2009.[43]

Prior to the 2008 update, the fixed-dose combination of zidovudine plus lamivudine was among the preferred agents for initial therapy in treatment-naïve HIV-infected individuals, in the DHHS guidelines. Recent studies have shown that tenofovir + emtricitabine and abacavir + lamivudine-containing regimens are more efficacious and/or better tolerated than zidovudine + lamivudine-containing regimens, thus the fixed dose combination if zidovudine + lamivudine is now listed as an alternative option for treatment-naïve patients.[44,45]

The most recent update of the DHHS guidelines lists abacavir plus lamivudine as an alternative to the preferred tenofovir plus emtricitabine NRTI backbone. This move came as a result of new concerns regarding the possibility of an increased risk of myocardial infarction (MI) in patients with high cardiac risk factors who were treated with abacavir in two large observational cohort studies; and concerns regarding virologic potency of abacavir in patient with viral loads greater than 100,000 (as described above).[1,44,47] Thus far, no increased risk of MIs has been shown in large randomized trials in which abacavir has been compared to other NRTIs; and no clear mechanism to confirm an increased risk attributable to abacavir has been described.[48,49] Nonetheless clinicians should be aware of the potential risk of MIs in patients with increased cardiac risk factors who are treated with abacavir and counsel patients toward strategies to reduce risk which may include use of agents other than abacavir.

When to Start HAART

The United States Department of Human Health Services (DHHS) guidelines, perhaps the most commonly referenced, recommends that patients who are symptomatic and/or have CD4 cell counts <350 cells/mm^3 be treated with antiretroviral therapy (Table 4). Increasingly, some clinicians have begun to move toward earlier initiation of therapy as more long-term data from cohort studies have suggested significant lower progression to AIDS and/or death in HIV-infected individuals who start ART at higher CD4 cell counts.[46,47] In addition a number of studies have

Table 4 DHHS recommendations on when to initiate antiretroviral therapy, 2008

Clinical condition and/or CD4 count	Recommendations
History of AIDS-defining illness CD4 + count <200 cells/mm^3 CD4 + count 200–350 cells/mm^3 Pregnant women Persons With HIV-associated nephropathy Persons coinfected with hepatitis B virus (HBC), when HBC treatment is indicated (Treatment with fully suppressive antiviral drugs active against both HIV and HBV is recommended.)	Antiretroviral therapy should be initiated
Patients with CD4 + count >350 cells/mm^3 who do not meet any of the specific conditions listed earlier	The optimal time to initiate therapy is asymptomatic patients with CD4 + count >350 cells/mm^3 is not well defined. Patient scenarios and comorbidities should be taken into consideration

From Ref. 1

shown that the incidence of drug-related toxicities such as peripheral neuropathy and lipoatrophy is lower in individuals who start therapy with higher CD4 cell counts. Furthermore, the currently available agents for initial therapy have significantly improved efficacy and tolerability compared with early ART regimens, and thus the benefits of early ART now outweigh the risks in many patients.

The challenge for clinicians is that many patients present for care late in the course of HIV disease. This is particularly true of African Americans and Hispanics. A study by the Centers for Disease Control and Prevention (CDC) reported that 56% of "late testers," – those who were diagnosed with AIDS within 1 year of HIV diagnosis – were black.[48] McNaghten et al. evaluated data from 4,379 HIV-infected patients participating in the Adult and Adolescent Spectrum of HIV Disease project between 1996 and 2000 to determine at which point in their illnesses they initiated antiretroviral therapy.[49] They found that the proportion of patients initiating HAART late (i.e., CD4 + cell count <200 cells/mm^3) increased from 37% in 1997 to 46% in 2000. Hispanics and blacks were 1.74 and 1.65 times, respectively, more likely to initiate HAART later than whites ($P < 0.0001$). In an effort to reverse this trend, the CDC has released recommendations that HIV testing be increased in all clinical settings. Specifically, the recommendation is that screening for HIV infection should be performed routinely for all patients aged 13–64 in an "opt-out" manner. That is, patients should be informed that HIV testing would be done unless they request refuse testing. This is an important step forward and may help identify more HIV-infected individuals at earlier stages of disease, thus providing an opportunity for early treatment. Of course, broader testing does not address the other factors that may lead to late treatment in African Americans and Hispanics, such as poorer access to care, lack of health insurance, and language barriers. Nonetheless identifying HIV-infected individuals sooner should allow more individuals to benefit from treatment.

Race/Ethnicity Effect Cohort Studies

Anastos et al. published one of the largest studies investigating the effect of race on HIV treatment outcomes. They examined 961 women who were initiating HAART and found that white women were significantly more likely to have treatment response and less likely to experience virologic rebound or death following initiation of HAART than African American women. This difference appeared to be driven by higher rates of treatment discontinuation among AA women. When women who had discontinued therapy were excluded from the analysis the racial difference was no longer present. This of course leads to the question of what drives AA women to discontinue therapy at higher rates? The impact of depression was examined in this study and found to be significantly associated with treatment discontinuation. However, although there was a higher prevalence of depression among AA and Hispanic women, race was a stronger predictor with white women half as likely to discontinue ART in comparison to AA or Hispanic women independent of depression. They also examined adherence and found no difference in adherence between racial or ethnic groups in a representative subset of subjects. Other factors such as stable treatment access and treatment toxicity may also play a role in excess treatment discontinuation among AA and Hispanic women.

Investigators at the Johns Hopkins University HIV Clinic have examined risk factors for virologic failure in a large urban clinic at several time points in the era of highly active antiretroviral therapy.[50] Repeatedly, these examinations have found that nonwhite or African American race is a risk factor for virologic failure in univariate analyses. Race consistently became a less significant risk factor when controlling for missed clinic visits, lower CD4 cell counts, and injection drug use. In comparison, a Danish study examined the impact of nonwhite origin on the outcome of HAART over 500 HIV-infected patients and found no difference in treatment outcomes.[51] Seventy-eight percent of nonwhites and 76% of whites achieved a viral load <500 copies/ml after 1 year of treatment. Nonwhites included in this cohort were primarily black Africans from sub-Saharan Africa. It is notable that in Denmark treatment for HIV and access to health facilities is free and comparabe proportions (>90%) of whites and nonwhites in the cohort were receiving HAART. The authors concluded that it was this broad access to health care that allowed race/ethnicity to be a nonfactor in the treatment outcomes on the cohort.[51] Investigators in the U.S. Military's Tri-Service AIDS Clinical Consortium Natural History Study Group came to a similar conclusion.[52] This group examined disease progression in the pre- and post-HAART eras in 991 AA and 911 European Americans and found no statistical difference between blacks and whites. Again, the authors noted that in a clinical setting where access to treatment was free and universally available, treatment outcomes were comparable by race/ethnicity. A smaller study of a military cohort found that African-American race and presence of a mental health diagnosis were associated with a greater risk of virologic failure despite comparable access care.[53]

However, in the broader population of HIV-infected individuals in the U.S., access to care and use of antiretroviral therapy is significantly different when stratified by race and ethnic group. A large study of ten HIV primary care centers from across the U.S. analyzed the association between use of antiretroviral therapy in 2001 and a variety of demographic and clinical characteristics of 10,905 individuals.[54] The study found that previously identified factors such as age more than 40 years and male gender were associated with greater use of HAART by multivariate analysis. However, African Americans, compared with Caucasians or Hispanics, were less likely to receive HAART (adjusted odds ratio of 0.83) even after adjusting for outpatient utilization. Thus, even after being engaged in HIV care, African American individuals were less likely to be prescribed antiretroviral therapy by their providers than the two other ethnic groups. These findings were similar to the findings reported in older literature from the late 1990s.[55,56] Although this particular study did not analyze treatment response, it is certainly likely that that lower utilization of HAART would be associated with poorer overall outcomes.

These cohort studies offer a wide-angle view of treatment responses by race and overall indicate that in circumstances where "racial" differences are identified they often reflect "race" as a surrogate for socioeconomic status and treatment access rather than true differences between racial or ethnic groups. Cohort studies in general are less effective at identifying subtle differences in outcomes particularly when the variable producing the outcome is heterogeneous (i.e., responses to "antiretroviral therapy" vs. response to a specific regimen) Clinical trials allow more detailed examination of responses to specific agents and/or regimens and allow comparisons of outcomes given a specific input.

Race and Ethnicity Effects: Clinical Trials

Historically few clinical trials have effectively examined racial differences in treatment responses to specific agents or treatment regimens. This may reflect lower participation of racial minorities in early clinical trials of HIV treatments. However, more recently some investigators have begun to examine treatment response to specific regimens by race, and a number of important observations have been reported. A retrospective review comparing responses to antiretroviral therapy in blacks vs. whites revealed that the time to virologic failure on EFV-based therapy was significantly shorter in blacks than in whites [422 vs. 1,400 days, Cox proportional hazard risk ratio = 2.42 (95% CI, 1.35–4.57; $P = 0.0027$)], although there was no difference between racial groups with regard to the time to failure on nelfinavir.[57] This study raised the possibility of a racial difference in response to EFV, but the study had several limitations: it was a retrospective study with few subjects ($n = 99$), it was not randomized, and it did not assess adherence as a possible factor affecting outcomes. This study did note the presence of differences in cytochrome P450 CYP2D6 genotypes between blacks and whites but was unable to correlate these differences with outcome.

ACTG 5095 was a large multicentered randomized double blind placebo-controlled clinical trial sponsored by the AIDS clinical trials group that compared three treatment regimens: zidovudine + lamivudine + EFV (three drugs) vs. zidovudine + lamivudine + abacavir (3-NRTI) vs. zidovudine + lamivudine + abacavir + EFV (four drugs) in treatment-naïve HIV-infected subjects. Virologic failure was defined as confirmed HIV-1 RNA ≥ 200 copies/ml at week 16 on study. The **three NRTI arms of the study were halted prematurely due to poorer responses rates in comparison with treatment arms that included EFV.[58] The more intriguing finding, however, was that among the subjects treated with EFV, blacks were 67% more likely to experience virologic failure than whites. Self-reported adherence was assessed at weeks 4, 12, and 24. Overall, there was no significant difference in adherence between racial groups. A post hoc analysis further explored associations between race, virologic failure, adherence, and quality of life. Notably that analysis found that blacks who were found to be nonadherent (missing ≥ 1 dose in past 4 days) at week 12 were significantly more likely to experience virologic failure (53% nonadherents failed vs. 25% adherents: $P < 0.001$).[59] However, there was no difference in the failure rate for adherent vs. nonadherent whites at the same time point. Thus, nonadherence in blacks had a greater effect than nonadherence in whites. The explanation for this finding is unclear. It could reflect different patterns of nonadherence among blacks compared with whites with one pattern leading to lower drug levels and greater failure risk.

Findings from a substudy of ACTG 5095 may also contribute to our understanding. In this study, a clear relationship was shown between race and EFV clearance. Study subjects included 89 (57%) European-Americans, 50 (32%) African-Americans, and 15 (10%) Hispanics. The CYP2B6 T/T genotype at position 516 (Gln172His) was more common in African Americans (20%) than in European-Americans (3%), and it was associated with significantly greater EFV plasma exposure.[60] The median EFV AUC (area under the curve) according to G/G, G/T, and T/T genotypes was 44, 60, and 130 μg h/ml, respectively ($P<0.0001$). The CYP2B6 T/T genotype was also associated with more central nervous system symptoms at week 1. Black and Hispanic HIV-infected persons had lower clearance rates of EFV (and therefore higher concentrations) than did whites. There was also a relationship between discontinuation of EFV and decreasing clearance rates (and, again, higher EFV concentration).[6] Thus, blacks were more likely to experience higher EFV blood levels, which may have led to more CNS toxicity. Could this lead to variable adherence or more frequent treatment discontinuation? The answer to this question is unknown, but it is clear that differences in drug metabolism could contribute to variations in treatment toxicity and as a result differences in treatment discontinuation and failure. Investigators at Moore Clinic at

John Hopkins examined racial differences in EFV discontinuation in a clinical practice setting.[61] In this study African Americans were twice as likely to discontinue an EFV-based ART regimen in the first year of therapy compared with non-Hispanic whites. However, there was no difference in the rate of discontinuation of ritonavir boosted PI regimens between NHW and AA in the control arm of this study. In contrast to this finding a recent study, ACTG a5142, prospectively compared EFV-based regimens to lopinavir/ritonavir-based regimens in treatment-naïve HIV-infected individuals. A third arm of this study compared a nucleoside-sparing regimen containing lopinavir/ritonavir and EFV to the two more standard regimens. The study found that blacks were 36% more likely to experience virologic failure than whites.[20] There was, however, no difference in response based upon treatment group, thus blacks responded similarly to EFV or lopinavir or the combination of both. The disparity in treatment response overall is concerning and thus far, not well understood.

Combined, these studies illustrate the clinical importance of some subtle differences in drug metabolism and underscore the need for diversity in clinical trial enrollment. It is important to note that genetic differences in metabolism may be relevant to many drugs other than EFV. Several studies have demonstrated differences in cytochrome P450 CYP2D6 and CYP3A4 activity and genetic polymorphisms in blacks compared with whites.[62,63] Studies have shown differences in multidrug resistance gene (MDR1 P-glycoprotein) polymorphisms in blacks compared with whites.[64–66] The clinical relevance of these differences has been suggested by studies showing racial differences between blacks and whites with regard to bioavailability and clearance of drugs, such as cyclosporine, fexofenadine, digoxin, and midazolam.[67,68] Considering the importance of these drug transporter and metabolic enzymes in drug metabolism in general and antiretroviral agents in particular, further investigation into the potential impact of cytochrome P450 and P-glycoprotein polymorphisms on antiretroviral treatment responses is needed.

Newer Agents

Over the past year, several new agents have been approved by the FDA for treatment of HIV disease. Frequently, the initial studies of new agents are performed primarily in treatment-experienced patients since these patients have the greatest need for new drugs to which they are not resistant. Historically many of the trials with treatment-experienced patients have lower enrollment of women and minorities, thus new agents are often approved with little data on women and minorities. While genetic differences in drug metabolism among racial groups have been described as a potentially effecting drug efficacy and tolerability less is known about the impact of genetic differences on the effectiveness of drugs that target host factors. Maraviroc, the first CCR5 inhibitor approved for treatment of HIV disease, is an agent that blocks the CCR5 coreceptor, thus interfering with the entry of the virus into the cell.[69] The CCR5 coreceptor is known to be vital to HIV entry, and genetic variation in CCR5 has been shown to influence HIV-1 transmission *and* disease progression. A 32-base pair (bp) deletion mutation in the beta-chemokine receptor *CCR5* gene has been associated with resistance to human immunodeficiency virus type 1 (HIV-1) infection and disease.[70,71] Large-scale studies conducted among Caucasians indicate that individuals who are homozygous for this deletion mutation (D32/D32) are protected against HIV-1 infection despite multiple high-risk exposures, whereas CCR5/D32 heterozygotes have a slower progression to acquired immunodeficiency syndrome (AIDS).[72] Prevalence of the Δ32 mutation varies among different racial groups. It is most common in whites, in whom the *Δ32 gene* frequency ranges from 4 to 16%, with roughly 20% of Caucasians found to be heterozygous for the Δ32 deletion and 1% homozygous for the deletion. The mutation is less common in African Americans and Hispanics.[73–75] Although there are significant differences in the distribution of the CCR5 D32 deletion among racial groups it is not clear that this will effect the efficacy of CCR5 inhibitors is different racial groups. CXCR4-trophic viruses are known to be capable of utilizing the CXCR4 coreceptor for viral entry and have been associated with more rapid disease progression.[76] Viruses that are X4 trophic are not suppressed CCR5 inhibitors. Are there racial differences in the frequency of CCR5-trophic viruses vs. CXCR4-trophic viruses by racial group? A recent ACTG study analyzed HIV-infected subjects who screened for participation in a study of an investigational CCR5 inhibitor involving treatment-experienced subjects.[77] Half of the subjects who screened for the study had R5-trophic virus; 46% of subjects had dual-trophic or mixed-trophic virus and 4% had X4-trophic virus. Of note, blacks were 70% more likely to have dual- or mixed-trophic virus than whites. Hispanic patients were comparable to whites. It is possible that some of the differences could have been driven from other factors such as CD4 cell count and duration of HIV infection; however, this information was not included in the publication. Further investigation into this finding is warranted.

The other new class of antiretroviral agents is the integrase inhibitor. Thus far, one agent in this class, raltegravir, has been FDA approved.[78] Raltegravir is metabolized primarily via UDP-glucuronosyltransferase 1 (UGT 1A1). Racial differences in the frequency of polymorphisms in the gene that encode for this enzyme have been described; however, it is unclear if these differences specifically impact the metabolism of this agent and no information has been published to date regarding treatment response by race to this agent.[79] Importantly the FDA has increasingly demanded that pharmaceutical companies provide data on use of new agents in women and minorities, thus more information in this area should become available in the near future.

Conclusion

Given many effective choices for initial HAART, we must individualize therapy based on the characteristics of each patient and the characteristics of each agent in the regimen. A good understanding of the patient's challenges, needs, and desires combined with detailed knowledge of a drug's attributes and liabilities is the foundation for making a good choice for initial therapy. There is little in the published literature to suggest that the treatment of choice for treatment-naïve patients should be determined by the patient's race or ethnic background. However, it is important to prioritize the inclusion of minorities and women in clinical trials in order to allow the research to remain relevant and applicable to all HIV-infected individuals.

References

1. Panel on Antiretroviral Guidelines for Adults and Adolescents. Guidelines for the use of antiretroviral agents in HIV-1-infected adults and adolescents. Department of Health and Human Services. November 3, 2008; 1–146. Available at http://www.aidsinfo.nih.gov/ContentFiles/AdultandAdolescentGL.pdf. Accessed April 2009.
2. Hammer SM, Eron JJ, Jr, Reiss P, et al. Antiretroviral treatment of adult HIV infection: 2008 recommendations of the International AIDS Society – U.S. Panel. JAMA 2008; 300(5):555–570.
3. Sustiva (efavirenz)[package insert]. Princeton NJ. Bristol Myers Squibb. March 2008.
4. Atripla (Efavirenz/tenofovir/emtricitabine) [package insert]. © 2006 Bristol-Myers Squibb & Gilead Sciences, LLC.
5. Taylor S, Allen S, Fidler S, White D, Gibbons S, Fox J, Clarke J, Weber J, Cane P, Wade A, Smit E, Back D. Stop Study: After discontinuation of efavirenz, plasma concentrations may persist for 2 weeks or longer. Program Abstr Conf Retrovir Oppor Infect 11th 2004 San Franc Calif. 2004 Feb 8–11; 11: abstract no. 131.
6. Haas D, Ribaudo H, Kim R, et al. Pharmacogenetics of efavirenz and central nervous system side effects: an Adult AIDS Clinical Trials Group study. AIDS 2004; 16:2391–400.
7. Little SJ, Holte S, Routy JP, Daar ES, Markowitz M, Collier AC, Koup RA, Mellors JW, Connick E, Conway B, Kilby M, Wang L, Whitcomb JM, Hellmann NS, Richman, DD. Antiretroviral-drug resistance among patients recently infected with HIV. N Engl J Med 2002; 347:385–394.
8. Shet A, Berry L, Mohri H, Mehandru S, Chung C, Kim A, Jean-Pierre P, Hogan C, Simon V, Boden D, Markowitz M. Tracking the prevalence of transmitted antiretroviral drug-resistant HIV-1: a decade of experience. J Acquir Immune Defic Syndr 2006 Apr 1; 41(4):439–446.
9. Paredes R., Lalama C., Ribaudo H., et al. Presence of minor populations of Y181C mutants detected by allele-specific PCR and risk of efavirenz failure in treatment-naïve patients: results of an ACTG 5095 case-cohort study. [Abstract #83]. Paper presented at the 15th Conference on Retroviruses and Opportunistic Infections. Boston: February 3–6, 2008.
10. Weinstock, Zaidi I, Heneine W, Bennett D, Garcia-Lerma JG, Douglas JM, Jr., LaLota M, Dickinson G, Schwarcz S, Torian L, Wendell D, Paul S, Goza GA, Ruiz J, Boyett B, Kaplan JE. The epidemiology of antiretroviral drug resistance among drug-naïve HIV-1-infected persons in 10 U.S. cities. J Infect Dis 2004; 189:12, 2174–2180.
11. Fundaro C, Genovese O, Rendeli C, Tamburrini E, Salvaggio E. Myelomeningocele in a child with intrauterine exposure to efavirenz. AIDS 2002 Jan 25; 16(2):299–300.
12. van Leth, Phanuphak P, Ruxrungtham K, Baraldi E, Miller S, Gazzard B, Cahn P, Lalloo U, van der Westhuizen I, Malan D. Comparison of first-line antiretroviral therapy with regimens including nevirapine, efavirenz, or both drugs, plus stavudine and lamivudine: a randomised open-label trial, the 2NN Study. Lancet 2004 Apr 17; 363(9417), 1253–1263.
13. Virammune (Nevirapine) [package insert]. Boehringer Ingelheim Pharmaceuticals, Inc. Ridgefield, CT. Revised November 2008.
14. Norvir (ritonavir) [package insert]. Abbott Laboratories. Ridgefield, CT. Revised October 2008.

15. Walmsley S, Bernstein B, King M, Arribas J, Beall G, Ruane P, Johnson M, Johnson D, Lalonde R, Japour A, Brun S, Sun E, the M98-863 Study Team. Lopinavir-ritonavir versus nelfinavir for the initial treatment of HIV infection. N Engl J Med 2002; 346:2039–2046.

16. Cohen C, Nieto-Cisneros L, Zala C, Fessel WJ, Gonzalez-Garcia J, Gladysz A, McGovern R, Adler E, McLaren C, on behalf of the BMS AI424-043 Study Group. Comparison of atazanavir with lopinavir/ritonavir in patients with prior protease inhibitor failure: a randomized multinational trial. Curr Med Res Opin 2005 Oct; 21(10):1683–1692.

17. Gathe JC Jr, Ive P, Wood R, Schurmann D, Bellos NC, DeJesus E, Gladysz A, Garris C, Yeo J. SOLO: 48-week efficacy and safety comparison of once-daily fosamprenavir/ritonavir versus twice-daily nelfinavir in naïve HIV-1-infected patients. AIDS 2004 Jul 23; 18(11):1529–1537.

18. Kempf DJ, Isaacson JD, King MS, Brun SC, Xu Y, Real K, Bernstein BM, Japour AJ, Sun E, Rode RA. Identification of genotypic changes in human immunodeficiency virus protease that correlate with reduced susceptibility to the protease inhibitor lopinavir among viral isolates from protease inhibitor-experienced patients. J Virol 2001; 75:7462–7469.

19. Kaletra (lopinavir/ritonavir) [package insert]. Abbott Laboratories. Ridgefield, CT. Revised July 2007.

20. Riddler SA, Haubrich R, DiRienzo AG, Peeples L, Powderly WG, Klingman KL, Garren KW, George T, Rooney JF, Brizz B, Lalloo UG, Murphy RL, Swindells S, Havlir D, Mellors JW, the AIDS Clinical Trials Group Study A5142 Team. Class-sparing regimens for initial treatment of HIV-1 infection. N Engl J Med 2008; 358:2095–2106.

21. Reyataz (Atazanavir) [package insert]. Princeton NJ. Bristol Myers Squibb. September 2008.

22. Molina J., Andrade-Villanueva J., Echevarria J., Efficacy and safety of once-daily atazanavir/ritonavir compared to twice-daily lopinavir/ritonavir, each in combination with tenofovir and emtricitabinein ARV-naive HIV-1-infected subjects: The CASTLE study, 48-week results. [Abstract #37]. Paper presented at the 15th Conference on Retroviruses and Opportunistic Infections. Boston: February 3–6, 2008.

23. Lexiva (Fosamprenavir) [package insert]. Research Triangle Park, NC. GlAxoSmithKline. Cambridge MA. Vertex Pharmaceuticals, Inc. October 2008.

24. Eron J Jr, Yeni P, Gathe J Jr, Estrada V, DeJesus E, Staszewski S, Lackey P, Katlama C, Young B, Yau L, Sutherland-Phillips D, Wannamaker P, Vavro C, Patel L, Yeo J, Shaefer M, KLEAN study team. The KLEAN study of fosamprenavir-ritonavir versus lopinavir-ritonavir, each in combination with abacavir-lamivudine, for initial treatment of HIV infection over 48 weeks: a randomised non-inferiority trial. Lancet. 2006 Aug 5; 368(9534):476–482.

25. Smith KY, Weinberg WG, Dejesus E, Fischl MA, Liao Q, Ross LL, Pakes GE, Pappa KA, Lancaster CT, the ALERT (COL103952) Study Team. Fosamprenavir or atazanavir once daily boosted with ritonavir 100 mg, plus tenofovir/emtricitabine, for the initial treatment of HIV infection: 48-week results of ALERT. AIDS Res Ther 2008 Mar 28; 5(1):5.

26. Prezista (darunavir) [package insert]. Tibotec Therapeutics, Division of Ortho Biotech Products, L.P., Raritan NJ. June 2006.

27. Clotet B, Bellos N, Molina JM, et al. Efficacy and safety of darunavir-ritonavir at week 48 in treatment-experienced patients with HIV-1 infection in POWER 1 and 2: a pooled subgroup analysis of data from two randomised trials. Lancet 2007 Apr 7; 369(9568):1169–1178.

28. Ortiz R, DeJesus E, Khanlou H, et al. Efficacy and safety of once-daily darunavir/ritonavir versus lopinavir/ritonavir in treatment-naïve HIV-1-infected patients at week 48. AIDS 2008; 22:1389–1397.

29. Truvada (tenofovir+emtricitabine) [package insert]. Gilead Sciences. November 2008.

30. Epzicom (abacavir+lamivudine) [package insert]. Research Triangle Park, NC. GlAxoSmithKline. March 2009.

31. De Silva TI, Post FA, Griffin MD, Cockrell DH. HIV-1 infection and the kidney: an evolving challenge in HIV medicine. Mayo Clin Proc 2007; 82:1103–1116.

32. Lucas GM, Mehta SH, Atta MG, et al. End-stage renal disease and chronic kidney disease in a cohort of African-American HIV-infected and at-risk HIV-seronegative participants followed between 1988 and 2004. AIDS 2007; 21:2435–2443.

33. Gardner LI, Klein RS, Szczech LA et al. Rates and risk factors for condition specific hospitalizations in HIV infected and uninfected women. J Acquir Immune Defic Syndr 2003; 32:203–209.

34. Atta MG and Fine DM. Editorial comment: tenofovir nephrotoxicity-the disconnect between clinical trials and real-world practice. The AIDS Reader 2009; 19(3): 118–119.

35. Gallant JE, Staszewski S, Pozniak AL, et al. Efficacy and safety of tenofovir DF vs stavudine in combination therapy in antiretroviral-naïve patients: a 3-year randomized trial. JAMA 2004; 292:191–201.

36. Izzedine H, Hulot JS, Vittecoq D, et al. Long-term renal safety of tenofovir disoproxil fumarate in antiretroviral-naïve HIV-1-infected patients: data from a double-blind randomized active-controlled multicentre study. Nephrol Dial Transplant 2005; 20:743–746.

37. Szczech LA. Tenofovir nephrotoxicity: focusing research questions and putting then into clinical context. J Infect Dis 2008; 197:7–9.

38. Becker S., Balu R., Fusco J., Beyond serum creatinine: identification of renal insufficiency using glomerular filtration: implications for clinical research and care. [Abstract #819]. Paper presented at the 12th Conference on Retroviruses and Opportunistic Infections. Boston: February 22–25, 2008.

39. Symonds W, Cutrell A, Edwards M, et al. Risk factor analysis of hypersensitivity reactions to abacavir. Clin Ther 2002 Apr; 24(4):565–573.

40. Hughes AR, Spreen WR, Mosteller M, et al. Pharmacogenetics of hypersensitivity to abacavir: from PGx hypothesis to confirmation to clinical utility. The Pharmacogenomics Journal 2008; 8(6):365–374.

41. Faruki H, Heine U, Brown T, Koester R, Lai-Goldman M. HLA-B*5701 clinical testing: early experience in the United States. Pharmacogenet Genomics 2007; 17:857–860.

42. Saag M, Balu R, Bachman P, et al. High sensitivity of HLA-B*5701 in whites and blacks in immunologically-confirmed cases of hypersensitivity. Clin Infect Dis 2008.

43. Smith K., Fine D., Patel P., et al. Efficacy and safety of abacavir/lamivudine compared to tenofovir/emtricitabine in combination with once-daily lopinavir/ritonavir through 48 weeks in the HEAT Study. [Abstract #774]. Paper presented at the 15th Conference on Retroviruses and Opportunistic Infections. Boston: February 3–6, 2008.

44. Sax P, et al. ACTG 5202: shorter time to virologic failure (VF) with abacavir/lamivudine (ABC/3TC) than tenofovir/emtricitabine (TDF/FTC) as part of combination therapy in treatment-naïve subjects with screening HIV RNA $\geq$ 100,000 c/mL. Seventeenth International AIDS Conference, Mexico City, abstract THAB0303, 2008.

45. Gallant JE, DeJesus E, Arribas JR, Pozniak AL, Gazzard B, Campo RE, Lu B, McColl D, Chuck S, Enejosa J, Toole JJ, Cheng AK, the Study 934 Group. Tenofovir DF, emtricitabine, and efavirenz vs. zidovudine, lamivudine, and efavirenz for HIV. N Engl J Med 2006; 354:251–260.

46. DeJesus E, Herrera G, Teofilo E, Gerstoft J, Buendia CB, Brand JD, Brothers CH, Hernandez J, Castillo SA, Bonny T, Lanier ER, Scott TR, for the CNA30024 Study Team. Abacavir versus zidovudine combined with lamivudine and efavirenz, for the treatment of antiretroviral-Naïve HIV-infected adults. Clin Infect Dis 2004; 39(7):1038–1046.

47. D:A:D Study Group. Use of nucleoside reverse transcriptase inhibitors and risk of myocardial infarction in HIV-infected patients enrolled in the D:A:D study: a multi-cohort collaboration. Lancet 2008 Apr 26; 371(9622), 1417–1426.

48. McComsey G, Smith KY, Patel P, et al. Similar reductions in markers of inflammation and endothelial activation after initiation of abacavir/lamivudine or tenofovir/emtricitabine: The HEAT Study. Program and abstracts of the 16th Conference on Retroviruses and Opportunistic Infections; February, 2009; Montreal, Canada. Abstract 732.

49. Cutrell, et al. Is abacavir (ABC)-containing combination antiretroviral therapy (CART) associated with myocardial infarction (MI)? No association identified in pooled summary of 54 clinical trials. XVII International AIDS Conference, Mexico City, abstract WEAB0106, 2008.

50. Centers for Disease Control and Prevention. Late versus early testing of HIV – 16 Sites, Unites States, 2002–2003. MMWR Morb Mortal Wkly Rep 2003; 52:581–586.

51. McNaghten A, Hanson DL, Kellerman S, et al. Factors associated with immunologic stage at which patients initiate antiretroviral therapy. Program and abstracts of the 9th Conference on Retroviruses and Opportunistic Infections; February 24–28, 2002; Seattle, Washington. Abstract 473-M.
52. CDC. Revised recommendations for HIV testing of adults, adolescents, and pregnant women in health-care settings. MMWR Recomm Rep 2006 Sep 22; 55(RR14):1–17.
53. Anastos K, Schneider MF, Gange SJ, et al. The association of race, sociodemographic, and behavioral characteristics with response to highly active antiretroviral therapy in women. J Acquir Immune Defic Syndr 2005 Aug 15; 39(5):537–544.
54. Lucas GM, Chaisson RE, Moore RD. Highly active antiretroviral therapy in a large urban clinic: risk factors for virologic failure and adverse drug reactions. Ann Intern Med 1999; 81–87.
55. Lucas GM, Chaisson RE, Moore RD. Survival in an urban HIV-1 clinic in the era of highly active antiretroviral therapy: a 5-year cohort study. J Acquir Immune Defic Syndr 2003 Jul 1; 33(3):321–328.
56. Jensen-Fangel S, Pedersen L, Pedersen C, et al. The effect of race/ethnicity on the outcome of highly active antiretroviral therapy for human immunodeficiency virus type-1 infected patients. Clin Infect Dis 2002; 35:1541–1548.
57. Silverberg MJ, Wegner SA, Milazzo MJ, et al. Effectiveness of highly-active antiretroviral therapy by race/ethnicity. AIDS 2006; 20:1531–1538.
58. Hartzell JD, Spooner K, Howard R, et al. Race and mental health diagnosis are risk factors for highly active antiretroviral therapy failure in a military cohort despite equal access to care. J Acquir Immune Defic Syndr 2007 April 1; 44(4):411–416.
59. Gebo KA, Fleishman JA, Conviser R, et al. Racial and gender disparities in receipt of highly active antiretroviral therapy persist in a multistate samples of HIV patients in 2001. J Acquir Immune Defic Syndr 2005; 38:96–103.
60. Cunningham WE, Markson LE, Andersen RM, et al. Prevalence and predictors of highly active antiretroviral therapy use in patients with HIV infection in the United States. HCSUS Consortium. HIV Cost and Services Utilization Survey. J Acquir Immune Defic Syndr 2000; 25:115–123.
61. Shapiro MF, Morton SC, McCaffrey DF, et al. Variations in the care of HIV-infected adults in the United States: results from the HIV Cost and Services Utilization Study. JAMA 1999; 281:2305–2315.
62. Wegner S, Vahey M, Dolan M, et al. Racial differences in clinical efficacy of efavirenz-based antiretroviral therapy. Program and abstracts of the 9th Conference on Retroviruses and Opportunistic Infections; February 24–28, 2002; Seattle, Washington. Abstract 428.
63. Gulick RM, Ribaudo HJ, Shikuma CM, et al. Triple-nucleoside regimens versus efavirenz-containing regimens for the initial treatment of HIV-1 infection. N Engl J Med 2004; 350:1850–1861.
64. Schackman BR, Ribaudo HJ, Krambrink A, et al. Racial differences in virologic failure associated with adherence and quality of life on efavirenz-containing regimens for initial HIV therapy: results of ACTG A5095. J Acquir Immune Defic Syndr 2007 Dec 15; 46(5):547–554.
65. Ribaudo HJ, Haas D, Tierney C. Pharmacogenetics of plasma efavirenz exposure after treatment discontinuation: an adult AIDS clinical trials group study. Clin Infect Dis 2006; 42(3):401–407.
66. Moore R, Keruly J, Gebo K, and Lucas G, Racial differences in efavirenz discontinuation in clinical practice. Abstract 619 12th Conference on Retroviruses and Opportunistic Infections. 2005.
67. Wandel C, Witte JS, Hall JM, Stein CM, Wood AJ, Wilkinson GR. Cyp3a in African American and European American men: population differences and functional effect of CYP3a4*1B5'-promoter region polymorphism. Clin Pharmacol Ther 2000; 68:82–91.
68. Wan YJ, Poland RE, Han G, et al. Analysis of the CYP2D6 gene polymorphism and enzyme activity in African Americans in Southern California. Pharmacogenetics 2001; 11:489–499.
69. Schaeffeler E, Eichelbaum M, Brinkmann U, et al. Frequency of C3435T polymorphism of MDR1 gene in African people. Lancet 2001; 358:383–384.

70. Ameyaw MM, Regateiro F, Li T, et al. MDR 1pharmecogenetics: frequency of C3435T mutation in Exon 26 is significantly influenced by ethnicity. Pharmacogenetics 2001; 11:217–221.

71. Kim RB, Leake BF, Choo EF, et al. Identification of functionally variant MDR 1 alleles among European Americans and African Americans. Clin Pharmacol Ther 2001; 7:189–199.

72. Stein CM, Sadeque AJ, Murray JJ, Wandel C, Kim RB, Wood AJ. Cyclosporine pharmacokinetics and pharmacodynamics in African American and white subjects. Clin Pharmacol Ther 2001; 69:317–323.

73. Min DI, Lee M, Ku YM, Flanigan M. Gender-dependent racial difference in disposition of cyclosporine among healthy African American and white volunteers. Clin Pharmacol Ther 2000; 68:478–486.

74. Selzentry (Maraviroc) [package insert]. Pfizer Labs, Division of Pfizer Inc, New York, NY. November 2008.

75. Samson M, Libert F, Doranz BJ, et al. Resistance to HIV-1 infection in Caucasian individuals bearing mutant alleles of the CCR-5 chemokine receptor gene. Nature 1996; 382:722–725.

76. Dean M, Carrington M, Winkler C, et al. Genetic restriction of HIV-1 infection and progression to AIDS by a deletion allele of the CKR5 structural gene. Science 1996; 273:1856–1862.

77. Tang J, Shelton B, Makhatadze NJ, Zhang Y, Schaen M, Louie LG, Goedert JJ, Seaberg EC, Margolick JB, Mellors J, Kaslow RA. Distribution of chemokine receptor CCR2 and CCR5 genotypes and their relative contribution to human immunodeficiency virus type 1 (HIV-1) seroconversion, early HIV-1 RNA concentration in plasma, and later disease progression. J Virol 2002 Jan; 76(2):662–72.

78. Martinson JJ, Chapman NH, Rees DC, Liu YT, Clegg JB. Global distribution of the CCR5 gene 32-base pair deletion. Nat Genet 1997; 16:100–103.

79. Philpott S, Burger H, Tarwater PM, et al. CCR2 genotype and disease progression in a treated population of HIV type 1-infected women. Clin Infect Dis 2004 Sep 15; 39(6):861–865. 2004 Aug 27.

80. Zimmerman PA, Buckler-White A, Alkhatib G, Spalding T, Kubofcik J, Combadiere C, Weissman D, Cohen O, Rubbert A, Lam G, Vaccarezza M, Kennedy PE, Kumaraswami V, Giorgi JV, Detels R, Hunter J, Chopek M, Berger EA, Fauci AS, Nutman TB, Murphy PM. Inherited resistance to HIV-1 conferred by an inactivating mutation in CC chemokine receptor 5: studies in populations with contrasting clinical phenotypes, defined racial background, and quantified risk. Mol Med 1997 Jan; 3(1):23–36.

81. Berkowitz DR, Alexander S, Bare C, et al. CCR5 and CXCR4-utilizing strains of human immunodeficiency virus type 1 exhibit differential tropism and pathogenesis in vitro. J Virol 1998 Dec; 72(12): 10108–10117.

82. Wilkin TJ, Zhaihui S, Kuritzkes DR, et al. HIV Type 1 Chemokine coreceptor use among antiretroviral-experienced patients screened for a clinical trial of a CCR5 inhibitor: AIDS Clinical Trial Group 5211. Clin Infect Dis 2007 Feb 15; 44(4):591–595.

83. Raltegravir (Isentress) [package insert]. MERCK & CO., INC., Whitehouse Station, NJ. Revised January 2009.

84. Fertrin KY, Gonalves MS, Saad STO, et al. Frequencies of UDP-glucuronosyltransferase 1 (UGT1A1) gene promoter polymorphisms among distinct ethnic groups from Brazil. Am J Med Genet 2002 Mar 1; 108(2):117–119.

Overcoming Challenges to Successful Treatment Outcomes in Minority Patients with HIV/AIDS

Valerie E. Stone

Introduction

Improved HIV/AIDS outcomes and decreased mortality due to treatment with highly active antiretroviral therapy (HAART) in the U.S. have not benefited minorities to the same extent as whites.[1,2] HIV/AIDS is one of the largest contributors to the gap in life expectancy between blacks and whites in the U.S., because of disproportionate HIV infection rates as well as higher HIV-related death rates, which have persisted in the post-HAART era.[1] Furthermore, HIV/AIDS is one of the key clinical areas in which disparities were found and documented in the Institute of Medicine report on health care disparities, "Unequal Treatment".[3]

In addition, many other challenges and barriers may impede and complicate efforts to provide optimal care for minority persons living with HIV/AIDS in the U.S. These include the competing life issues of patients who are living in poverty, such as joblessness and housing instability. For many women, the challenges can include domestic violence as well. Mental health issues and substance abuse also are prevalent in patients with HIV/AIDS and often serve as major barriers to effective treatment.

It is these facts: (1) HIV/AIDS epidemiology showing a disproportionate infection rate in minority communities and (2) the documented pattern of disparities in HIV/AIDS care for minorities, and (3) numerous co-morbidities and life circumstances that can make treatment challenging, which make efforts to improve (and ideally optimize) the treatment of minorities with HIV/AIDS particularly pressing.

V.E. Stone
Divisions of Infections Diseases and General Medicine,
Department of Medicine, Massachusetts General Hospital, Harvard Medical School,
Boston, MA, U.S.
E-mail: vstone@partners.org

V. Stone et al. (eds.), *HIV/AIDS in U.S. Communities of Color*.
DOI: 10.1007/978-0-387-98152-9_4, © Springer Science + Business Media, LLC 2009

It is hoped that effective efforts to optimize the treatment provided to minorities with HIV/AIDS will result in improved outcomes. Key challenges to HIV care will be reviewed here, and recommendations for improving and potentially optimizing the HIV care provided to U.S. minorities will be outlined and discussed.

Disparities in HIV/AIDS

Earlier chapters of this book and recent data from the U.S. Centers Disease Control and Prevention have documented the disproportionate rates of HIV infection and AIDS among U.S. minority individuals and communities.[1,4] These disparities in incidence and prevalence are compounded by even higher rates of HIV/AIDS-related deaths among minorities than expected based on their infection rates, in comparison to U.S. whites. While all of the factors that contribute to these higher HIV-related death rates have not been elucidated, it is well documented that these disparities are due in part to the consequences of disparities in HIV/AIDS treatment and care.

Disparities in HIV/AIDS Care

Since early in the HIV epidemic, there has been evidence of disparities in the care provided to minority patients. Specifically, minority patients have reported more problems getting the HIV/AIDS care they needed, and studies show they have been less likely to receive medications to treat their HIV/AIDS.[5–7] Numerous studies have documented that these disparities have persisted into the HAART era.[8–16] These studies have shown that minorities have a longer average delay after diagnosis until receipt of HIV/AIDS care, and once in care for HIV/AIDS, they are less likely to receive HAART. Several of these studies have also shown that women are also less likely to receive HAART.[8,11] However, among women with HIV/AIDS, black women are even less likely than other women to be treated with HAART.[14] One study has shown that black patients with racially concordant providers (e.g. black providers) do not experience a delay in the receipt of HAART compared to white patients, while the black patients with white providers experienced a much longer wait for the receipt of HAART compared to white patients.[10]

A recent study by Losina and colleagues confirms the role that suboptimal care plays in HIV/AIDS outcomes for minority patients.[17] In their analysis, which used a transition-state model, they found that the average person with HIV/AIDS in the U.S. loses 9.6 years of life because of HIV. However, additional years of life are lost by minorities, particularly minority women (Fig. 1) largely due to late presentation (and thus late initiation of HAART) and premature discontinuation of HAART.

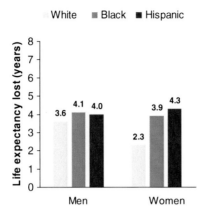

Losina E,Schackman B, Sadownik, et al. *Disparities in survival attributable to suboptimal HIV care in the U.S.: influence of gender and race/ethnicity [Abstract #142]. Presented at the 14th CROI,* Los Angeles, February 25-28, 2007.

Fig. 1 Life expectancy years lost by race and gender, U.S., 2007

As stated earlier, there are clearly other issues besides disparities in the receipt of HAART that contribute to the differences in mortality rates seen between minorities and whites with HIV/AIDS. A recent analysis of the HIV Outpatient Study (HOPS) showed that HAART use is now nearly equal by race/ethnicity.[18] However, despite this apparent similar HAART use in their cohort, in a multivariate analysis of the predictors of mortality, blacks were found to have a 50% higher mortality rate (OR = 1.52) than whites. Latinos did not have a statistically significant higher rate of mortality; the only other significant predictors of death were older age, public insurance, and initial lower CD4 count.[18] Of note, many of the deaths were non-AIDS related and were due to preventable comorbid illnesses. A similar finding of higher mortality despite receipt of HIV care, was reported by Lemly et al. in an analysis of outcome data from a Tennessee clinic cohort.[19] In this cohort of 2605 persons with HIV all receiving their care in the same site, black patients (OR = 1.3) and female patients (OR = 1.5) had significantly higher mortality. Importantly, the use of HAART (but not the percent who received any HAART) differed significantly by race ethnicity in this cohort: proportion of time on HAART was significantly lower in blacks compared to whites (47% vs. 76%). Of note, the proportion of time on HAART was also significantly lower in women compared to men (57% vs. 71%). Similar to the HOPS analysis, Latinos did not have a statisticallysignificant higher rate of mortality; the only other significant predictors of death were older age and initial lower CD4 count.[19]

Taken together, these studies suggest that minorities may be on HAART less time than others and this may contribute to their poorer outcomes. However, these studies also suggest that there may be other factors that contribute to minority patients' poorer outcomes with HIV/AIDS. These may include factors about the care experience (e.g. whether it is continuous vs. discontinuous, timely vs. late, and provider characteristics) and may also include non-care-related factors such as socioeconomic status (poverty and factors related to poverty), disparate rates of other comorbidities such as depression and other mental illnesses, substance abuse, hepatitis C, or coronary heart disease.

HIV/AIDS Care and Its Cultural and Social Context

The cultures and nationalities of minority individuals affected by HIV are quite diverse. Blacks include African Americans, as well as blacks from numerous African and Caribbean countries with diverse cultural and religious traditions. Hispanics affected by the HIV/AIDS epidemic also reflect a diversity of cultures including Puerto Ricans, Dominicans, Mexicans, and others, all of whom may have varying levels of acculturation, differing cultural norms, and English language skills. Thus, while this book and many other publications refer to "minority HIV/AIDS patients," it is not a homogenous group, but represents a diversity of cultures, nationalities, lifestyles and cultural norms, as well as varying levels of education and socioeconomic status. Therefore, any effort to enhance the care and outcomes of minorities living with HIV/AIDS in the U.S. should be mindful of this diversity, and advance strategies that acknowledge and respect group and individual differences, including cultural diversity as a critical part of the HIV/AIDS care process.

Many minority patients approach the health care system and providers with distrust and suspicions. This distrust among African Americans is often reported as stemming from research abuses, the most notorious of which occurred during the Tuskegee Syphilis Trial. However, several authors have recently detailed centuries of medical abuses dating back to slavery which probably serve as the more complete historic basis of distrust in medicine and research among African Americans.[20–22] Distrust may also be an issue for other racial/ethnic minorities, especially Hispanics. These feelings of distrust among Hispanics often stem from a history of personal or family difficulties with the health care system, and from a similar history of abuses in past research studies such as those examining the efficacy of oral contraceptive pills.[23]

HIV/AIDS and its complex baggage in minority communities magnify these distrust issues because of beliefs regarding HIV/AIDS and its advent being a result of a "conspiracy" of some type, beliefs which are held by nearly half of the African Americans.[24,25] In addition to these broader contextual beliefs, some minority HIV/AIDS patients may believe on a personal level that their HIV is some type of "punishment," either because of culture, religion or personal belief systems.[26,27]

Stigma has negatively affected the lives of countless individuals with HIV/AIDS from the beginning of this epidemic. Importantly though, HIV-related stigma may be greater in minority communities. On the basis of a survey of the general U.S. population, African Americans and Latinos perceive there to be more stigma and discrimination against those with HIV/AIDS than are white Americans.[28] For those living with HIV, stigma has a powerful negative impact on self-esteem and self-acceptance. Patients are seen and see themselves as "contaminated and linked to stereotypes of promiscuity, drug use and homosexuality that characterize HIV".[29] On the basis of a recent study by Sayles and colleagues, this leads to one of the two coping mechanisms: denial/social isolation or internal change and self-acceptance.[29] Those who utilize the denial/isolation coping strategy are clearly at risk for poor engagement in HIV/AIDS care or may avoid seeking HIV-related care at all. These patients may therefore only be seen urgently – when they become sick and seek emergency care or when they require hospitalization. Stigma may also at times characterize patients' experience with the health care system. Many persons with HIV infection report that they have suffered discrimination and fear of contagion when obtaining health care, resulting in fear of disclosing their HIV status in personal settings in the future, and fear of disclosing their status in future health care encounters.[29]

Strategies to Optimize the Care of Minorities with HIV/AIDS

With this backdrop, the goal of the remainder of this chapter is to review and highlight those areas in which minority HIV/AIDS patients have documented challenges or barriers to optimal care, and those areas in which minority patients' HIV/AIDS care has been documented to be less than optimal. In each of these areas, specific suggestions and strategies are provided which can be implemented at the individual and clinical care site level to improve the minority HIV/AIDS patients' care and outcomes.

Provide Culturally Competent HIV/AIDS Care

In light of the many complex sociocultural issues that minority patients bring into the clinical encounter in addition to their HIV/AIDS, it is critically important for the HIV/AIDS provider to be aware of these issues and have a strategy for building trust and for optimizing the initial patient–provider encounter. Therefore, it is important for the clinician to be aware of the particular health-related cultural beliefs, including stigma, within the predominant minority groups in his or her HIV/AIDS practice. It is likely, given the cultural diversity of those affected by HIV/AIDS and the limited number of minority HIV/AIDS providers, that most HIV/AIDS patient–provider encounters will be cross-cultural ones. Therefore, it is important that each HIV/AIDS provider be comfortable and skilled in eliciting the personal and cultural views and perspectives of each individual patient and applying a cultural competency framework on each visit.[27] The strength of the framework outlined by Carrillo is that it does not require the clinician to memorize the cultural beliefs and practices of numerous different groups. Instead, the framework relies upon a structured dialogue between the provider and patient which elicits key issues of importance to the individual patient, whether these are due to culture, lifestyle, religion or other factors. As a result, this framework avoids reliance on labels or assumptions which can lead to stereotyping and fuel misunderstandings and miscommunications between the patient and provider.

A recent article has discussed and outlined strategies that providers and care sites can use to reduce or eliminate racial/ethnic disparities.[30] The chapter by Dionne-Odom et al. in this book outlines strategies for providing culturally competent HIV/AIDS care. A variety of additional resources including courses and training opportunities exist in this important area as well.

Enhancing Communication in Clinical Care

Several studies have found that minority patients are less satisfied with their HIV/AIDS care than other patients.[31,32] While many issues may contribute to this lower satisfaction, one issue that comes up repeatedly is patient–provider communication. Minority patients are more likely to experience communication difficulties such as having trouble in understanding their doctor, feeling like their doctor did not listen to them, or did not ask the questions they would have wanted or expected. Minority patients feel less involved in decisions regarding their health care than do others, and they report needing more time with their provider to make treatment decisions.[33,34] Time spent with the medical provider has recently been found to be a key predictor of patients' satisfaction with the health care they receive.[35]

Several strategies are suggested by these findings: Providers should endeavor to spend more time with their minority HIV/AIDS patients, and should spend more of that time listening to the patient. When the provider is doing the talking, he or she should endeavor to enhance the patient's comprehension and retention of what has been said by asking the patient about his/her understanding in a way that is sensitive and not condescending. This can be done by asking "Does that make sense to you?" or requesting that the patient repeat the agreed upon treatment plan aloud to you – the "teach back" approach. Providing follow-up written materials that are appropriate for the patient's literacy level and language may also serve to enhance comprehension. Having nonphysician staff such as nurses, physician assistants, case managers or peer counselors spend more time with the patient and answering patients' questions may also be particularly useful. The important role that these nonphysician staff play in enhancing patient's satisfaction with HIV/AIDS care has data to support it – patients, who have and can identify a primary nurse or case manager, have been found to be more satisfied with their HIV care.[7,31] Medical interpreters should be an essential component of the care of minority patients who are not fluent in English, because communication is markedly compromised if there is a language barrier between the patient and provider.

Diversify the Clinical Staff

An analysis from the HCSUS study has recently found that racial concordance between HIV/AIDS patient and provider essentially eliminates the disparity in time to receive HAART for black patients.[10] This study provides compelling evidence of the potential benefit of diversifying our HIV/AIDS clinical staff. However, very few HIV/AIDS physicians are racial/ethnic minorities; thus, efforts to diversify the clinical staff may appear futile. While it may be nearly impossible to recruit a clinical staff, especially a physician staff, that reflects the diversity of the patients, small steps in this direction may make a substantial difference to minority patients. No matter how welcoming an HIV/AIDS care site is, minority patients will feel even more comfortable if some of the providers are of their own racial/ethnic background. In addition, care sites should also endeavor to employ other staff, such as medical assistants, front desk staff and others who reflect the diversity of the community being served.[30,36] Meanwhile, it should be a goal that all the staff in HIV care settings receive comprehensive training in cross-cultural care to improve the effectiveness of the care that minority patients receive from all staff members.

Enhance Engagement in Treatment and Care

Poor engagement in care has been found to be a predictor of higher mortality among those living with HIV/AIDS. Patients with poor retention in care have been found to have approximately 50% higher mortality.[37] Furthermore, one of the most important predictors of adherence to antiretroviral therapy is adherence with visits and engagement in care.[38,39]

The quality of the patient–provider relationship is often cited as one of the most important factors in a patient's engagement in care. Having a provider with whom the patient feels comfortable and can communicate effectively and frankly is key in developing an effective relationship.[40,41] A care site in which providers are able to devote sufficient time in addressing the needs of each patient is also quite important in promoting engagement in care.[42] Ideally, the site should provide a setting in which provider accessibility and scheduling, and a team approach to care make these goals achievable. Also, with respect to time, a long wait time from the patient's request to schedule an initial appointment for HIV care until the date of the initial HIV medical visit has been shown to be one predictor of decreased engagement in care.[43] This study also found that, unfortunately, minority patients are less likely to keep initial HIV care appointments than are nonminority patients; hence, the need for the strategies outlined in this chapter.

Optimizing Treatment with HAART of Minorities

HIV/AIDS providers should be familiar with the data regarding disparities in receipt of HAART and utilize strategies in the clinical setting to optimize the likelihood that minority patients will be offered, prescribed, and actually take antiretroviral medications. Such strategies include working to build trust in the patient–provider relationship, ensuring that the patient participates in decisions about their own care, providing enough time and information for them to make an informed decision, and by efforts to enhance adherence to HAART.[11,44]

Optimizing Minority Patient's Adherence to HAART

Once it became apparent how important adherence was to the success of treatment with HAART, HIV/AIDS providers became interested in strategies to optimize patient adherence in order to maximize the likelihood of treatment success. There was also an interest in whether patients' adherence to HAART could be predicted and whether certain patients were more at risk for nonadherence than others. While several key studies showed that providers were generally unable to predict or estimate their own patients' adherence to HAART,[45] this data did not deter providers from trying to predict adherence nonetheless. Nor did it convince them that their predictions were inaccurate. Unfortunately, the predictions of poor adherence were more likely to be focused on minority patients than other patients. And, thus, there were early stereotypes circulated among HIV/AIDS providers that minority patients were less likely to be adherent to HAART than other patients, and even the lay press reported that HAART was at times withheld from minority patients because of these preconceptions regarding their ability to adhere.[46] Surveys of HIV providers have confirmed that these biases and stereotypes do affect providers' treatment decisions and result in failure to treat some minority patients for whom HAART is indicated.[47–49] Moreover, longer time in receiving HAART and lower likelihood of receiving HAART among minority and women patients in HCSUS,[8] were found to be in large part because of providers' failure to prescribe perceptions based on the patients' adherence, including future adherence.[49]

Statistically being of minority race is not associated with lower adherence to most well-designed studies that control for confounders such as substance abuse, low health literacy, depression, nondisclosure of HIV, and homelessness/chaotic life situation.[50–56] Most of the studies have found that minority patients have similar adherence to HAART as others, when controlling for other key factors known to be predictors of poorer adherence. In "real life", a given minority patient living with

HIV/AIDS is in fact more likely to have one or more of these factors associated with poor adherence than are white patients, and thus, at higher risk for poor adherence to HAART. Some of this has to do with who from the minority community acquires HIV/AIDS – challenges such as poverty, distrust of the medical system, stigma, denial (and associated nondisclosure) are much more prevalent among minorities than among whites in the U.S. living with HIV/AIDS. Each of these challenges makes consistent adherence less likely or more difficult. Given this, having a strategy that is as evidence based as possible for optimizing minority patients' adherence to HAART is essential for optimizing their outcome/success on HAART. It should be noted, however, that there have been a few notable exceptions – excellent studies that have in fact found that African Americans and Latinos have lower adherence to HAART even after controlling for these key confounders.[50,51]

Assess Readiness for HAART

The first step in a plan to optimize a patient's adherence to HAART is assessing readiness for HAART. A lot has been written about readiness assessment, including recent studies on how to improve readiness. Briefly, the key issues to examine in any readiness assessment are:[57–60] (1) Does the patient feel ready to begin HAART now? Why or why not? What would it take for them to feel ready? (2) Does the patient believe that he/she will be able to consistently take and adhere to the prescribed HAART regimen? This question relates to the patient's self-efficacy. (3) Does the patient believe that the medications are effective and will make a difference for his/her health and in his/her life? What do they think about medications to treat HIV/AIDS – their helpfulness, toxicity and whether they have other beliefs about these medications. This question relates to the patient's belief in the efficacy of the medications. It is very important to assess the patient's beliefs about HAART in this way before beginning treatment, since minority patients may hold a wide range of misperceptions about medications to treat HIV.[24,25,44] Both adherence-related self-efficacy and the patient's belief in the efficacy of the prescribed HAART regimen are critically important components of readiness.[60] In addition, the readiness assessment should include an evaluation for depression, active substance abuse, and determination of health literacy. Finally, it is important to become familiar with the patient's social situation, the stability of the patient's social and living situation, and their psychosocial supports and key people in their life. The presence and/or absence of supportive friends and family (and whether they are aware of the patient's HIV) are critical factors that will influence (or detract from) adherence and treatment success.

Strategies for assisting the patient in the development of more positive attitudes and beliefs about HAART include the use of support groups, peer educators, or a treatment buddy. Building a high-quality and trusting therapeutic relationship before beginning HAART medications will also serve to enhance adherence.[53] Three key studies examining adherence have shown that the quality of the patient–provider relationship may be one of the most important predictors of adherence, particularly among minorities and women with HIV/AIDS.[39–41,44] Patients who are disclosed to their most important family members, friends, and/or intimate partners gain substantial social support and encouragement with HIV treatment and adherence. Thus, HIV care sites and providers should proactively assist newly diagnosed patients with HIV/AIDS with the disclosure process before they start HAART.[39]

Depression has been found to be the most consistent predictor of poor adherence to HAART.[53] Many persons living with HIV have concurrent depression, substance abuse, alcohol abuse, or two or more of these issues.[61,62] While we do not have evidence that depression is more prevalent in minority HIV patients, it may be more difficult to diagnose[61,62] because minority patients may have atypical or unusual presenting symptoms of depression such as anger or increase in energy level. In addition, flat affect or decreased verbal communication due to depression in minority patients may be mistaken by providers for a cultural style or norm. Treatment of depression can improve patient's quality of life and it can result in improved adherence to HAART, thus, it is essential that patients with depression be identified early and treated for depression to optimize their well-being and their ability to adhere to HIV treatment.[63] Thus, routinely screening all HIV/AIDS patients for depression, especially minority patients, before initiating HAART is essential. Substance abuse is highly prevalent in patients with HIV/AIDS and is probably second only to depression in terms of its negative effect on adherence to HAART.[64–67] The range of substances that persons with HIV may use or abuse is extensive, with alcohol leading the list, but also includes crack cocaine, methamphetamines, injected illicit drugs and prescription pain relievers. Given this, all patients with HIV should be screened for substance abuse and alcohol abuse, not just those who acquired HIV through injection drug use. Many experts advocate attempting to treat or at least have a management plan in place for these issues before initiating HAART, because of the high likelihood of poor adherence to HAART if they go unaddressed. The HIV/AIDS care provider and the mental health or drug treatment professional should aim to collaborate on behalf of the patient to optimize his or her HIV treatment as well as their mental health outcomes.

A variety of treatment strategies, including directly observed therapy for HAART and colocating HIV primary care with methadone treatment programs, have been found to enable successful HIV treatment and improved outcomes for active substance abusers.[68–70] Therefore, identifying those with substance abuse is essential for clarifying the best concurrent approach to their HIV medical care and substance abuse management. Without such special efforts, their adherence to HAART and engagement in HIV care is at the risk of being quite poor.[70]

Assessment or at least awareness of each patient's health literacy is an important component of the readiness assessment. Most minority patients living with HIV will have low health literacy.[52] Providers and care sites should plan all educational sessions for patients, carefully choose written materials for distribution, and verbal explanations with this in mind. Because many providers cannot accurately estimate patients' understanding of medication-related instructions, it is often helpful to utilize a "checking in approach" to assess what patients have understood from these explanations. As mentioned earlier, a "teachback" approach can often be very effective in this regard and also is perceived by patients as nonjudgmental. The teachback approach just means that the provider asks the patient to repeat the dosage (or other medication related directions) to the provider to determine the accuracy of what was heard by the patient.

Additional key components of low literacy strategies include using pictures, visuals or analogies to assist with understanding while avoiding medical jargon. Provide small bite size amounts of information and repeat this information often. Focus on "key messages" about HAART medications and HIV treatment goals and success and repeat these often, while making sure that the messages are consistent. Personalize the medication related education to the patient, build and individualize the information around their life, routine, personal barriers and supports.

Logistical supports can also be quite helpful in enhancing patients' adherence, especially medication organizers, and have been reviewed extensively elsewhere.[58] Medication organizers are particularly useful in enhancing patient's adherence even when they have simple regimens to take.

Summary

In addition to being disproportionately affected by the HIV/AIDS epidemic in terms of incidence, prevalence and death rates, minority patients' HIV/AIDS care is often characterized by numerous challenges and barriers. These challenges include disparities in HIV/AIDS care, distrust of the health care system, stigma, poverty, challenges engaging in care, and barriers to adhering to HAART. Unfortunately, these challenges often impede and negatively impact the care that minority patients receive for their HIV/AIDS. It is, therefore, critically important for providers and care sites to have a strategy which proactively seeks to address and reduce these challenges and optimize care and treatment for racial/ethnic minorities with HIV/AIDS. This chapter has reviewed and detailed the most important of these strategies which only serve as "first steps" in ensuring that we deliver the best care possible and thus, improve the outcomes of minorities with HIV/AIDS.

References

1. Centers for Disease Control and Prevention, HIV/AIDS Surveillance Report. 2006; 18: 1–56
2. Wong MD, Shapiro MF, Boscardin WJ, Ettner SL. Contribution of major diseases to disparities in mortality. N Engl J Med 2002; 347(20): 1585–1592
3. Smedley BD, Stith AY, Nelson AR. Institute of Medicine. Unequal Treatment: Confronting Racial and Ethnic Disparities in Health Care. National Academy Press, Washington, D.C., 2002
4. Centers for Disease Control and Prevention. Racial/ethnic disparities in diagnoses of HIV/AIDS – 33 states, 2001–2005. MMWR 2007; 56(09): 189–193

5. Moore R, Stanton D, Gopalan R, et al. Racial differences in the use of drug therapy for HIV disease in an urban community. N Engl J Med 1994; 330(11): 763–768
6. Weissman JS, Makadon HI, Seage GR, et al. Changes in insurance status and access to care by persons with AIDS in the Boston Health Study. Am J Public Health 1994; 84: 1997–2000
7. Mor V, Fleishman JA, Dresser M, et al. Variation in health service among HIV infected patients. Med Care 1992; 30(1): 17–29
8. Shapiro MF, Morton SC, McCaffrey DF, et al. Variations in the care of HIV-infected adults in the United States. JAMA 1999; 281: 2305–2315
9. Turner BJ, Cunningham WE, Duan N, et al. Delayed medical care after diagnosis in a U.S. national probability sample of persons infected with HIV. Arch Intern Med 2000; 160: 2614–2622
10. King WD, Wong MD, Shapiro MF, et al. Does racial concordance between HIV-positive patients and their physicians affect the time to receipt of protease inhibitors? J Gen Intern Med 2004; 19: 1146–1153
11. Stone VE, Steger KA, Hirschhorn LR et al. Access to Treatment with Protease Inhibitor Containing Regimens: Is it Equal For All? [Abstract #42305] Paper presented at the 12th World AIDS Conference. Geneva, Switzerland: June 28–July 3, 1998
12. Anastos K, Schneider ME, Gange SJ, Minkoff et al. Association of race, sociodemographic, and behavioral characteristics with response to HAART in women. J Acquir Immune Defic Syndr 2005; 39(5): 537–544
13. Anderson RM, Bozzette AM, Shapiro MF, et al. Access of vulnerable groups to antiretroviral therapy among persons in care for HIV disease in the U.S. Health Serv Res 2000; 35(2): 389–416
14. Cohen MH, Cook JA, Grey D, et al. Medically eligible women who do not use HAART: The importance of abuse, drug use, and race. Am J Public Health 2004; 94(7): 1147–1151
15. Cunningham WE, Mardson LW, Andersen RM, et al. Prevalence and predictors of highly active antiretroviral therapy use in patients with HIV infection in the United States. J Acquir Immune Defic Syndr 2000; 25(2): 115–123
16. Gebo KA, Fleishman JA, Conviser R, et al. Racial and gender disparities in receipt of highly active antiretroviral therapy persist in a multistate sample of HIV patients in 2001. J Acquir Immune Defic Syndr 2005; 38(1): 96–103
17. Losina E, Schackman B, Sadownik S, et al. Disparities in Survival Attributable to Suboptimal HIV Care in the U.S.: Influence of Gender and Race/Ethnicity [Abstract #142]. Paper Presented at the 14th Conference on Retroviruses and Opportunistic Infections. Los Angeles: February 25–28, 2007
18. Pallela F, Baker R, Chmiel J, et al. Higher Adjusted Mortality Rates Among Publicly Insured Patients and Blacks in the HIV Outpatient Study [Abstract #530]. Paper Presented at the 15th Conference on Retroviruses and Opportunistic Infections. Boston: February 3–6, 2008
19. Lemly D, Shepherd B, Hulgan T, et al. Race and Sex Differences in HAART Use and Mortality Among HIV-Infected Persons in Care [Abstract #810]. Paper Presented at the 15th Conference on Retroviruses and Opportunistic Infections. Boston: February 3–6, 2008
20. Byrd WM, Clayton LA. An American health dilemma. Volume I: A Medical History of African Americans and the Problem of Race – Beginnings to 1900. Routledge, New York, 2000
21. Corbie-Smith G, Thomas SB, St. George DMM. Distrust, race, and research. Arch Intern Med 2002; 162: 2458–2463
22. Armstrong K, Ravenell KL, McMurphy S, Putt M. Racial/ethnic differences in physician distrust in the United States. Am J Public Health 2007; 97(7): 1283–1288
23. Guendelman SW, Denny C, Mauldon J, Chetkovich C. Perceptions of hormonal contraceptive safety and side effects among low-income Latina and non-Latina women. Matern Child Health J 2000; 4(4): 233–239
24. Thomas SB, Quinn SC. The Tuskegee Syphilis Study: Implications for HIV education and AIDS risk education programs in the black community. Am J Public Health 1991; 81: 1497–1504

25. Gant LM, Green W, Stewart PA, Wheeler DP, Wright EM. HIV/AIDS and African Americans: assumptions, myths and realities. In: Gant LM, Stewart PA, Lynch VJ, eds. Social Workers Speak out on the HIV/AIDS Crisis. Praeger, Westport, CT, 1998, pp. 1–12

26. Safren SA, Radomsky AS, Otto MW, and Salomon E. Predictors of psychological well-being in a diverse sample of HIV-positive patients receiving highly active antiretroviral therapy. Psychosomatics 2002; 43(6): 478–485

27. Carrillo JE, Green AR, Betancourt JR. Cross-cultural primary care: a patient-based approach. Ann Intern Med 1999; 130: 829–834

28. Henry J. Kaiser Family Foundation. African Americans and HIV/AIDS, 2001, Washington, DC

29. Sayles JN, Ryan GW, Silver JS, Sarkasian CA, Cunningham WE. Experiences of social stigma and implications for healthcare among a diverse population of HIV positive adults. J Urban Health 2007; 84(6): 814–828

30. Washington DL, Bowles J, Saha S, et al. Transforming clinical practice to eliminate racial-ethnic disparities in healthcare. J Gen Intern Med 2008; 23(5): 685–691

31. Stone VE, Weissman JS, Cleary P. Satisfaction with ambulatory care of persons with AIDS: Predictors of patient ratings of quality. J Gen Intern Med 1995; 10: 239–245

32. Stein MD, Fleishman J, Mor V, Dresser M. Factors associated with patient satisfaction among symptomatic HIV-infected persons. Med Care 1993; 31: 182–188

33. Collins KS, Hughes DL, Doty MM. Diverse communities, common concerns: Assessing health care quality for minority Americans. The Commonwealth Fund, New York, 2002

34. Cooper-Patrick L, Gallo JJ, Gonzales JJ, et al. Race, gender and partnership in the patient–physician relationship. JAMA 1999; 282: 583–589

35. Warde C. Time is of the essence. J Gen Intern Med 2001; 16: 712–713

36. Angelino A, Willard S. The need for sociocultural awareness to maximize treatment acceptance and adherence in individuals initiating HIV therapy. J Int Assoc Physicians AIDS Care 2008; 7(Suppl 1): S17–S21

37. Giordana TP, Gifford AL, White AC, et al. Retention in care: A challenge to survival with HIV infection. Clin Infect Dis 2007; 44: 1493–1499

38. Lucas GM, Chaisson RE, Moore RD. Highly active antiretroviral therapy in a large urban clinic: risk factors for virologic failure and adverse drug reactions. Ann Intern Med 1999; 131: 81–87

39. Bakken S, Holzemer WL, Brown MA, et al. Relationships between perception of engagement with health care provider and demographic characteristics, health status, and adherence to therapeutic regimen in persons with HIV/AIDS. AIDS Patient Care and STDs 2000; 14: 189–197

40. Schneider J, Kaplan SH, Greenfield S, Li W, Wilson IB. Better physician-patient relationships are associated with higher reported adherence to antiretroviral therapy in patients with HIV infection. J Gen Intern Med 2004; 19: 1096–1103

41. Malcolm SE, Ng JJ, Rosen RK, Stone VE. An examination of HIV/AIDS patients who have excellent adherence to HAART. AIDS Care 2003; 15: 251–261

42. Dugdale DC, Epstein R, Pantilat SZ. Time and the patient–physician relationship. J Gen Intern Med 1999; 14(Suppl 1): S34–S40

43. Mugavera MJ, Lin H, Allison JJ, et al. Failure to establish HIV care: characterizing the "no show" phenomenon. Clin Infect Dis 2007; 45: 127–130

44. Stone VE, Clarke J, Lovell J, et al. HIV/AIDS patients' perspectives on adhering to regimens containing protease inhibitors. J Gen Intern Med 1998; 13(9): 586–593

45. Bangsberg DR, Hecht FM, Clague H, et al. Provider assessment of adherence to HIV antiretroviral therapy. J Acquir Immune Defic Syndr 2001; 26(5): 435–442

46. Sontag S. Doctors withhold potent HIV treatments from some. New York Times. March 17, 1997, pp. 1A, 34A

47. Bogart LM, Catz SL, Kelly JA, Benotsch EG. Factors influencing physicians' judgements of adherence and treatment decisions for patients with HIV. Med Decis Making 2001; 21: 28–36

48. Bogart LM, Kelly JA, et al. Impact of medical and nonmedical factors on physician decision making for HIV/AIDS antiretroviral treatment. J Acquir Immune Defic Syndr 2000; 23(5): 396–404

49. Wong MD, Cunnigham WE, Shapiro MF, et al. Disparities in HIV treatment and physician attitudes about delaying protease inhibitors for non-adherent patients. J Gen Intern Med 2004; 19(4): 366–374

50. Golin CE, Liu H, Hays RD, et al. A prospective study of predictors of adherence to combination antiretroviral medication. J Gen Intern Med 2002; 17(10): 756–765

51. Silverberg M, Leyden W, Quesenberry C, Horberg M. Influence of Race/Ethnicity on Adherence to and Effectiveness of Antiretroviral Therapy in Patients with Access to Care [Abstract WePeB107]. Abstract Presentation at the 4th IAS Conference on HIV Pathogenesis, Treatment and Prevention. Sydney, July 25, 2007.

52. Kalichman SC, Ramachandran B, Catz S. Adherence to combination antiretroviral therapies in HIV patients of low literacy. J Gen Intern Med 1999; 14(5): 267–273

53. Turner BJ. Adherence to antiretroviral therapy by HIV infected patients. J Infect Dis 2002; 185(Suppl 2): S143–S151

54. Vervoot S, Borleffs, Hoepelman A, Grypdonck MHF. Adherence in antiretoviral therapy for HIV: a review of qualitative studies. AIDS 2009; 21(3): 271–281

55. Wong MD, Sarkisian CA, Davis C, Kinsler J, Cunningham WE. The association between life chaos, health care use, and health status among HIV-infected persons. J Gen Intern Med 2007; 22: 1286–1291

56. Stone VE. Strategies for optimizing adherence to highly active antiretroviral therapy (HAART). Clin Infect Dis 2001; 33(6): 855–872

57. Department of Health and Human Services. Guidelines on Treatment of HIV/AIDS in Adults and Adolescents. Updated January 28, 2008. Accessed online at http:www.hivatis.org

58. Simoni JM, Pearson CR, Pantalone DW, Marks G, Crepaz N. Efficacy of interventions in improving highly active antiretroviral therapy adherence and HIV-1 RNA viral load. J Acquir Immune Defic Syndr 2006; 43(Suppl 1): S23–S35

59. Willard S, Angelino, A. The need for sociocultural awareness to maximize treatment acceptance and adherence in individuals initiating HIV therapy. J Int Assoc Physicians AIDS Care 2008; 7(1): S17–S21

60. Enriquez M, Gore PA, O'Connor MC, McKinsey DS. Assessment of readiness for adherence by HIV positive males who had previously failed treatment. J Assoc Nurses AIDS Care 2004; 15: 42–49

61. Treisman GJ, Angelino AF, Hutton HE. Psychiatric issues in the management of patients with HIV infection. JAMA 2001; 286: 2857–2864

62. Angelino AF, Treisman GJ. Management of psychiatric disorders in patients infected with human immunodeficiency virus. Clin Infect Dis 2001; 33: 847–856

63. Horberg MA, Silverberg MJ, Hurley LB, et al. Effects of depression and selective serotonin reuptake inhibitor use on adherence to highly active antiretroviral therapy and on clinical outcomes in HIV-infected patients. J Acquir Immune Defic Syndr 2008; 47(3): 384–390

64. Turner BJ, Laine C, Cosler L, Hauck WW. Relationship of gender, depression, and health care delivery with antiretroviral adherence in HIV-infected drug users. J Gen Intern Med 2003; 18: 248–257

65. Lucas GM, Cheever LW, Chaisson RE, et al. Detrimental effects of continued illicit drug use on the treatment of HIV-1 infection. J Acquir Immune Defic Syndr 2001; 27: 251–259

66. Arnsten JH, Demas PA, Grant RW, et al. Impact of active drug use on antiretroviral therapy adherence and viral suppression in HIV-infected drug users. J Gen Intern Med 2002; 17: 377–381

67. Cook RL, Sereika SM, et al. Problem drinking and medication adherence among persons with HIV infection. J Gen Intern Med 2001; 16(2): 83–88

68. Altice FL, Maru DS, Bruce RD, Springer SA, Friedland GH. Superiority of directly administered antiretroviral therapy among HIV-infected drug users: a prospective, randomized, controlled trial. Clin Infect Dis 2007; 45(6): 770–778

69. Mitty JA, Stone VE, Sands M, Macalino G, Flanigan T. Directly observed therapy for the treatment of people with human immunodeficiency virus infection: a work in progress. Clin Infect Dis 2002; 34: 984–990

70. Flanigan TP, Mitty JA. The good, the bad and the ugly: providing highly active antiretroviral therapy when it is most difficult. Clin Infect Dis 2006; 42: 1636–1638

Access to Culturally Competent Care for Patients Living with HIV/AIDS

Jodie Dionne-Odom, Loida Bonney, and Carlos del Rio

Cultural competence is a term that has been increasingly used over the past decade to outline a certain principle of care often deemed as lacking in the American system of medical care. Although there is no agreed upon definition, the American Medical Association defines cultural competence as:

> Knowledge and interpersonal skills that allow providers to understand, appreciate, and work with individuals from cultures other than their own. It involves an awareness and acceptance of cultural differences; self-awareness; knowledge of patient's culture; and adaptation of skills.[1]

The principles of culturally competent care have been derived from a vast body of knowledge in medical anthropology outlining the relationship between illness, culture, and the individual. Some experts in this field have expressed concern about the "medicalization" of cultural competence into a set of skills and list of behaviors that need to be memorized to be practiced effectively. Because the topic is complex and unique to each patient, it is not well suited to rote memorization and can be difficult to teach. But within the HIV research community many insightful studies have been performed that outline disparities in care for minority populations and propose mechanisms to help bridge the divide between patient and provider and to inform the discussion of how best to teach cultural competence.

Barriers to culturally competent HIV care include issues that impact access, retention in care, and the provision of ancillary services. Although some barriers are socioeconomic in nature, others are interpersonal and only need to be recognized to be changed. Both barriers to care and training issues specific to cultural competency will be addressed.

Carlos del Rio (✉)
Department of Medicine, Division of Infectious Diseases, Emory University School of Medicine, Atlanta, GA, U.S.
E-mail: cdelrio@emory.edu

V. Stone et al. (eds.), *HIV/AIDS in U.S. Communities of Color*.
DOI: 10.1007/978-0-387-98152-9_5, © Springer Science + Business Media, LLC 2009

Access to Care

We understand access to care as the ability of a patient to gain entry into the health care system. Ideally, health care would be close to home, affordable, and easy to navigate. Unfortunately, the current state of medical care in the U.S. is far from ideal, and access is challenging even for those who are educated and can pay or have insurance. For HIV care, access is complicated even more by the sheer stigma and discrimination, which are prevalent and pervasive in most communities surrounding HIV disease.[2] It is further complicated by unique individual character-istics related to socioeconomics, immigration status, homelessness, substance abuse, racism, and mental illness. The challenge that minority persons with HIV infection face in accessing care is underscored by the CDC statistics showing that 47% of new cases of AIDS in 2006 occurred among African Americans (who comprise 13% of the U.S. population).[3] The CDC statistics also show that HIV continues to be the leading cause of death in African American males aged 35–44 despite dra-matic drops in mortality observed for HIV as a result of highly active antiretroviral therapy (HAART).[4]

The U.S. Department of Health and Human Services released its first Report of the Secretary's Task Force on Black and Minority Health in 1985. This report outlined the disparities of care based on race in the U.S. and documented the poorer state of health among minority populations. As a marker of their difficulty in access-ing the healthcare system, ethnic minorities were less likely to have an identifiable care provider and more likely to lack health insurance.[5] Since that time, disparities in care have become only more obvious and pronounced in several studies from many areas of medicine. For example, African Americans with significant heart dis-ease have repeatedly been shown to be less likely to undergo coronary angiography and coronary artery bypass graft surgery than white patients (32% less likely in one study) and African American females with breast cancer have 37% higher mortality than white women despite a lower incidence of disease.[6–8] Naturally, HIV patients are not immune to these racial disparities in care.[9]

HIV Testing and Entry into Care

The first hurdle in accessing HIV care is making the diagnosis. CDC estimates that approximately 25% of those living with HIV infection in the U.S. do not know their serostatus, yet they account for approximately 55% of the 40,000 new infections that occur each year.[10] Furthermore, a significant number of those who are diagnosed with HIV are diagnosed when their disease is already advanced. In the U.S., 38% of African Americans diagnosed with AIDS in 2006 had their first positive HIV test less than 12 months before their AIDS diagnosis.[3] To decrease the number of people who are unaware of their infection or who are diagnosed late in the course of HIV disease, the CDC made broad recommendations in September 2006 to simplify the testing process and advised routine screening for all adults, adolescents, and pregnant women.[11]

On the basis of data from the 1999 National Health Interview Survey (NHIS), 30.9% of adults in the U.S. have been tested for HIV (excluding testing for blood donation), an increase from 5% in 1987 and 26% in 1995. In the late 1980s, rates of HIV testing (excluding testing for blood donation) were slightly higher for blacks (7%) and Hispanics (7%) than for whites (5%). The 1999 data indicated a higher rate of HIV testing among minority populations (blacks 52%, Hispanics 40%, and whites 44% "ever tested").[12] One CDC outreach to high-risk populations (National HIV Behavioral Surveillance System) included cross-sectional HIV testing in 5 of 17 cities that report data. Of 1,767 MSM participants, 27% were Hispanic, 25% were black, and 450 (25%) tested positive. Despite programs such as these, a substantial number of persons at risk for HIV have never been tested.[13]

The current barriers to implementation of the new HIV testing recommendations made by the CDC include local and state laws that dictate HIV testing and frequently mandate written informed consent for testing, pre and posttest counseling, as well as the discussion about finding an appropriate payer source for these additional screening tests not yet recommended by the U.S. Preventive Services Task Force. Ongoing studies are examining the utility of rapid testing in emergency rooms, inpatient settings, and primary care offices across the country to help close these gaps.

Diagnosing HIV infection, while important, is not sufficient. Once the diagnosis of HIV infection is made, it is imperative that the patient be linked to care and prevention services. Linkage to care not only benefits the patient, but it is also a good public health practice. Unfortunately, linkage to care after confirmation of HIV diagnosis is not automatic.[14] An estimated 40% of patients who receive a diagnosis of HIV delay their entry into care for more than a year.[15] One study investigating factors associated with delay into care found that men and the uninsured waited longer than women and those with insurance to enter care.[16] Linkage to care requires familiarity with the available HIV services in the community and can be complicated particularly in the rural setting where services may be sparse and transportation to distant providers unavailable. There are several other potential barriers at this linkage step, including language, substance abuse, lack of housing, and psychiatric disease, each of which defines a marginalized population that may be at particular risk of HIV infection. Risk factors associated with poorer access include ethnic minorities, less severe illness, less education, more substance abuse, younger patients, and those with a history of incarceration.[16]

Although most studies are inclusive of only those patients who are successful in accessing care, a few have tried to focus upon those who are not. One multisite outreach program targeted 610 underserved, hard to reach HIV patients for analysis. The study population was 61% African American and 20% Latino, and 85% had an annual income of less than $10,000. A majority (82%) had known of their HIV infection for more than 3 years; many had mental health visits in the past 6 months (59%), and 76% were currently using cocaine or heroin. Surprisingly, 93% reported having insurance and, on multivariate analysis, this was significantly associated with accessing ambulatory care (AOR 2.5, 95% CI 1.02–5.9) along with case management (AOR 4.8, 95% CI 3.8–6.2) and taking mental health medications (AOR 7.5, 95% CI 2.8–19.8).[17]

One multisite intervention study of linkage to care published in 2005, called the Antiretroviral Treatment and Access Study (ARTAS), randomized 316 patients to standard of care (educational pamphlets and contact information for a local HIV care provider) or intervention arm (strengths-based case management). The primary outcome of two care visits within 12 months was met by 49% in the control group and 64% in the intervention group ($p = 0.0005$). Those most likely to meet the primary outcome were older than 40, Hispanics, diagnosed with HIV within the past 6 months, and were less likely to use crack cocaine.[18] The ARTAS intervention was pivotal in the design of a case management intervention by the CDC that is now recognized as "best practice" by the Division of HIV/AIDS at CDC.

Engagement/Retention in Care

Although linkage to care is crucial, it cannot have an impact on quality of life or decrease mortality unless the patient remains "linked" and continues on antiretroviral therapies (ARVs.) The Ryan White Comprehensive AIDS Resources Emergency (CARE) Act was first funded by Congress in 1990 as a payer of "last resort." In spite of this designation, funds are distributed widely and help to provide care for more than 500,000 people annually ($2.06 billion in fiscal year 2006). In 2004, 59% of those covered by this funding were ethnic/racial minorities.[19, 20]

A 2002 analysis of HIV services funded nationally by the Ryan White CARE Act showed that women, members of ethnic minority groups, uninsured, and low-income patients often postponed medical care due to illness or lack of transportation. They also interviewed patients and health care providers in California about reasons for poor adherence and found that African American patients often did not trust their provider, had limited or conflicting information about the benefits of HAART and were concerned about drug side effects. Hispanic patients more often noted language barriers, concern about immigration procedures, and they cited a cultural preference to not discuss disease. Ethnic minorities, uninsured patients, women, and IV drug abusers also waited longer before they were prescribed new therapies (NNRTI/PI regimens), often due to the fact that providers had concerns about their potential for nonadherence. This has been cited as a partial explanation for the lower CD4 counts among minority patients than among white patients.[21, 22]

Engagement with HIV care is predicated on a strong relationship between the provider and patient. Turner et al. specifically analyzed factors that predict staying in care and found that they included having a care provider prior to the time of diagnosis, having Medicaid insurance, and having "a lot of trust" in their provider.[23] Given the powerful role of the provider in this situation, it is all the more devastating when providers are perceived as introducing stigma into the relationship. One prospective study of 223 patients living with HIV in Los Angeles County found that a quarter of them reported perceived stigma from a health care provider in the past.

These patients noted several behaviors in their providers, varying from "treating me as inferior" and "preferring to avoid me" to "refusing to serve me." Although the study authors did not attempt to verify these behaviors, they acknowledged that perceived stigma is a barrier to care irrespective of the provider's intention.[2]

While solutions for poverty and lack of insurance are beyond the capabilities of individual providers, the provision of culturally competent care is something that must happen at the level of each nurse, nurse practitioner, physician assistant, and physician. Thus, the value of teaching this type of care to students and residents is enormous and will be addressed later in the chapter. Although providers often focus on the HIV itself and medical complications that inevitably arise, many patients (when asked about their specific needs) request access to consultative services in other specialties or ancillary services, including emotional counseling (33%), benefits advocacy (43%), and substance abuse treatment (28%), and addressing these needs is a key component to retaining patients in care.[21]

Patients may be reluctant to ask for additional services from their providers although they may have a significant impact on retention and medication compliance. Homeless patients and those with a history of crack cocaine use have the most unmet needs, but those with access to a case manager are much more likely to have their service needs met. One example of an effective intervention is an HIV clinic in Atlanta that noticed the high "no-show" rate for their female patients and decided to pilot the implementation of on-site daycare in the women's clinic. The "no-show" rate fell precipitously and the pilot project was converted into an ongoing service for patients.

Simply put, perhaps one of the best ways to solve the problem of poor retention is to ask the patient what services they need. Females are more likely than males to report barriers to care such as long wait times, concern about denial of treatment, fear of loss of custody of their children, difficulty in communicating their needs to their provider, and worrying that family and friends do not want them to receive services.[24,25]

Several studies have analyzed the role of ancillary services with respect to retention in care. One observational study in Chicago of 2,647 patients showed that 85% of patients had need for services and that providing case management, mental health services, and transportation allowed patients to stay in regular care with their providers ($p = 0.0003$) and corroborated the data showing that female patients have the greatest need of services.[25] Another study of patients receiving care funded by the Ryan White CARE Act ($n = 29,153$) found mental health and substance abuse treatment, companion services, client advocacy, and respite care to be most associated with retention in care.[26] These and other studies make it clear that the service needs of the population vary greatly from clinic to clinic but that meeting the specific needs of the patient will improve engagement in care.[27]

A retrospective cohort study of 2,619 HIV-infected men in the VA system (54% African American) allowed for a unique analysis of retention in care since patients in their system should have high levels of access independent of insurance carrier and socioeconomic status. The authors used multivariate regression modeling to show stepwise higher mortality in the 4-year follow-up period among those patients with fewer than four appointments in 12-months time. The adjusted hazard ratio of death was 1.42 for patients with visits during three quarters of the year and 1.95 for those patients with visits in only one quarter of the year. This was also highly associated with adherence to ARV. Patients with lower CD4 and older age had better retention, while alcohol abuse, hepatitis C coinfection, and use of illicit substances were independently associated with worse retention (race and ethnicity were not considered as variables in this study). In this setting with minimal barriers to health care access, there was no association seen with socioeconomic status.[28]

Need for Cultural Competency

Given the significance of the HIV epidemic in U.S. minority populations and the issues associated with access to care and retention in care, cultural competence among care providers is crucial. Once patients are linked to care, it is clear that many will remain engaged only if they have trust in their provider. This is something that can be built into the patient–provider relationship over time and is fostered by active listening, patient advocacy, and a sense of teamwork toward common goals.

Based on the principle of Maslow's hierarchy of needs that outlines stages of development like building blocks (with physiological needs at the base and self-actualization at the summit), there are several components inherent to cultural competency that can be ordered from the most basic tenets to the most sophisticated. One of the most fundamental requirements of culturally competent care is language. Census data from 2000 reveals that 47 million Americans (nearly one-fifth of the population) speak a language other than English at home, a majority of whom (60%) speak Spanish. The provision of interpreter services is relevant to every clinical setting and has been mandated by law. In 1964, the Civil Rights Act was written to prohibit discrimination on the basis of race, color, and national origin in federally funded programs and activities. Title VI specifically outlined the need for patients with limited English proficiency to have access to language services when receiving medical care.

Despite the national laws written over 40 years ago, one of five Spanish speakers recently surveyed reported delaying or refusing care secondary to language barriers with their provider.[29] In one study in a Los Angeles County emergency room, language concordant providers (those who speak the same language as the patient) were more likely to give their patients referrals for follow-up care.[30] Provision of interpreter services is beneficial, but not sufficient in creating a strong patient–provider relationship,[31] which may be in part due to the fact that communication involves more than language skills alone. Communication between provider and patient can be derailed by inappropriate nonverbal cues, as well as language differences.

This has been studied among Asian/Pacific Islander Americans (APIA), whom as a group comprise 49 different ethnicities in which more than 100 languages and dialects are spoken. For example, nodding of the head does not always signify comprehension or agreement, nor does silence always signify that the patient has no questions to ask. Often, these nonverbal cues are assumed to be universal, but are found to have significant and often conflicting meanings necessitating help from others who are more familiar with the cultural context.[32]

The next level of competent care in this proposed hierarchy involves the maintenance of an open line of communication between patient and provider. Even English-speaking patients often complain that their providers do not really listen to them. Since HIV is intimately associated with sensitive topics of conversation related to sexuality and substance abuse, the onus is on the care provider to establish a rapport that is nonjudgmental and allow the patient to ask questions and express concerns freely. This can be particularly challenging in a busy clinical setting with patients of varied backgrounds and is often compounded by competing issues such as homelessness, substance abuse, and a general sense of distrust toward the medical profession. Time is implicit to this relationship, since patient satisfaction with their provider is correlated with their sense that "sufficient" time was spent with them.[33]

Higher yet on this scale of cultural competence is gaining a fund of knowledge about the patient's personal history and cultural beliefs. These may be rooted in ethnicity, country of origin, gender, sexual orientation, and/or religious beliefs (among others) and generally require both time and sensitivity to explore. The inclusion of partners and family members in this care can be helpful in understanding the community surrounding patients with HIV infection. Community outreach programs for HIV have been found to be effective in "meeting patients where they are" in order to link them to care as well as to keep them engaged.[17]

Providers who come from communities that are similar to their patients are often the most effective, yet the low numbers of minority HIV providers do not afford all patients this type of access. One study found that racial concordance between physician and patient decreased the length of time to receipt of first protease inhibitor (461 days for African American patients with white providers vs. 342 days for African American patients with African American providers, $p < 0.001$).[34] Increasing the training of minority HIV providers is a priority that has been recognized by multiple groups including the HIVMA/IDSA, which recently launched a minority clinical fellowship program.[35] Short of knowing the culture personally, providers can indeed be trained in a variety of exercises about how to deliver culturally competent care. These exercises should be introduced early and often as providers adopt their practice style in caring for patients with HIV.[36]

Training Needs

Dr. David Satcher, the U.S. Surgeon General from 1998 to 2002, has repeatedly called attention to the objectives stated in "Healthy People 2010," which includes the ambitious goal of eliminating racial and ethnic health disparities. He cites culturally competent health care teams as critical to reaching these goals and describes mechanisms for funding the necessary training programs.[37]

If we are convinced of the relevance of clinical competency in the provision of care to HIV patients, we must have mechanisms in place to teach it to existing and upcoming providers. Therein lies the difficulty, as cultural competence cannot be boiled down to a set of concrete skills or a formula that applies to every patient encounter. Some would simplify cultural competency training into a set of characteristics common among members of a certain ethnic group, but this would paradoxically increase the stereotyping that is inherent to cultural incompetence. We tend to use age, country of origin, race, and gender to classify patients into subsets and can sometimes make the mistake of assuming to understand certain things about our patients based upon these characteristics. This is often a subconscious process, which can help to explain some of the prejudice that can exist between patient and provider.

Because the health care encounter involves meeting a number of different people, this training would be relevant to everyone who comes into contact with the HIV patient, from the outpatient office assistant to the inpatient critical care intensivist to the case manager assigned to the patient on hospital discharge. Although we will focus on training programs for health care professionals, the underlying principles have been developed by experts from a number of cross-disciplinary settings and can be broadly applied.

U.S. medical schools and residency training programs are obvious places for the introduction of such topics, and policies have been laid out for this to occur. Beginning in 2000, the Liaison Committee on Medical Education (LCME) added the following to its long list of standards for medical school accreditation:[38]

> ED 21. The faculty and students must demonstrate an understanding of the manner in which people of diverse cultures and belief systems perceive health and illness and respond to various symptoms, diseases, and treatments.
>
> Clarification: The objectives for clinical instruction should include student understanding of demographic influences on health care quality and effectiveness, such as racial and ethnic disparities in the diagnosis and treatment of diseases. The objectives should also address the need for self-awareness among students regarding any personal biases in their approach to health care delivery.
>
> ED 22. Medical students must learn to recognize and appropriately address gender and cultural biases in themselves and others, and in the process of health care delivery.
>
> Clarification: All instruction should stress the need for students to be concerned with the total medical needs of their patients and the effects that social and cultural circumstances have on their health. To demonstrate compliance with this standard, schools should be able to document objectives relating to the development of skills in cultural competence, indicate where in the curriculum students are exposed to such material, and demonstrate the extent to which the objectives are being achieved.

Toward the end of assisting medical schools in meeting these objectives, the Association of American Medical Colleges (AAMC) has developed a self-administered assessment tool, called the Tool for Assessing Cultural Competence Training (TACCT), which helps with curriculum analysis to determine what is already being taught that might fall under the rubric of cultural competency. The goals of this curriculum are broken down into specific knowledge, skills, and attitudes that fall into one of five domains. Schools are expected to utilize this information to identify gaps in their cultural competency curriculum and to create a program that is not only seamless and well integrated but one that encompasses learning in all 4 years of medical school.[39]

Barriers to this teaching are many, including the lack of a unified curriculum and sparse outcomes of research delineating the precise relationship between teaching cultural competence and its effect on health care disparities.[40] Perhaps an even more significant hurdle is the sense among teachers and students alike that these lessons are "soft" science and secondary to the overriding curricular goals of medical education. Some teachers surveyed in the United Kingdom expressed ambivalence about the necessity to test student ability in cultural competence although most agreed that students would be more likely to take the subject seriously if they were evaluated. Another barrier is the lack of agreement about methods of teaching and evaluation, although objective structured clinical examinations (OSCEs) are used by medical schools widely. Yet another barrier cited is that medical students often lack the broad background in social and behavioral sciences that form the underpinnings of cultural competence work.[41]

Many studies of medical education cite the power of the "unwritten curriculum," which students learn on the wards from their residents during the latter 2 years of medical school. Residents taking care of inpatients with HIV are not always fully conscious of their position as role model for the students assigned to their team. As a consequence, their beliefs and attitudes may impact the student's treatment of HIV patients. In addition to attention at the medical school level, graduate medical education has become increasingly inclusive of cultural competence over the past 10 years. One study of residency training programs from 2000 to 2003 noted an increase in those with curriculum devoted to cultural competence from 36 to 51%. In addition, approximately one-fifth offered language instruction during this time and nearly a quarter offered lessons on complementary medicine.[42]

Some have investigated whether or not newly minted physicians see a need for this significant increase in cultural competency training. When interviewed, residents in one study equated cultural competence with language proficiency alone. When asked specifically about the value of teaching cultural competence, many residents responded that it was "a waste of time" since they already knew how to talk to patients. In addition to the language constraints they cited time and "patient shortcomings" as the biggest barriers to effective communication. Both residents and faculty pointed to problems using interpreter services. When patients were interviewed as part of this qualitative study, their suggestions to improve communication included the following: "listen carefully to the patient," "take patients seriously," and "don't make assumptions about patients based on their skin color or surname."[43]

In considering again the role of the resident as a teacher in addition to that of a provider, there is much room for improvement in modern-day curriculum. Given the increasing number of requirements for both undergraduate and graduate medical residents, the acuity of patients admitted to the hospital, and work hour restrictions, there is a sense of urgency in many clinical settings today. The addition of a language barrier or cultural misunderstanding can make the encounter unpleasant in the mind of both patient and provider despite the best of intentions on both sides.

How to Meet Training Needs

For health care systems providing HIV care, a number of techniques previously described by Brach and Fraser can be applied to the clinical setting to increase cultural competence in the care of minority patients.[44] These include provision of interpreter services, recruitment and retention of ethnically diverse staff (ideally representative of the community being served), the recognition of the vital role of traditional healers in many communities, the use of community health workers, culturally appropriate health promotion pamphlets and activities (in various languages), inclusion of the family and community in care, and administrative/organizational accommodations to address the specific needs of the HIV patient.[45]

None of these alone is sufficient nor are all fully inclusive of a culturally sensitive environment, but they provide guidance for steps in the right direction. Although there is some available funding for clinics, more still is needed if cultural competence is our standard for providing effective HIV care. One health policy report funded by the Commonwealth Fund in 2002 explored the link between cultural competence and health care disparities and looked for models of care in the U.S. It was one of a few analyses to include the private sector and it highlighted Kaiser Permanente in San Francisco and Sunset Park Family Health Center Network in Brooklyn for their successful community oriented, culturally competent approaches.[46]

To meet the training needs specific to medical providers, there are the guidelines previously mentioned laid out by the LCME, as well as the addition of six general competencies in 2002 for resident development by the ACGME (Accreditation Council for Graduate Medical Education). Cultural competence falls under the competency entitled "professionalism," and residents are expected to be evaluated specifically based upon their abilities in this area. Because these guidelines offer little provision as to exactly how the training should happen, there are a variety of models being used across the country. Despite ongoing local evaluation, there are a few published studies to help determine which models are most effective.[47]

The Society of General Internal Medicine Health Disparities Task Force has recently published recommendations for teaching about racial and ethnic disparities that are directly relevant to training needs for delivering culturally competent HIV care. They recommend starting with an exploration of attitudes unique to the provider as related to caring for patients from a variety of backgrounds. Authors of the recommendations are candid about the barriers to this type of small group discussion, not the least of which is discomfort in exploring reasons for discrimination in health care settings.[48]

The next learning objective is the acquisition of knowledge about health care disparities to which one could easily add lessons about varied cultural norms and their relationship with beliefs about health and illness. Finally, a set of skills is outlined to facilitate the elicitation of patient beliefs, their accommodation, and the treatment of all patients with respect. There is mention of the relevance of effective training for the teachers of these sessions as well, since they are the key to facilitating discussion and keeping the group engaged with the material. Teachers will also act as role models in setting the example of a practitioner who values cultural competence and is able to articulate its significance in the everyday clinical setting.[49]

Another commonly cited approach to teaching cultural competence is that outlined by Carrillo several years ago. It involves five modules each covering a specific theme[50]:

1. Basic concepts – disease, culture, and attitudes are defined and explored
2. Core cultural issues – case presentations of cross-cultural issues
3. Meaning of illness – explanatory model studied via actor interviews
4. Social context – relationship of social factors to health status
5. Negotiating across cultures – acknowledgment of unique belief systems

Most medical schools and residency programs rely on a combination of facilitated small group settings, patient actors, and objective structured clinical exams as mechanisms to both teach and evaluate students in their grasp of cultural competency issues. Until there are studies showing the superiority of one method over another, this blend will continue as it allows each institution to call on its particular strengths and faculty experience. In addition to the focus on medical students and residents, there is a need to expand the scope to practitioners in all communities with HIV-infected patients in their panel. Lessons on cultural competency could easily be added to continuing medical education efforts nationwide to have a significant and direct impact on patients being treated today as well as tomorrow.

Conclusion

Culturally competent care for minority HIV patients is the goal of many health care providers and the right of every patient, despite the fact that it is difficult to teach and cumbersome to measure. Given the increasing diversity both in the U.S. and in those diagnosed with HIV infection, it is imperative to have clarity about the administrative and training needs implicit in reaching these goals as well as the necessary funding to do so.

Ideally, patients would receive a timely diagnosis of HIV in one of a number of settings and they would immediately be linked to a local experienced provider. HIV clinics would have a diverse staff able to cater to patients from a variety of backgrounds, and interpreter services would be widely available as well as teaching materials in the necessary languages. Patients would be provided with ancillary services on an as-needed basis, including case managers, transportation, and referral for mental health services and substance abuse programs.

All providers would receive cultural competency training integrated into medical school and residency curricula that would involve awareness of health care disparities, the significance of culture in medical practice, and guidance in fostering effective communication styles. Curricula would be evidence and outcome based, and students would take the bar from their teachers in recognizing the relevance of cultural competency in the provision of effective medical care.

The barriers to this ideal state are many and not limited to the fragmented system of care in the U.S., the complicated lives of many patients with HIV, and the frenzied pace of training in our residency programs. Nonetheless, we should strive toward the best practices and move beyond the simple documentation of disparities and barriers to care toward the implementation of new and effective strategies for patient care and teaching. The delivery of culturally competent care to minorities with HIV is integral to effective medical care of these patients.

Acknowledgments Supported in part by an HIVMA/IDSA Minority Clinical Fellowship Award to Dr. Loida Bonney and by the NIH/NIAID Grant No. 2P30 AI 50409-09 (Emory Center for AIDS Research).

References

1. Davis BJ and Voegtle KH. Culturally Competent Health Care for Adolescents: A Guide for Primary Health Care Providers. Chicago, IL. American Medical Association, 1994.
2. Kinsler JJ, Wong MD, Sayles JN, et al. The Effect of Perceived Stigma from a Health Care Provider on Access to Care Among a Low-Income HIV-Positive Population. AIDS Patient Care and STDs 2007, 21(8):584–592.
3. CDC 2008. HIV/AIDS Surveillance Report 2006. vol 18. Table 1. http://www.cdc.gov/hiv/topics/surveillance/resources/reports/
4. National Center for Health Statistics. National Vital Statistics Report 2002; vol 50(16):30.
5. Executive Summary Report of the Secretary's Task Force on Black and Minority Health. 1985. Vol 1. http://www.omhrc.gov/assets/pdf/checked/ANDERSON.pdf
6. Mayberry RM, Mili F, and Ofili E. Racial and Ethnic Differences in Access to Medical Care. Medical Care Research and Review 2000;57:108–45.
7. Smigal C, Jemal A, Ward E, et al. Trends in Breast Cancer by Race and Ethnicity: Update 2006. CA: A Cancer Journal for Clinicians 2006;56:168–83.
8. Peterson ED, Shaw LK, DeLong ER, et al. Racial Variation in the Use of Coronary-Revascularization Procedures – Are the Differences Real? Do They Matter?. NEJM 1997;336:480–6.
9. Shapiro MF, Morton SC, McCaffrey EF, et al. Variations in the Care of HIV-Infected Adults in the United States. JAMA 1999;281:2305–15.
10. Marks G, Crepaz N and Janssen RS. Estimating sexual transmission of HIV from persons aware and unaware that they are infected with the virus in the U.S. AIDS 2006;20:1447–50.
11. CDC Revised Recommendations for HIV Testing of Adults, Adolescents and Pregnant Women in Health Care Settings. MMWR 2006;55:1–17.
12. CDC HIV Testing Among Racial/Ethnic Minorities – U.S. 1999. MMWR 2001;50:1054–8.
13. Sifakis F, Flynn CP, Metsch L, et al. HIV Prevalence, Unrecognized Infection, and HIV Testing Among Men Who Have Sex with Men – Five U.S. Cities, June 2004–April 2005. MMWR 2005;54:597–601.
14. Mugavero MJ, Lin HY, Allison JJ, et al. Failure to Establish HIV Care: Characterizing the "No Show" Phenomenon. CID 2007;45:127–130.

15. CDC Advancing HIV Prevention Fact Sheet. August 2006. http://www.cdc.gov/hiv/topics/prev_prog/AHP/resources/factsheets/pdf/ARTASII.pdf
16. Milberg J, Sharma R, Scott F, et al. Factors Associated with Delays in Accessing HIV Primary Care in Rural Arkansas. AIDS Patient Care and STDs 2001;15:527–32.
17. Cunningham CO, Sohler NL, Wong MD, et al. Utilization of Health Care Services in Hard-to-Reach Marginalized HIV-Infected Individuals. AIDS Patient Care and STDs 2007;21:177–86.
18. Gardner LI, Metsch LR, Anderson-Mahoney P, et al. For the Antiretroviral Treatment and Access Study (ARTAS) Study Group. Efficacy of a Brief Case Management Intervention to Link Recently Diagnosed HIV-Infected Persons to Care. AIDS 2005;19:423–31.
19. CARE Act Overview. U.S. Department of Health and Human Services. July 2006. http://hab.hrsa.gov
20. Parham D and Conviser R. A Brief History of the Ryan White CARE Act in the U.S. and its Implications for Other Countries. AIDS Care 2002;14:S3–6.
21. McKinney MM and Marconi KM. Delivering HIV Services to Vulnerable Populations: A Review of CARE Act-Funded Research. Public Health Reports 2002;117:99–113.
22. Wood E, Montaner JS, Chan K, et al. Socioeconomic Status, Access to Triple Therapy, and Survival from HIV-Disease since 1996. AIDS 2002;16:2065–72.
23. Turner BJ, Cunningham WE, Duan N, et al. Delayed Medical Care After Diagnosis in a U.S. National Probability Sample of Persons Infected With Human Immunodeficiency Virus. Archives of Internal Medicine 2000;160:2614–22.
24. Mundy LM, Kalluri P, Meredith K, et al. Women with HIV Infection: A Model of University-Based Care, Training and Research. AIDS Care 2002;14:S95–107.
25. Sherer R, Stieglitz K, Narra J, et al. HIV Multidisciplinary Teams Work: Support Services Improve Access to and Retention in HIV Primary Care. AIDS Care 2002;14:S31–44.
26. Ashman JJ, Conviser R, and Pounds MB. Associations between HIV-positive Individuals' Receipt of Ancillary Services and Medical Care Receipt and Retention. AIDS Care 2002;14:S109–118.
27. Conviser R and Pounds MB. The Role of Ancillary Services in Client-Centered Systems of Care. AIDS Care 2002;14:S119–131.
28. Giordano TP, Gifford AL, White AC, et al. Retention in Care: A Challenge to Survival with HIV Infection. Clinical Infectious Diseases 2007;44:1493–9.
29. Anderson LM, Scrimshaw SC, Fullilove MT, et al. Culturally Competent Healthcare Systems. American Journal of Preventive Medicine 2003;24:68–79.
30. Sarver J and Baker D. Effect of Language Barriers on Follow Up Appointments After an Emergency Department Visit. Journal General Internal Medicine 2000;15:256–64.
31. Baker DW, Hayes R and Fortier JP. Interpreter Use and Satisfaction with Interpersonal Aspects of Care for Spanish-Speaking Patients. Medical Care 1998;36:1461–70.
32. Chng CL and Collins JR. Providing Culturally Competent HIV Prevention Programs. American Journal of Health Studies 2000;16:24–33.
33. Federman AD, Cook EF, Phillips RS. Intention to Discontinue Care Among Primary Care Patients 2001;16:668–74.
34. King WD, Wong MD, Shapiro MF, et al. Does Racial Concordance Between HIV positive Patients and Their Physicians Affect the Time to Receipt of a Protease Inhibitor? Journal of General Internal Medicine 2004;19:1146–53.
35. HIVMA Awards New Minority Clinical Fellowships. IDSA News Summer 2007. http://www.idsociety.org/newsArticle.aspx?id=4870.
36. Stone, VE. Optimizing the Care of Minority Patients with HIV/AIDS. Clinical Infectious Diseases 2004;38:400–404.
37. Satcher, D. Ethnic Disparities in Health: The Public's Role in Working for Equality. PLoS medicine 2006;3:1683–5.
38. Functions and Structure of a Medical School. Liaison Committee on Medical Education. June 2007. http://www.lcme.org/functions2007jun.pdf
39. Cultural Competence for Medical Students. American Association of Medical Colleges 2005. http://www.aamc.org/meded/tacct/culturalcomped.pdf

40. Betancourt JR, Green AR, Carrillo JE, and Park ER. Cultural Competence and Health Care Disparities: Key Perspectives and Trends. Health Affairs 2005;24:499–505.

41. Dogra N and Wass V. Can We Assess Students' Awareness of Cultural Diversity? A Qualitative Study of Stakeholders' Views. Medical Education 2006;40:682–90.

42. Brotherton SE, Rockey PH, and Etzel SI. U.S. Graduate Medical Education, 2003–2004. JAMA 2004;292:1032–37.

43. Shapiro J, Hollingshead J, and Morrison EH. Primary Care Resident, Faculty and Patient Views of Barriers to Cultural Competence, and the Skills Needed to Overcome Them. Medical Education 2002;36:749–59.

44. Brach C and Fraser I. Can Cultural Competency Reduce Racial and Ethnic Health Disparities? A Review and Conceptual Model. Medical Care Research and Review 2000;57:181–219.

45. Rapp DE. Integrating Cultural Competency into the Undergraduate Medical Curriculum. Medical Education 2006;40:704–10.

46. Betancourt JR, Green AR, and Carrillo JE. Cultural Competence in Health Care: Emerging Frameworks and Practical Approaches. Field Report for the Commonwealth Fund. October 2002.

47. Godkin MA and Savageau JA. The Effect of a Global Multiculturalism Track on Cultural Competence of Preclinical Medical Students. Medical Student Education 2001;33:178–86.

48. Smith WR, Betancourt JR, Wynia MK, et al. For the Society of General Internal Medicine Health Disparities Task Force. Recommendations for Teaching about Racial and Ethnic Disparities in Health and Health Care. Annals of Internal Medicine 2007;147:654–665.

49. Rogers J. Competency-Based Assessment and Cultural Compression in Medical Education: Lessons from Educational Anthropology. Medical Education 2005;39:1110–17.

50. Carrillo JE, Green AR, and Betancourt JR. Cross-Cultural Primary Care: A Patient-Based Approach. Annals of Internal Medicine 1999;130:829–34.

Women of Color and HIV/AIDS Epidemiology, Clinical Aspects, and Management

Bisola O. Ojikutu, Valerie E. Stone, and Arlene Bardeguez

Introduction

A growing number of women in the U.S. have been diagnosed with HIV/AIDS since the beginning of the epidemic. The proportion of new HIV/AIDS cases in women has increased from 8% of all cases in 1985 to 27% in 2005.[1] Women of color have borne the brunt of this shift in epidemiology. African Americans and Hispanic women account for more than 80% of new HIV/AIDS diagnoses in women.[2] In 2005, the rate of AIDS diagnosis for black women (45.5/100,000) was 23 times higher than the rate for white women (2.0/100,000). The rate for Hispanic women (11.2/100,000) was more than five times higher than that for their white counterparts.[1] A myriad of psychosocial, socioeconomic, and health system factors, including poverty, higher rates of other sexually transmitted diseases, drug and alcohol use, low perception of risk, sexual inequality, and lack of access to care and treatment have led to the disparate rise in HIV infection in women of color.[3-5] For similar reasons, increasing numbers of HIV cases have also been noted in women worldwide. Globally, women represent more than one-half of all infections amongst adults and are the fastest growing population living with HIV.[6]

Much of the HIV/AIDS information that was published early in the epidemic was based on data collected from male-predominant cohorts.[7,8] As the demographics of the epidemic changed, so did the need for research studies investigating the impact of HIV on women. In the early 1990s, research cohorts comprising women were formed.[9,10] Prospective studies from these longitudinal cohorts and independent research have contributed to an improved understanding of gender-based differences in HIV infection. We now have a better understanding of the environmental factors that impact disease progression in women, gender-specific side effects and toxicities caused by highly active antiretroviral therapy (HAART), and the gynecologic

B.O. Ojikutu (✉)
Massachusetts General Hospital, Office of International Programs, Division of AIDS, Harvard Medical School, Boston, MA, U.S.
E-mail: bojikutu@partners.org

V. Stone et al. (eds.), *HIV/AIDS in U.S. Communities of Color*.
DOI: 10.1007/978-0-387-98152-9_6, © Springer Science + Business Media, LLC 2009

manifestations specific to HIV. Our knowledge of the unique impact that HIV has on women, particularly on women of color, must continue to evolve. As new therapeutics become available, gender differences in efficacy and pharmacokinetics must be determined. As HIV-infected women live longer, the effect of HIV on menopause and on the development of chronic diseases associated with age deserves further investigation. Clearly, many questions remain.

This chapter will serve as a reference tool to provide clinical guidance to providers caring for women living with HIV infection. Risk factors for acquiring HIV will be reviewed as will the natural history of HIV infection with and without treatment. Clinical management strategies will be discussed, and the unique aspects of caring for women living with HIV, including the management of women on HAART, will be outlined. The gynecologic manifestations of HIV will be reviewed. An overview of reproductive challenges that women living with HIV face and the management of HIV in pregnancy will be reviewed in detail in a separate chapter.

Sex and HIV Risk

Most women contract HIV through high-risk heterosexual contact (sex with a male known to have or to be at risk for HIV infection).[1] This represents a reversal in dominant transmission mode in the U.S. In 1988, nearly 60% of newly diagnosed women reported injection drug use (IDU) as their risk factor.[11] Heterosexual transmission was reported as a distant second risk factor. By 2005, 80% of new infections in all U.S. women were attributed to high-risk heterosexual sex and only 19% were due to IDU. These rates are similar for black women. The rate of IDU as a reported risk factor for HIV infection is slightly higher in Hispanic women (29%).[1]

Biologically, women are more vulnerable to HIV infection than men during vaginal intercourse. Five-hundred and sixty-three discordant couples were followed in the European Study Group on Heterosexual Transmission of HIV, and it was found that the rate of male-to-female transmission was almost twice that of female to male. Stage of infection in the HIV-infected partner, age of female over 45, and concomitant anal sex were significantly associated with HIV transmission in that study.[12] Women are more susceptible because the area exposed to HIV is larger in women (vagina, cervix, and uterus) than in men (head of the penis, exposed urethra). In addition, women are exposed to a larger quantity of infectious fluid (ejaculate) than men (vaginal fluids which contain less HIV on average than semen). Overall, receptive vaginal intercourse with an infected partner carries a 0.1–0.2% risk per episode vs. 0.06% per episode for the insertive partner.[13, 14]

Unprotected anal intercourse is well established as a high-risk behavior associated with HIV seroconversion. Per episode risk to the receptive partner is approximately 0.1–3.0%.[13] Adolescent and younger women in all demographic groups have been found to engage in anal sex at a higher rate than those who are older.[15] Drug use, low HIV risk perception, and the desire to avoid pregnancy may play a role.[16]

Though oral sex poses minimal risk for HIV infection, there have been a few case reports of transmission to receptive partners.[17, 18] Female to female transmission has also been reported via oral route and through the use of shared sex toys.[19, 20]

HIV is more efficiently transmitted to sexually active younger women (ages 20 and under).[21, 22] Multiple factors lead to higher rates of transmission within this age group. Biologically, younger women have a larger area of cervical ectopy (the area of the cervix lined by columnar epithelium, which is highly vascular and fragile). The nature of this lining provides a lower mucosal barrier to sexually transmitted infections (STIs) and easier access to the blood stream and the lymphatic system.[23, 24] From a behavioral perspective, young women may also be at higher risk secondary to lower condom use, transactional sex (trading sex for money or drugs), and history of other sexually transmitted diseases.[25, 26] Age may also impact transmission rates later in life. Perimenopausal or postmenopausal women may have increased genital mucosal fragility secondary to hormonal changes typical of that stage of life, which may increase the risk of HIV transmission.[12]

Other Sexually Transmitted Diseases and HIV Risk

Both ulcerative (Herpes Simplex Virus, syphilis, chancroid) and nonulcerative (gonorrhea, chlamydia, and trichomonas) STIs have been associated with increased HIV transmission.[27] In a retrospective cohort study of patients attending an STI clinic, women with either ulcerative or nonulcerative STIs had a significantly increased risk of HIV seroconversion [hazard ratio 5.0; 95% confidence interval (1.9–13.0)].[28] Ulcerative STIs can provide a portal of entry for HIV and recruit HIV target cells to sites of epithelial infection. Nonulcerative STIs enhance the risk of HIV transmission through inflammation of the epithelium of the urethra, cervix, or penis.[27]

Herpes simplex virus is the most common cause of genital ulcer disease. According to NHANES data (1999–2004), overall HSV-2 prevalence in the U.S. is estimated to be 17%, down from 21% noted in a prior analysis. Infection with HSV-2 doubles the risk for HIV infection and may accelerate HIV progression. Though overall HSV-2 rates have decreased, significant differences in prevalence exist by race, ethnicity, and gender. Seroprevalence is highest amongst non-Hispanic blacks (40.3%), followed by non-Hispanic whites (13.7%), and Mexican-Americans (11.9%). HSV-2 seroprevalence was also noted to be twice as high among females suggesting that women may be more susceptible to HSV-2 infection than men.[29] Approximately one-half of all genital herpes infections are caused by HSV-1, which was previously primarily associated with oral, mucosal lesions.[30] This finding may be attributed to an increase in oral-genital sexual activity.

When examining rates of gonorrhea, chlamydia, and syphilis, disparities by race and ethnicity also exist. In 2005, the rate of gonorrhea in African American women aged 15–19 years was 14 times higher than that in their white counterparts. The rate amongst Hispanics was twice as high. Rates of chlamydia were three times and five times as high in Hispanic and African American women, respectively. Though the rate of syphilis is considerably lower than that of other genital ulcer diseases in all women, African Americans and Hispanics still experience a higher burden of infection.[31]

Other Factors Contributing to HIV Risk

It is well established that host factors such as high viral load increase the rate of HIV transmission.[32,33] Additional factors that may confer risk specifically to women have also been studied. There is evidence to suggest that sexual intercourse during menstruation increases the rate of transmission from females to males, most likely due to the higher amount of HIV viral particles noted in menstrual blood versus vaginal fluid.[34] Trauma incurred during intercourse causing vaginal tears might also diminish the mucosal barrier to transmission.[35] Studies have also explored the role that hormonal contraception may have on HIV transmission to male partners and HIV acquisition. Increased cervical and vaginal inflammation, increased genital tract expression of the HIV-1 coreceptor CCR5, higher levels of HIV-1 DNA in the genital tract, and increases in cervical ectopy noted during hormonal contraception use have all been postulated as mechanisms.[36–39] However, to date, there are no conclusive data to suggest that hormonal contraception use leads to increased HIV risk.

Data on potential risk of HIV transmission associated with intrauterine device (IUD) use are inconsistent.[40,41] It is clear that IUDs provide no protection against HIV infection. However, women using IUDs may have a higher risk of pelvic inflammatory disease.[42] HIV-infected women who are at low risk for contracting other STDs can safely use IUDs.[43]

Natural History

Our understanding of the natural history of HIV disease in women has evolved over the years. Initial studies suggested that there might be a difference in disease progression by gender. More recent studies have demonstrated no difference between men and women in progression to AIDS and death when matched by socioeconomic status, race, and HIV risk factor.[44] The previously noted gender disparities were most likely due to late presentation and poor access to care due to poverty, transportation difficulty, cultural and language barriers, and other issues.[45,46]

Mortality rates amongst both African American women and men are significantly higher than that amongst whites. The same is true for Latino men and women living with HIV. In a recent analysis, African American women in all age groups had a 13-times greater risk of dying from HIV compared with white women of the same age, and African American women aged 65–74 years had more than 20-times greater risk than white women of the same age.[47] This study included both a pre-HAART and post-HAART analysis, and based on these analyses, the authors postulated that differences in access to HAART led to this disparity in mortality. Other studies have concurred that significant disparities in access to care and treatment have led to increased mortality by race and gender.[48]

Women have been noted to have lower viral loads than men at similar CD4 counts. In a study of the ALIVE (AIDS Linked to the Intravenous Experience) cohort, which is 95% African American, the initial median viral load was 0.5 $\log_{10}$ (3.16 times) lower for women than it was for men. Multivariate proportional hazard model stratified by sex and controlling for initial CD4 cell count and age showed no significant difference between men and women in the risk of progression to AIDS in 5 years of follow-up, despite women starting with lower HIV RNA loads. Thus, although the relative viral load has a similar predictive value for progression to AIDS for men and women, the same absolute viral load seems to confer different risk of progression to AIDS between the sexes.[49]

Because HIV-infected women tend to progress to AIDS and death in a time course similar to that for men, women apparently progress to these end points with lower initial viral loads. Of note, the U.S. Department of Health and Human Services recommends the same guidelines for HAART initiation for both men and women, using CD4 count thresholds for HAART initiation, not HIV RNA viral load.[50]

Nongynecologic Manifestations of HIV in Women

Malignancies

Kaposi's sarcoma occurred more frequently in men than in women in both the pre-HAART and post-HAART eras. Overall incidence declined post-HAART in both males and females.[51,52] Though the incidence is lower, there is some evidence to suggest that Kaposi's sarcoma might manifest as a more severe disease in women. In a study of 162 (54 women and 108 men) HIV-infected patients with Kaposi's sarcoma in Italy, it was found that the disease occurred at an earlier age ($p = 0.001$), was associated with a more severe immunodeficiency ($p = 0.03$), more advanced stages of HIV disease ($p = 0.05$), and had more aggressive presentation and course in women than in men.[53] A second study in Zimbabwe also found that women were more likely to report associated symptoms (fever, weight loss, pain) suggesting more severe disease.[54] The reason for more aggressive clinical behavior is unclear.

The rate of AIDS related non-Hodgkins lymphoma (NHL) also declined in the post-HAART era. The risk of NHL declined by 57.5% between 1990–1995 and 1996–2002 for all patients living with HIV.[55] The NHL incidence rate among women in both the pre-HAART and post-HAART era was lower than that noted in men within the same racial category. Among white women the incidence was noted to be 13.8/100,000 in 1998. Among black women the incidence was noted to be slightly lower at 9.1. Rates for white and black men were 19.0 and 12.9 in 1998, respectively.[52]

Several studies have noted an increased rate of lung cancer in HIV-infected persons. In a study that included 48,949 women (57% black and 21% Hispanic), lung cancer was the most commonly noted non-AIDS defining cancer.[56] However, the rate of smoking was also higher in the study population. The association of lung cancer risk and HIV has been further evaluated in a recent study of 2,086 HIV-infected patients. After adjusting for age, sex, smoking status, and calendar period, HIV infection was associated with increased lung cancer risk (hazard ratio, 3.6; 95% confidence interval, 1.6–7.9).[57]

Several studies have noted a decrease in the incidence of breast cancer in women living with AIDS compared with the general population.[58–60] Further study should be undertaken to understand the underlying factors mediating this decreased risk and to uncover any confounding variables that might have led to these findings.

Pneumocystis Pneumonia

Pneumocystis pneumonia (PCP) remains the most common opportunistic infection found in HIV-infected patients in the U.S.[61] Men and women appear to have equivalent risk of infection.[62] Although one study noted a lower rate of PCP in African Americans, other studies have disputed this finding.[63–65]

Hematologic Complications

Anemia is a common finding in women presenting with HIV. Women of color may be particularly impacted.[66] Iron deficiency, food insecurity, IDU, CD4 count <200 cells/ml^3, and other underlying illnesses, particularly renal disease, predispose women with HIV to anemia.[67,68] In addition, antiretroviral medications (most commonly AZT) can lead to anemia in patients. Thrombocytopenia is also a frequent occurrence in people living with HIV. In a medical record survey including over 30,000 patients, clinical and immunological AIDS, history of injecting drug use, anemia, lymphoma, and black race were significantly associated with thrombocytopenia, but gender was not.[69]

Gynecologic Issues and Clinical Manifestations in Women with HIV Infection

Early manifestations of HIV disease in women are often gynecological in nature. These are most commonly recurrent herpetic or candidal infections, pelvic inflammatory disease, and cervical cytologic abnormalities. Prevalence data from early in the epidemic and those reported more recently in the post-HAART era document this frequent clinical phenomenon.[70–73] Thus, it is imperative that women who present with or report a history of frequent recurrences of these problems, without other predisposing factors, be tested for HIV infection. In general, the treatment of STIs, pelvic inflammatory disease, and other genital infections among HIV-uninfected and HIV-infected women is the same; however, the clinical presentation may be more severe and/or more varied among women with HIV infection.[74] Menstrual abnormalities, particularly amenorrhea, are frequently seen in women living with HIV/AIDS. However, a recent prospective cohort analysis using the HERS and WIHS cohorts found no association between HIV infection alone and menstrual disorders. However, there was a correlation found between increasing likelihood of these disorders and lower CD4 counts and higher HIV viral loads.[75] In addition, the higher frequency of menstrual disorders among the women with HIV was associated with other factors related to their health status, including weight loss, chronic disease, substance abuse, and use of psychoactive medications.

Bacterial Vaginosis

Bacterial vaginosis (BV) is one of several nonulcerative STIs that have been found to confer a higher risk of acquiring HIV when a woman has sexual contact with an infected partner, as mentioned previously.[28,76,77] In addition, however, the prevalence of this infection in women living with HIV is higher than in uninfected controls with estimates ranging from 18 to 42%.[68] This infection also persists longer in HIV-infected women, and the tendency to persist and the severity of BV increase with lower CD4 counts.[70,77] Treatment of BV in HIV-infected women is the same as in other women – metronidazole 500 mg by mouth twice a day (po bid) for 7 days or metronidazole 0.75% vaginal gel qd for 5–7 days.

Trichomonas Vaginalis Infections

Overall, the prevalence of genital Trichomonas vaginalis is higher among African American women in the U.S. than among other races. This is of concern, since this infection is strongly associated with increased risk of HIV acquisition.[28,78–80] However, surprisingly, this infection does not have a higher prevalence, incidence, or persistence in HIV-infected women than in high-risk uninfected controls.[81] There are no changes to general treatment recommendations for this infection for HIV-infected women. Most women can be effectively treated with metronidazole 500 mg po bid for 7 days.

Candidal Vaginal Infections

Many women may first be diagnosed with HIV infection because of recurrent vulvovaginal candidiasis. HIV-infected women have been found to have a higher incidence and greater persistence of candidal vaginal infections.[70,73,77] While the severity has not been found to be greater among women with HIV in carefully controlled studies, lower CD4 counts and other predisposing factors may together worsen the severity of vaginal candidiasis in a given patient (e.g., use of antibiotics or corticosteroids, obesity, diabetes mellitus). Many HIV-infected women may require longer oral treatment courses with fluconazole or longer courses of topical antifungal agents such as clotrimazole or miconazole to effectively treat an episode of vaginal candidiasis. Usually a week-long course of topical agents should be used. Alternatively sequential doses of fluconazole 150 mg po given for several days, or fluconazole 200 mg on day 1 and then 100 mg po qd to complete a 5–7-day course is effective.

Gonorrhea and Chlamydia

The prevalence and incidence rates of gonorrhea and chlamydia in HIV-infected women are essentially the same as those in similar HIV-uninfected women. The clinical manifestations and management of these STIs in HIV-infected women do not differ from those for HIV-uninfected women.[70]

Syphilis Infections in HIV-Infected Women

Syphilis is also much more prevalent in African American and Hispanic women than in their white counterparts, irrespective of HIV status.[31] Primary syphilis, with its associated ulcerative chancre, is well known to greatly increase a patient's risk of acquiring HIV when exposed.[27] Management of patients with serologic and/or clinical evidence of syphilis is generally the same irrespective of gender and HIV status. However, current guidelines recommend that HIV-infected patients with RPR titers of 1:32 or greater have a CSF evaluation done prior to treatment to rule out CNS infection (e.g., neurosyphilis).[82]

Herpes Simplex Virus Infections

Genital herpes simplex infection is the most common cause of genital ulcers in the U.S. Most genital herpes is caused by HSV-2 (60–95%), and the age-adjusted prevalence of HSV-2 infection is significantly higher in women than in men.[83]

Genital HSV infection has been found to confer a higher risk of acquiring HIV when exposed.[27,84] Genital herpes is highly prevalent in HIV-infected women. Episodes of genital herpes in HIV-infected women tend to be more frequent and prolonged. They may often appear atypical (for example, with confluent large ulcers) particularly in those with lower CD4 counts. HIV-infected women often require higher doses and longer courses of anti-virals to effectively treat an episode of genital HSV. Those who have frequent recurrences should be offered suppressive therapy. HSV prophylaxis during pregnancy has also been recommended to prevent perinatal transmission to the fetus for both HIV-negative and HIV-infected women.[85–87] This is a critically important recommendation, since a recent study found higher mother-to-child HIV transmission among infants born to HSV/HIV coinfected women.[88]

Human Papilloma Virus Infection and Cervical Cytologic Abnormalities

The rates of abnormal Pap smear, human papilloma virus (HPV) coinfection, and invasive cancer are higher among HIV-infected women than among their seronegative counterparts.[89–91] The reported rates of low-grade squamous intraepithelial lesions (LGSIL) are 1.6% among the general population, but 7.3–13.7% among HIV-infected women. The rates of high-grade intraepithelial lesions (HGSIL) are 0.45% in the general population, but markedly higher at 2.5–13.3% among HIV-infected women.[92–94] The associated risk factors for abnormal Pap smear and invasive cervical cancer include advanced immunosuppression, AIDS, low CD4 count, high viral load, and coinfection with HPV virus.[89,91,92] Although some studies suggest that initiation of HAART is associated with reversion of LGSIL, this observation has not been consistently found and may reflect elimination of HPV infection in women with better immune status.[93]

The optimal management of abnormal Pap smears among HIV-infected women is uncertain since they tend to have greater rates of recurrences and faster progression than their HIV-negative counterparts. Age, HPV type, presence of cofactors for cervical cancer such as smoking, and future reproductive plans should all be taken into consideration in making management decisions. Current recommendations are that all HIV-infected women should have a cervical Pap smear performed twice during the first year after diagnosis and, if the results are normal, annually thereafter.[82] Rapid referral for colposcopy, biopsy, and treatment should be provided for any woman found to have concerning abnormalities on Pap smear (ASCUS, LGSIL, HGSIL). For review of the current recommendation for surveillance and management of abnormal cervical cancer screening the reader is referred to standard guidelines and the 2006 consensus guidelines and the U.S. Public Health Service (USPHS) guidelines for screening and treatment of opportunistic infections.[95]

HPV infections are responsible for most premalignant cervical lesions as well as cervical cancer.[96,97] It is hoped that early vaccination of adolescents and young women (<27-years old) prior to acquisition of infection could lead to a dramatic reduction in the number of cervical cancer cases reported in the U.S. and globally.[98] Despite increased rates of Pap smear screening in the U.S. over the last decade, African American and Hispanic women and those living in the southern U.S. continue to have higher cervical cancer rates.[96,99] As has been stated already, these are the same subpopulations of women with the highest HIV-seroprevalence rates in our nation. It is thus imperative to ascertain the safety, tolerability, and response of HPV vaccination among HIV-infected adolescents and women. Several studies are ongoing and the interested reader could monitor the results of those studies in the scientific literature or as their findings are incorporated to the U.S. PHS recommendations for opportunistic infections.

Vulvar intraepithelial neoplasia (VIN) is also caused by HPV, and increased incidence of these lesions as well as VIN-related cancer has been reported among young women in recent decades.[100] VIN lesions have a high rate of recurrence and invasion frequently requiring multiple biopsies or surgical resection and potentially decreasing quality of life for those affected.[100,101] Sporadic case reports of high-grade VIN as well as invasive vulvar carcinoma among HIV-infected women have been reported in the literature.[102,103] In a study conducted prior to the HAART era by Jamieson et al. the authors observed higher prevalence rates of vulvar, vaginal, and perianal intraepithelial neoplasia among HIV-infected women than among their seronegative counterparts.[104] The incidence of these lesions was statistically significant when these groups were compared [1.96 per 100 person years and 0.26 per 100 person years, $p = 0.03$].[104] Thus, prevalence of this complication as well as its response to local resection or prevention among women who receive HPV vaccination with or without antiretroviral treatment is of tremendous ongoing interest and concern.

Contraception

Discussion of contraception options should be a priority for providers caring for HIV-infected women. The role of contraception in this population serves two purposes: avoidance of unwanted pregnancy and prevention of transmission to the woman's sexual partner. For the latter, barrier contraception, such as male or female condoms, is the best option. However, these methods are not so effective in pregnancy prevention for a number of reasons: (1) inconsistent use, (2) the need to use them with spermicide to increase their effectiveness, (3) the need to have their use linked to the timing of sexual intercourse, and (4) the need to have the male partner agree to their use. On the other hand, hormonal contraception is controlled by the female patient who has the option of nondisclosure of its use to her partner, and the level of efficacy is close to 99% with perfect use. Nonetheless, there are concerns of systemic adverse events or drug interactions, particularly among women on both oral hormonal contraception and HAART, with the potential for decreased effectiveness of the contraceptive agent, HAART regimen, or both.

At this point, the available information regarding effectiveness of hormonal contraception for HIV-infected women on HAART is incomplete. Studies are underway to attempt to provide more optimal information. For now, what we do know is that use of Depo-Provera in HIV-infected women on NNRTI or protease inhibitor-based regimens has documented effectiveness and lack of significant interactions.[105] Furthermore, a recent study comparing the use of oral contraceptives, Depo-Provera, and condoms for pregnancy prevention in HIV-infected women found that the overall risk of pregnancy was lower with injectable contraception (Depo-Provera) than with oral contraception.[106] Certainly, the greater effectiveness of the injectable contraceptive could be due to differences of adherence, but there also may be fewer drug interactions with HAART medications. An additional concern regarding oral contraception in HIV-infected women that has been raised by some studies is increased genital HIV shedding and more rapid HIV disease progression.[107,108] Another option, the IUD, has also been shown to be a safe and acceptable method for HIV-infected women and could avert drug interactions with other HIV-related drugs needed by these patients. Finally, for women who do not desire any additional children, surgical sterilization could be the optimal contraceptive approach.[109] Providers need to be judicious regarding this approach in young patients as they tend to have the highest level of regret. Several sterilization approaches are feasible including tubal sterilization, hysteroscopically inserted microinsert, or male sterilization (vasectomy).[109]

In summary, the optimal contraceptive approach must be clearly individualized to address patient choice, provide highest possible effectiveness, avert adverse effects and drug interactions and take into account the need for reversibility of the method. For patients uncertain of their choice, barrier method with Plan B (the morning after pill) as an option might be a reasonable approach if they engage in unprotected intercourse. Further studies to ascertain the efficacy and safety of contraception among HIV-infected women are needed to confirm or dismiss the concern of faster disease progression among women on hormonal contraceptives.

HIV and Older Women

HIV in older patients is often unrecognized.[110] Approximately 10–15% of all those living with HIV in this country are over 50 years of age.[111] The rate of new diagnoses within that age group is rising. In addition, since the advent of HAART, more patients with HIV are living longer. Therefore, many women with HIV are or will be experiencing menopause. Unfortunately, there are few studies characterizing menopause in HIV-infected women. Those that have been published have noted an earlier mean age of menopausal onset (46 years vs. 49 years).[112] Drug use may also contribute to this finding.[113] In addition, symptoms of menopause, hot flashes and vaginal dryness, may be more severe.[114] Whether older age and estrogen decline translate into differences in treatment response or clinical progression is unclear.

Both untreated HIV and HIV treated with HAART are associated with bone dem-
ineralization with increased prevalence of osteoporosis and osteopenia. Menopause
may add to the predisposition for these disorders in women. In a study of 31 HIV-
infected African American and Hispanic women, a 43% prevalence of osteoporosis
of the spine versus 23% in historical controls was noted.[115]

Providing Care for Women of Color with HIV/AIDS

Providing clinical care for women of color with HIV/AIDS is in most ways similar
to providing care for others living with HIV/AIDS. To optimize the care of women
of color with HIV, attention should be paid to several key issues: (1) ensuring that
the clinical care site is oriented to the needs and concerns of women and to the
specific cultures being served, (2) optimizing access to HAART, and (3) optimizing
adherence to HAART.

The diversity of individuals living with HIV/AIDS in the U.S. is striking, encom-
passing men who have sex with men (MSMs), injection drug users of both genders,
and men and women who have acquired HIV heterosexually. In each of these groups
(MSMs, IDUs, and heterosexuals without other risks) there can also be tremendous
racial, ethnic, and cultural diversity as well. Given this, clinicians and others who
endeavor to structure HIV/AIDS clinical care programs to meet the needs of all the
patients being served in a given site face tremendous challenges. For this reason,
many care sites have simply structured the program around the needs of the predominant group being served – often nonminority MSMs. Other clinical care sites
are not structured to meet the needs of any one particular type of patient.

However, to ideally engage women of color in care (and >80% of women living with HIV/AIDS are women of color), clinical care sites should demonstrate
in multiple small ways that they are there to welcome and care for women living
with HIV/AIDS. These approaches can include, but are not limited to employing staff who are women and who are of the same culture as the patients being
served, having magazines and educational materials of interest to women of color
in the waiting room, and displaying art and flyers that are of interest to women, and
making the environment appear more inviting and appealing. In addition, clinical
care sites should host celebrations at special times of the year (such as holidays
and World AIDS Day) that are fun and include foods from the cultures of the
patients being served. Most importantly, clinical programs should be developed and
offered that meet the special (and frequent) needs and concerns of women living
with HIV/AIDS. These include ensuring on-site (or easy access to) social workers, mental health services, substance abuse services, gynecologic care especially
colposcopy, dermatology, and nutritionists, as well as other weight-related care services. Finally, educational programs focused on the needs of the women who come
to the clinical care site should be offered on an intermittent (e.g., monthly) basis,
and support groups should be available for women to decrease social isolation and

to promote social support through contact with staff and with others living with HIV/AIDS.[116, 117]

Optimizing access to HAART and receipt of HAART should be a priority in the care of women living with HIV infection. Numerous studies have found that women are less likely to receive HAART when indicated than are men with HIV infection.[118, 119] And, a series of more recent studies have found that minority women, particularly black women, are even less likely than other women to receive HAART when indicated.[120] The reasons for this disparity in the receipt/use of HAART have not been clearly elucidated. Contributing factors to this disparity in the receipt of HAART may include (1) provider–patient encounter factors (e.g., miscommunications and misunderstandings in the clinical care setting), (2) medical comorbidities such as hepatitis C infection, depression, or substance abuse that cause the patient or her provider to delay prescribing HAART, and (3) competing life circumstances such as unstable living situation, personal relationship problems such as domestic violence, or needs of children, partners, parents, or others for which the patient serves as a caregiver. Finally, women may choose to discontinue HAART due to side effects more often than men do.[121, 122] While the causes are not entirely clear (and may be myriad), what is clear is that this disparity is one of the largest contributors to the disparity in death rates due to HIV/AIDS among minority women than among others.[111]

Given this, providers should proactively encourage women who meet current U.S. Department of Health and Human Services Guidelines indications for HAART to start HAART and to stay on HAART. Strategies such as the use of peer counselors and treatment buddies can be helpful in enhancing the patient's acceptance of HAART and engagement in treatment. The quality of the patient's relationship with her HIV primary provider has been found to be critically important for acceptance of treatment and adherence to treatment.[123, 124] Efforts to spend time with the patient, getting to know her, having relatively frequent visits, and spending some time during visits on nonclinical conversation can contribute to this goal. Having a second or third provider with whom the patient is consistently connected and can turn to in the primary provider's absence such as a primary nurse or case manager is also quite effective in building trust and enhancing engagement in care.[125, 126]

Many women living with HIV/AIDS may have one or more of the documented barriers to adherence to HAART such as depression, substance abuse, alcohol abuse, low literacy, chaotic living situation, or nondisclosure of HIV status to family. Providers and care sites should therefore have a set of strategies that they consistently utilize to proactively optimize adherence and thereby optimize outcome of women of color on HAART. Please refer to "Challenges in the Treatment of Minorities with HIV-infection, Chapter 4" for detailed strategies for enhancing adherence.

References

1. Centers for Disease Control and Prevention (CDC). HIV/AIDS Surveillance Report. 2005;17:1–54.
2. Centers for Disease Control and Prevention (CDC). Racial/ethnic disparities in diagnoses of HIV/AIDS-33 states, 2001–2005. MMWR Weekly Report. 2007;56:189–193.
3. Adimora AA, Schoenbach VJ, Martinson FE, et al. Social context of sexual relationships among rural African Americans. Sex Trans Dis. 2001;28:69–76.
4. Moreno CL, El-Bassel N, Morrill AC. Heterosexual women of color and HIV risk: sexual risk factors for HIV among Latina and African American women. Women Health. 2007;45:1–15.
5. Forna FM, Fitzpatrick L, Adimora AA. A case-control study of factors associated with HIV infection among black women. J Natl Med Assoc. 2006;98(11):1798–804.
6. UNAIDS and World Health Organization. AIDS Epidemic Update. December 2007. Available at: http://data.unaids.org/pub/EPISlides/2007/2007_epiupdate_en.pdf. Accessed: January 15, 2008.
7. Ginzburg HM, Fleming PL, Miller KD. Selected public health observations derived from Multicenter AIDS Cohort Study. JAIDS. 1988;1:2–7.
8. Ledergerber B, von Overbeck J, Egger M. The Swiss HIV Cohort Study: rationale, organization and selected baseline characteristics. Soz Praentivmed.1994;39:387–94.
9. Barkan S, Melnick S, Preston-Martin S. The Women's interagency HIV Study. Epidemiology. 1998;9:117–125.
10. Smith DK, Warren DL, Vlahov D. Design and baseline participant characteristics of the Human Immunodeficiency Virus Epidemiology Research (HER) Study: a prospective cohort study of human immunodeficiency virus infection in U.S. women. Am J Epidemiol. 1997;146:459–69.
11. Hader S, Smith DK, Moore JS, et al. HIV Infection in Women in the United States: status at the Millennium JAMA. 2001;9:1186–92.
12. European Study Group on Heterosexual Transmission of HIV. Comparison of female to male and male to female transmission of HIV in 563 stable couples. BMJ. 1992;304:809–813.
13. Mastro TD, de Vincezzi I. Probabilities of sexual HIV transmission. AIDS. 1996;10(Suppl A):S75–82.
14. Vittinghoff E, Douglas J, Judson F, et al. Per-contact risk of human immunodeficiency virus transmission between male sexual partners. Am J Epidemiol. 1999;150:306–11.
15. Jaffe LR, Seehaus M, Wagner C, et al. Anal intercourse and knowledge of acquired immunodeficiency syndrome among minority-group female adolescents. J Pediatr. 1988;112:1005–7.
16. Houston AM, Fang J, Husman C, et al. More than just vaginal intercourse: anal intercourse and condom use patterns in the context of "main" and "casual" sexual relationships among urban minority adolescent females. J Pediatr Adolesc Gynecol. 2007;20:299–304.
17. Lifson AR, O'Malley PM, Hessol NA, et al. HIV seroconversion in two homosexual men after receptive oral intercourse with ejaculation: implications for counseling concerning safe sexual practices. Am J Public Health. 1990;80:1509–11.
18. Rothenberg RB, Scarlett M, del Rio C, et al. Oral Transmission of HIV. AIDS 1998;12:2095–2105.
19. Rich JD, Buck A, Tuomala RE, et al. Transmission of human immunodeficiency virus infection presumed to have occurred via female homosexual contact. Clin Infect Dis. 1993;17:1003–5.
20. Kwakwa HA, Ghobrial MW. Female-to-female transmission of human immunodeficiency virus. Clin Infect Dis. 2003;36(3):e40–1. Epub 2003 Jan 10.
21. Sarkar K, Bai B, Mukherjee R, et al. Young age is a risk factor for HIV among female sex workers-An experience from India. J Infect. 2006;53:4;255–259.
22. Bulterys M, Chao A, Habimana P, et al. Incident HIV-1 infection in a cohort of young women in Butare, Rwanda. AIDS 1994;8:1585–1591.

23. Moscicki AB, Ma Y, Holland C, et al. Cervical ectopy in adolescent girls with and without human immunodeficiency virus infection. J Infect Dis. 2001;183:865–70.
24. Moss GB, Clemetson D, D'Costa L, et al. Association of cervical ectopy with heterosexual transmission of human immunodeficiency virus: results of a study of couples in Nairobi, Kenya. J Infect Dis. 1991;164:588–91.
25. Heffernan R, Chiasson MA, Sackoff JE. HIV risk behaviors among adolescents at a sexually transmitted disease clinic in New York City. J Adolesc Health. 1996;18:429–34.
26. Clark RA, Kissinger P, Bedimo AL, et al. Determination of factors associated with condom use among women infected with human immunodeficiency virus. Int J STD AIDS. 1997;8:229–33.
27. Fleming DT, Wasserheit JN. From epidemiological synergy to public health policy and practice: the contribution of other sexually transmitted diseases to sexual transmission of HIV infection. Sex Transm Infect. 1999;75:3–17.
28. Hanson J, Posner S, Hassig S, et al. Assessment of sexually transmitted diseases as risk factors for HIV seroconversion in a New Orleans sexually transmitted disease clinic, 1990–1998. Ann Epidemiol. 2005;15:13–20.
29. Xu F, Sternberg MR, Kottri BJ, et al. Trends in Herpes Simplex Virus Type 1 and Type 2 Seroprevalence in the United States. JAMA. 2006;296:964–973.
30. Gupta R, Warren T, Wald A. Genital herpes. Lancet. 2007;370:2127–37.
31. Centers for Disease Control and Prevention. Health Disparities in HIV/AIDS, Viral Hepatitis, Sexually Transmitted Disease and Tuberculosis in the United States. Available at: http://www.cdc.gov/NCHHSTP/healthdisparities/docs/NCHHSTPHealthDisparitiesReport1107.pdf. Accessed: February 3, 2008.
32. Ragni MV, Faruki H, Kingsley LA. Heterosexual HIV-1 transmission and viral load in hemophilic patients. J Acquir Immune Defic Syndr Hum Retrovirol. 1998;17:42–5.
33. Pedraza MA, Del Romero J, Roldan F, et al. Heterosexual transmission of HIV-1 is associated with high plasma viral load levels and a positive viral isolation in the infected partner. J Acquir Immune Defic Syndr. 1999;2:120–5.
34. Tanfer K, Aral SO. Sexual intercourse during menstruation and self-reported sexually transmitted disease history among women. Sex Transm Dis. 1996;23:395–40.
35. Guimaraes MD, Vlahov D, Castilho EA. Postcoital vaginal bleeding as a risk factor for transmission of the human immunodeficiency virus in a heterosexual partner study in Brazil. Rio de Janeiro Heterosexual Study Group. Arch Intern Med. 1997;157:1362–8.
36. Baeten JM, Nyange PM, Richardson BA, et al. Hormonal contraception and risk of sexually transmitted disease acquisition: results from a prospective study. Am J Obstet Gynecol. 2001;185:380–5.
37. Moss GB, Clemetson D, D'Costa L, et al. Association of cervical ectopy with heterosexual transmission of human immunodeficiency virus: results of a study of couples in Nairobi, Kenya. J Infect Dis. 1991;164:588–91.
38. Ghanem KG, Shah N, Klein RS, et al. Influence of sex hormones, HIV status, and concomitant sexually transmitted infection on cervicovaginal inflammation. J Infect Dis. 2005;191:358–66.
39. Prakash M, Kapembwa MS, Gotch F, et al. Oral contraceptive use induces upregulation of the CCR5 chemokine receptor on CD4(+) T cells in the cervical epithelium of healthy women. J Reprod Immunol. 2002;54:117–31.
40. Kapiga SH, Lyamuya EF, Lwihula GK. The incidence of HIV infection among women using family planning methods in Dar es Salaam, Tanzania. AIDS. 1998;12:75–84.
41. Daly CC, Helling-Giese GE, Mati JK. Contraceptive methods and the transmission of HIV: implications for family planning. Genitourin Med. 1994;70:110–7.
42. Meirik O. Intrauterine devices – upper and lower genital tract infections. Contraception. 2007;75(Suppl 6):S41–7.
43. Stringer EM, Kaseba C, Levy J, et al. A randomized trial of the intrauterine contraceptive device vs hormonal contraception in women who are infected with the human immunodeficiency virus. Am J Obstet Gynecol. 2007;197:144.e1–8.

44. Chaisson RE, Keruly JC, Moore RD. Race, sex, drug use and progression of human immunodeficiency disease. N Eng J Med. 1995;331:751–6.
45. Melnick SL, Sherer R, Louis TA, et al. Survival and disease progression according to gender of patients with HIV infection. The Terry Beirn Community Programs for Clinical Research on AIDS. JAMA. 1994;2727:1915–21.
46. Squires K. Gender difference in the diagnosis and treatment of HIV. Gend Med. 2007;4:294–307.
47. Levine RS, Briggs NC, Kilbourn BS. Black–white mortality from HIV in the United States before and after introduction of highly active antiretroviral therapy in 1996. Am J Pub Health. 2007;97:1884–92.
48. Gebo KA, Fleishan JA, Conviser R, et al. Racial and gender disparities in receipt of highly active antiretroviral therapy persist in a multistate sample of HIV patients in 2001. J Acquire Immune Defic Syndr. 2005;38:96–103.
49. Sterling TR, Vlahov D, Astemborski J, et al. Initial plasma HIV-1 RNA levels and progression to AIDS in women and men. N Engl J Med 2001;344:720–5.
50. Panel on Antiretroviral Therapy Guidelines for Adults and Adolescents. Guidelines for the use of antiretroviral agents in HIV-1 infected adults and adolescent. Department of Health and Human Services. January 29, 2008;1–128. Available: http://aidsinfo.nih.gov/contentfiles/AdultandAdolescentGL.pdf. Accessed on July 12, 2008.
51. Cooley TP, Hirschhorn LR, O'Keane JC. Kaposi's sarcoma in women with AIDS. AIDS. 1996;10:1221–5.
52. Eltom MA, Jemal A, Mbulaiteye SM, et al. Trends in Kaposi's sarcoma and non-Hodgkin's lymphoma incidence in the United States From 1973 through 1998. J Natl Cancer Inst. 2002;94:1204–1210.
53. Nasti G, Serraino D, Ridolfo, A, et al. AIDS-Associated Kaposi's Sarcoma Is More Aggressive in Women: A Study of 54 Patients. AIDS. 1999;20:337–341
54. Meditz AL; Borok M; MaWhinney S, et al. Gender differences in AIDS-associated Kaposi sarcoma in Harare, Zimbabwe. J Acquir Immune Defic Syndr.2007; 44:306–308.
55. Engels E; Pfeiffer RM; Goedert JJ, et al. Trends in cancer risk among people with AIDS in the United States 1980–2002. AIDS. 2006;20:1645–1654.
56. Frisch M, Biggar RJ, Engels E, et al. Association of cancer with AIDS-related immunosuppression in adults.JAMA. 2001;285:1736–1745.
57. Kirk GD, Merlo C, Driscoll P, et al. HIV infection is associated with an increased risk for lung cancer, independent of smoking. Clin Infect Dis. 2007;45:103–10.
58. Goedert JJ, Schainer C, McNeel TS, et al. Risk of breast, ovary, and uterine corpus cancers among 85 268 women with AIDS. Br J Cancer. 2006;95:642–648.
59. Frisch M, Biggar RJ, and Engels EA, et al. Association of cancer with AIDS-related immunosuppression in adults. JAMA. 2001;4;285:1736–45.
60. Herida M, Mary Krause M, Kaphan R, et al. Incidence of non-AIDS-defining cancers before and during the highly active antiretroviral therapy era in a cohort of human immunodeficiency virus-infected patients. J Clin Oncol. 2003;15;21:3447–53.
61. Morris A, Lundgren JD, Masur H, et al. Current epidemiology of pneumocystis pneumonia. Emerg Infect Dis. 2004;10:1713–1720.
62. Kaplan JE, Hanson DL, Navin TR, et al. Risk factors for Pneumocystis carinii pneumonia in human immunodeficiency virus infected adolescents and adults in the United States: reassessment of indications for chemoprophylaxis. J Infect Dis. 1998;178:1126–32.
63. Stansell JD, Osmond DH, Charlebois E, et al. Predictors of Pneumocystis carinii pneumonia in HIV-infected persons. Pulmonary Complications of HIV Study Group. AM J Respir Crit Care Med. 1997;155:60–6.
64. Chan IS, Neaton JD, Saravolatz LD, et al. Frequencies of opportunistic diseases prior to death among HIV-infected persons. Community Programs for Clinical Research on AIDS. AIDS. 1995;9:1145–51.
65. Jones JL, Hanson DL, Dworkin MS, et al. Surveillance for AIDS-defining opportunistic illnesses, 1992–1997. MMWR CDC Surveill Summ. 1999;48:1–22.

66. Wills TS, Nadler JP, Somboonwit C, et al. Anemia prevalence and associated risk factors in a single-center ambulatory HIV clinical cohort. AIDS Read. 2004;14:305–10, 313–5.
67. Semba RD. Iron-deficiency anemia and the cycle of poverty among human immunodeficiency virus-infected women in the inner city. Source: Clin Infect Dis. 2003;37(Suppl 1) 2–11.
68. Sullivan PS, Hanson DL, Chu SY, et al. Epidemiology of anemia in human immunodeficiency virus (HIV)-infected persons: results from the multistate adult and adolescent spectrum of HIV disease surveillance project. Blood. 1998;91:301–8.
69. Sullivan PS, Hanson DL, Chu SY, et al. Surveillance for thrombocytopenia in persons infected with HIV: results from the multistate adult and adolescent spectrum of disease project. JAIDS. 1997;14:374–9.
70. Cu-Uvin, S Hogan JW, Warren D, et al. Prevalence of lower genital tract infection among HIV-seropositive and high risk seronegative women. HIV Epidemiology Research Study (HERS) Group. Clin Infect Dis. 1999;29:1145–1150.
71. Minkoff HL, Eisenberger-Matityahu D, Fedman J, et al. Prevalence and incidence of gynecologic disorders among women infected with human immunodeficiency virus. Am J Obstet Gynecol. 1999;180:824–836.
72. Frankel RE, Selwyn PA, Mexger J, Andrews S. High prevalence of gynecologic disease among hospitalized women with human immunodeficiency virus infection. Clin Infect Dis. 1997;25:706–712.
73. Duerr A, Heilig CM, Meikle SF, et al. Incident and persisistent vulvovaginal candidiasis among human immunodeficiency virus infected women: risk factors and severity. Obstet Gynecol. 2003;101:548–556.
74. Irwin KL, Moorman AC, O'Sullivan MJ, et al. Influence of Human Immunodeficiency virus infection on pelvic inflammatory disease. Obstet Gynecol. 2000;95:525–34.
75. Harlow SD, Cohen M, Ohmit SE, Schuman P, Cu-Uvin S, Lin X, et al. Substance abuse and psychotherapeutic medications: a likely contributor to menstrual disorders in women who are seropositive for human immunodeficiency virus. Am J Obstet Gynecol. 2003;188:991–996.
76. Cu-Uvin S, Hogan JW, Caliendo AM, et al. HIV Epidemiology Research Study (HERS) Group. Association between bacterial vaginosis and expression of Human immunodeficiency virus type 1 RNA in the female genital tract. Clin Infect Dis. 1999;29:1145–1150.
77. Greenblatt RM, Bacchetti P, Barkan S, et al. Lower genital tract infections among HIV-infected and high risk uninfected women: findings of the Womens' Interagency HIV Study (WIHS) Sex Transm Dis. 1999;26:143–151.
78. Sutton M, Sternberg M, Koumans EH. The prevalence of Trichomonas vaginalis infection among reproductive-age women in the United States, 2001–2004. CID. 2007;45:1319–26.
79. Van Der Pol B, Kwolk C, Pierre-Louis B, et al. Trichomonas vaginalis infection and human immunodeficiency virus acquisition in African women. JID. 2008;197:548–54.
80. Miller M, Liao Y, Gomez AM, et al. Factors associated with the prevalence and incidence of Trichomonas vaginalis infection among African American women in New York city who used drugs. JID. 2008;197:503–9.
81. Cu-Uvin S, Ko H, Jamieson DJ, et al. Prevalence, incidence and persistence or recurrence of trichomonasis among HIV-positive women and among HIV negative women at high risk for HIV infection. Clin Infect Dis. 2002;34:406–11.
82. Aberg JA, Gallant JE, Anderson J, Oleske JM, Libman H, Currier JS, Stone VE, Kaplan JE. Primary care guidelines for the management of persons infected with human immunodeficiency virus: Recommendations of the HIV Medicine Association of the Infectious Disease Society of America. Clin Infect Dis. 2009; in press.
83. Xu F, Schillinger JA, Sternberg MR, et al. Seroprevalence and co-infection with Herpes simplex virus type 1 and type 2 in the U.S., 1988–1994. J Infect Dis. 2002;185:1019–1024.
84. Heng M, Heng S, Allen S. Coinfection and synergy of HIV-1 and HSV. Lancet. 1994; 343:255–258.
85. Little SE, Caughey AB. Acyclovir prophylaxis for pregnant women with a known history of herpes simplex virus: A cost-effectiveness analysis. Am J Obstet Gynecol. 2005;193:1274–9.

86. Brown ZA, Gardlla C, Wald A, et al. Genital Herpes Complicating Pregnancy. Obstet Gynecol. 2005;106(4):845–56.
87. Sheffield JS, Hill JB, Hollier LM, et al. Valacyclovir prophylaxis to prevent recurrent herpes at delivery. A randomized clinical trial. Obstet Gynecol. 2006;108:141–7.
88. Chen KT, Segu M, Lumey LH, et al. Genital herpes virus infection and perinatal transmission of Human Immunodeficiency Virus. Obstet Gynecol. 2005;106:1341–8.
89. Herad I, Tassie J, Schmitz V, Mandelbrot L, Kazatchkine MD, Orth G. Increased Risk of Cervical Disease Among Human Immunodeficiency Virus-Infected Women with severe Immunosuppression and High Human Papillomavirus Load. Obstet Gynecol. 2000;96:403–9.
90. Stratton P, Gupta P, Riester K. Cervical dysplasia on cerivcovaginal papanicolaou smear among HIV-1-infected pregnant and non-pregnant women. JAIDS. 1999;20(3):300–307.
91. Klein RS, Ho GYF, Vermund SH, Fleming I, Burk RD. Risk factors for squamous intraep-ithelial lesions on pap smear in women at risk for human immunodeficiency virus infection. J Infec Dis. 1994;170:1404–9.
92. Stanberry LR, Rosenthal SL, Mills L, et al. Longitudinal risk of herpes simplex virus (HSV) type 1, HSV type 2, and cytomegalovirus infections among young adolescent girls. CID. 2004;39:1433–8.
93. Massad LS, Riester KA, Anatos KM. Prevalence and predictors of squamous cell Abnormal-ities in Papanicolaou Smears from Women Infected with HIV-1. JAIDS. 1999;21(1):33–41.
94. Delmas M, Larsen C, van Benthem B, et al. Cervical squamous intraepithelial lesions in HIV-infected women: prevalence, incidence and regression. AIDS. 2000;14:1775–1784.
95. Wright TC, Massad LS, Dunton C, et al. for the 2006 American Society for Colposcopy and Cervical pathology (ASCCP) Sponsored Consensus Conference. 2006 Consensus Guidelines for the Management of Women with abnormal cervical cancer screening tests. Am L Obstet Gynecol. 2007;197:340–355.
96. Saraiya M, Ahmed F, Krishnan S, et al. Cervical cancer Incidence in a Prevaccine era in the United States, 1998–2002. Obstet Gynecol. 2007;109:360–70.
97. Wallin K, Wiklund F, Angstrom T, et al. Type-specific persistence of human papillomavirus DNA before the development of invasive cervical cancer. N Engl J Med. 1999;341:1633–8.
98. Human Papillomavirus Vaccination. ACOG Committee Opinion Number 344, September 2006. Obstet Gynecol. 2006;108:699–705.
99. Benard VB, Coughlin SS, Thompson T, et al. Cervical cancer incidence in the United States by area of residence, 1998–2001. Obstet Gynecol. 2007;110:681–6.
100. Jones RW, Rowan DM, Stewart AW. Vulvar Epithelial Neoplasia. Obstet Gynecol. 2005;106:1319–26.
101. Conley LJ, Ellerbrock TV, Bush TJ. HIV infection and risk of Vulvovaginal and Perianal Condylomata Accuminata and Intraepithelial Neoplasia: A prospective cohort study. Lancet 2002;359:108–13.
102. Taube JM, Nichols AD, Bornman DM, et al. Langerhans cell density and high grade vulvar intraepithelial neoplasia in women with human immunodeficiency virus infection. J Cutan Pathol. 2007;34:565–70.
103. Elit L, Voruganti S, Simunovic M. Invasive vulvar cancer in a women with human immun-odeficiency virus: Case report and review of the literature. Gynecol Oncol. 2005;98:151–4.
104. Jamieson D, Paramsothy P, Cu-Uvin S, et al. for the HIV Epidemiology Research Study Group. Vulvar, vaginal, and Perineal Intraepithelial Neoplasia in women with or at risk for Human immunodeficiency Virus. Obstet Gynecol. 2006;107:1023–8.
105. Cohn SE, Park J-G, Watts DH, et al. Depo-medroxyprogesterone in women on antiretroviral therapy:Effective contraception and lack of clinically significant interactions. Nature.com. 2007;81(2):222–2227.
106. Steiner MJ, Kwok C, dominik R, et al. Pregnancy risk among oral contraceptive pill, injectable contraceptive, and condom users in Uganda, Zimbabwe, and Thailand. Obstet Gynecol. 2007;110:1003–9.

107. Stinger EM, Kaseba C, Levy J, et al. A randomized trial of the intrauterine contraceptive devise versus hormonal contraception in women who are infected with the human immunodeficiency virus. Am J Obstet Gynecol. 2007;197:144.e1–144.e8.
108. Baeten JM, Lavreys L, Overbaugh J. The influence of hormonal contraceptive use on HIV-1 transmission and Disease progression. CID. 2007;45:360–9.
109. Peterson HB Sterilization Obstet Gynecol. 2008;111(1):189–202.
110. El-Sadr W, Gelttler J. Unrecognized Human Immuno-deficiency virus infection in the elderly. Arch Intern Med. 1995;155:184–86.
111. Centers for Disease Control and Prevention, HIV/AIDS Surveillance Report. 2006;18:1–56.
112. Cejtin HE. Gynecologic issues in the HIV-infected woman. Obstet Gynecol Clin North Am. 2003;30(4):711–29.
113. Santoro N, Arsten JH, Buono D, et al. Impact of street drug use, HIV infection, and highly active antiretroviral therapy on reproductive hormones in middle-aged women. J Womens Health (Larchmt). 2005;14:898–905.
114. Fantry LE, Zhan M, Taylor GH, et al. Age of menopause and menopausal symptoms in HIV-infected women. AIDS Patient Care STDs. 2005;19:703–711.
115. Yin M, Dobkin J, Brudney K, et al. Bone mass and mineral metabolism in HIV+ postmenopausal women. 2005;16:1345–52. Epub 2005 March 8.
116. Washington DL, Bowles J, Saha S, et al. Transforming clinical practice to eliminate racial-ethnic disparities in healthcare. J Gen Intern Med. 2008;23(5):685–91.
117. Angelino A, Willard S. The need for sociocultural awaremness to maximize treatment acceptance and adherence in individuals initiating HIV therapy. J Int Assoc Physicians AIDS Care. 2008;7(Suppl 1):S17–S21.
118. Shapiro MF, Morton SC, McCaffrey DF, et al. Variations in the care of HIV-infected adults in the United States. JAMA. 1999;281:2305–2315.
119. Gebo KA, Fleishman JA, Conviser R, et al. Racial and gender disparities in receipt of highly active antiretroviral therapy persist in a multistate sample of HIV patients in 2001. J Acquir Immune Defic Syndr. 2005;38(1):96–103.
120. Cohen MH, Cook JA, Grey D, et al. Medically eligible women who do not use HAART: The importance of abuse, drug use, and race. AM J Pub Health. 2004;94(7):1147–1151.
121. Hirschhorn LR, Boswell SL, Stone VE. Discontinuation (D/C) of Protease Inhibitor (PI) Therapy: Reasons and Risk Factors. Presented at the 12th World AIDS Conference, Geneva Switzerland, June 28–July 3, 1998.
122. Losina E, Schackman B, Sadownik S, et al. Disparities in survival attributable to suboptimal HIV care in the U.S.: influence of gender and race/ethnicity [Abstract #142]. Paper Presented at the 14th Conference on Retroviruses and Opportunistic Infections. Los Angeles, CA: February 25–28, 2007.
123. Malcolm SE, Ng JJ, Rosen RK, Stone VE. An examination of HIV/AIDS patients who have excellent adherence to HAART. AIDS Care. 2003;15:251–61.
124. Stone VE, Clarke J, Lovell J, et al. HIV/AIDS patients' perspectives on adhering to regimens containing protease inhibitors. J Gen Intern Med. 1998;13(9):586–593.
125. Stone VE, Weissman JS, Cleary P. Satisfaction with ambulatory care of persons with AIDS: Predictors of patient ratings of quality. J Gen Intern Med. 1995;10:239–245.
126. Stein MD, Fleishman J, Mor V, Dresser M. Factors associated with patient satisfaction among symptomatic HIV-infected persons. Med Care. 1993;31:182–88.

Management of Pregnancy in HIV-Infected Women and Prevention of Mother-to-Child Transmission

Arlene D. Bardeguez

Introduction

Although the HIV/AIDS cases worldwide continue to increase, the U.S. and other developed countries have witnessed an enhanced survival of chronically infected individuals, a decrease in mother-to-child transmission (MTCT) of HIV infection, and a growing number of medical and behavioral interventions that can decrease new infections. In spite of the amazing progress over the last two decades we still face challenges in empowering our patients to know their HIV diagnosis and that of their partner prior to conception, in the management of HIV-infected pregnant women based on their age, chronic illness, and behavioral risk patterns. We also face the dilemma of how to support discordant or concordant couples who desire to conceive in a financially challenged environment as the demographic profile of this population evolves and long-term survival is feasible.

Since the beginning of the HIV epidemic through 2006, nearly 9,000 infants have been diagnosed with AIDS that was acquired through perinatal transmission. As can be seen from Fig. 1, there has been a dramatic decline in new perinatal transmissions of HIV in the U.S. over the past 10 years. This decline has been the culmination of a variety of important public health interventions that will be reviewed in this chapter. It is important to note that just as most women living with HIV in the U.S. are black or Latino, the vast majority of infants who acquire HIV perinatally in the U.S. are children of color. Specifically, of the perinatally infected infants living with HIV as of 2006, 66% were black and 20% were Hispanic, resulting in population rates that are more than ten and three times higher than that of whites, respectively. Given this disproportionate impact of MTCT of HIV on U.S. children of color, enhancing our efforts to prevent perinatal transmission in these populations is particularly pressing.[1]

A.D. Bardeguez
Department of Obstetrics and Gynecology and Women's Health, UMDNJ-New Jersey Medical School, Newark, NJ
E-mail: bardeead@umdnj.edu

V. Stone et al. (eds.), *HIV/AIDS in U.S. Communities of Color*.
DOI: 10.1007/978-0-387-98152-9_7, © Springer Science + Business Media, LLC 2009

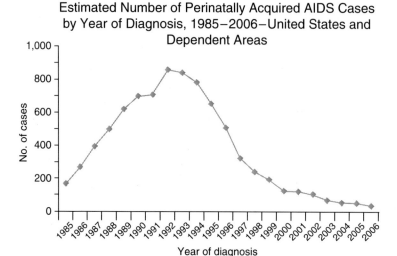

Fig. 1 Estimated number of perinatally acquired AIDS cases by year of diagnosis, 1985–2006, U.S. and dependent areas

Our challenge as health care providers is to optimize therapy prior, during, and after pregnancy to improve women's health, reduce maternal and fetal toxicities, decrease pregnancy-related complications of HIV infection or its treatment, safeguard future reproductive potential, improve maternal survival, and decrease HIV MTCT. Thus, in this section we will address management options, as well controversies and dilemmas regarding reproductive health for HIV-infected women through the age spectrum.

HIV Diagnosis and Characteristics of the HIV-Infected Pregnant Women in the U.S.

Counseling and testing for HIV-1 infection during pregnancy or the peripartum period has been the cornerstone strategy for decreasing MTCT globally.[2] The U.S. Public Health Task Force develops and regularly updates national guidelines for use by clinicians and health care institutions related to HIV testing in health care settings.[3] The last published update (July 2008) emphasizes that (1) HIV testing should be incorporated with other routine prenatal workup done during pregnancy after patient notification (opt out testing), (2) repeat HIV testing should be done in the late third trimester in high-prevalence areas to screen for seroconversion during pregnancy, which could increase the risk of MTCT transmission, and (3) implementing algorithms for rapid testing during labor at any facility caring for pregnant women is essential to ascertain HIV status of all women prior to delivery to maximize reduction of HIV transmission.[3,4]

Patients who decline HIV testing should be counseled regarding the risks and benefits of their decision and provided adequate support and counseling if fear or anxiety plays a role in that decision. A recent publication by Centers for Disease Control and Prevention highlights that as many as 31% of the pregnant women in the U.S. do not know their HIV status. Because lack of knowledge leads to lack of prevention, up to 25% of their children could acquire HIV infection perinatally.[3] Thus, to decrease HIV infection all health care providers of women of reproductive age should incorporate HIV testing into their routine health assessment in accordance with national guidelines by CDC and as stipulated by their state regulations. To familiarize themselves with such regulations, providers can contact their local or state Health Department officials or review a Compendium of State HIV Testing Laws kept by the University of California, San Francisco (UCSF) as a living document at http://www.nccc.ucsf.edu.

The Enhanced Perinatal Surveillance Report[5] conducted between 1999 and 2001 in 24 areas of the U.S. showed that most HIV-infected pregnant women in the U.S. (88%) received prenatal care, and the majority (90%) of them received their diagnosis during or prior to pregnancy. Eighty-three percent of the patients were less than 35-years old but there was also a significant group of women at the extremes of age, with 7% of them being adolescents and 10% over 35-years old. These two populations frequently represent a higher challenge for the provider due to their behavioral risk factors, concomitant illness, or unique age-related challenges. Eighty-five percent of the women were blacks or Hispanics with a greater burden of the disease in the former group (69% and 16%, respectively). Fifty-eight percent of these patients were born in the U.S.; 1–4% was born in the Caribbean or other Hispanic countries, and for 34% of the patients the place of birth was not documented. Most patients (nearly 80%) were exposed to HIV by heterosexual contact with an infected partner, and injection drug use accounted only for 12% of the reported cases. Also of note was the high rate of exposure to STIs among HIV-infected women, including Chlamydia, syphilis, and herpes as well as other infectious diseases such as hepatitis B and C. This observation is consistent with reported health disparities among racial/ethnic minorities in the U.S. and emphasizes the importance of early access to care to provide treatment and prevent perinatal or partner transmission of these infections.[6] The Enhanced Perinatal Surveillance also showed that as many as 20% of HIV-infected pregnant women who delivered in the U.S. had used illicit drugs during pregnancy.[5] While other investigators have previously reported a high prevalence of HIV infection among substance abusing parturients without prenatal care,[7] this observation highlights the need for counseling regarding the pregnancy complications associated with substance use such as preterm delivery (PTD), abruption of placenta, fetal growth restriction, and increased rate of HIV MTCT for all HIV-infected women receiving prenatal care. For a list of recommended laboratories and assessments the reader is referred to Table 1.

One-third of the women in the Enhanced Perinatal Surveillance Report delivered by elective cesarean delivery (CD), which is slightly higher than reported national CD rates in the general population. Nonetheless, neither the clinical indication for such management nor if the CD was primary or a repeat was reported. The rates of

Table 1 Routine Prenatal Laboratories and Timelines for Testing

Laboratary Catogory	Timelines
Hematologic	
CBC and differential	Entry to care and third trimester
Type and Screen	Entry to care
Hemoglobin electrophoresis	Entry to care
Metabolic	
Hepato-renal profile	
GCT	3rd trimester*
Infections screening	
STI's (Syphilis, GC, Chlamydia)	Entry to care and third trimester
UC & S	Entry to care and as indicated
Pap smear	Entry to care
Hepatitis B ag	Entry to care
Hepatitis C	Entry to care
PPD	Entry to care
GBS culture	late third trimester (usually 36 weeks)
Genetic Screening	
First Trimester	Nuchal translucency
Quad screen	15–20 weeks**
Routine or Target Sonogram**	Entry to care, for Obstetrical indications
HIV related	
Genotypic resistant testing	Entry to care, poor adherence, viral reboundor inability to suppress viral load
CD4	Entry to care, every trimester (every 3 months)
HIV Viral load	entry, 4 weeks after initiation of therapy every trimester***

* Usually 24–28 weeks; if suspicious of GDM, High BMI or protease based regimen >12 months do also at entry to care
** earliest as possible is preferable to ascertain risk fetal anomalies
*** last one should be at least 34–36 weeks

repeat CD have increased in country; therefore, this observation could be compatible with national trends or reflect an increase in operative delivery solely to decrease MTCT. Because this information is pertinent to maternal health and their future reproductive capacity, future reports should collect information regarding indication for this procedure.

A disturbing trend observed in this report was the lower percentage of black women who received antiretroviral therapy during pregnancy or labor when compared with those belonging to White race or of Hispanic origin.[5] This observation confirmed reports by other investigators regarding a lower receipt of zidovudine (ZDV) chemoprophylaxis among women who belong to minority groups and among substance users.[8,9] Indeed, Anderson et al. demonstrated a higher rate of awareness among reproductive-aged women in the U.S. of the survival benefits of antiretroviral use than of its merits for decreasing MTCT transmission.[10] These observations emphasize the need to increase HIV-related health literacy among women belonging to racial/ethnic minority groups and their communities.[11] It is also essential to address other financial, social, behavioral, or cultural barriers that hinder optimization of care for underserved populations.

Antiretroviral Therapy During Pregnancy and Prevention of MTCT

Antiretroviral therapy is recommended for all HIV-infected women during pregnancy; some of these women will be receiving therapy for their own health and also to reduce MTCT, while others will receive therapy only for the later objective. While the readers are advised to review updated information regarding preference of specific antiretrovirals during pregnancy as well as potential drug interactions and adverse events at AIDSinfo.nih.gov, this section will review current specific considerations for pregnant women.

The principles used for the treatment of HIV-infected adolescents and adults are also applicable to the HIV-infected pregnant woman, with some caveats.[12,13] A summary of antiretroviral agents and their use in pregnancy can be found in Table 2. Please refer to the most recent U.S. PHS Guidelines for more detailed antiretroviral therapy recommendations for the treatment of pregnant women.

Table 2 Recommended ART for Perinatal Use: Public Health Service Task Force July 2008

	PIs	NNRTIs	NRTIs	Other
Recommended	Lopinavir/r	Nevirapine	Zidoudine* Lamivudine*	
Alternative	Indinavir/r Nelfinavir Ritonavir Saquinavir-HGC/r		Abacavir didanosine Emtricitabine Stavudine	
Insufficient data	Amprenavir Atazanavir Fosamprenavir Darunavir Tipranavir		Tenofovir	Enfuvirtide Maraviroc Raltegravir
Not recommended		Efavirenz Delavirdine	Zalcitabine	

* ZDV and 3TC are included as a fixed-dose combination in Combivir®

U.S. Public Health Task Force Recommendations for Use of Antiretroviral Drugs in Pregnant HIV-infected Women for Maternal Health and Interventions to Reduce Perinatal HIV Transmission in the United States; July 8, 2008; http://AIDSinfo.nih.gov

Pregnancy is a unique physiologic state associated with dramatic changes in blood volume, renal clearance, circulating binding proteins, drug absorption, and a new compartment that includes the fetus.[14] Other authors also documented upregulation of the cytochrome P 450 during pregnancy.[15] It is therefore not surprising that the metabolism and clearance of many HIV drugs is altered during this period.

In general, studies done with selective nucleoside reverse transcriptase (NRTI) and nonnucleoside reverse transcriptase inhibitors (NNRTI) such as ZDV, lamidivine (3TC) didanosine (DDI), d4T, abacavir, and nevirapine (NEV) achieve similar areas under the curve (AUCs) in pregnant women as in nonpregnant counterparts; therefore, no dose adjustment is needed during pregnancy. These drugs readily cross the placenta (ZDV, DDI, 3TC, d4T, and abacavir), can accumulate in the amniotic fluid (ZDV, DDI, 3TC), be detected in compartments such as the genital tract (ZDV), and even achieve measurable concentrations in the newborn (ZDV, 3TC, NEV), which can partly explain the success of these agents to reduce MTCT.[16–21] However, these same attributes could increase the risk for fetal toxicities or teratogenicity on the unborn child. For example, animal data, retrospective published cases, and reports to the Antiretroviral Pregnancy Registry (APR) suggest that transplacental passage of efavirenz is feasible and associated with an increased risk of neural tube defects (NTD) in the unborn child when this drug is used in early pregnancy.[22–24] This observation led to a change in FDA classification for this drug to category D and the recommendation to avert efavirenz exposure in the first trimester or throughout pregnancy if alternative regimens are feasible. Women of reproductive age receiving this antiretroviral should use effective contraception and if they conceive while on treatment they should be offered screening for neural tube defect and a modification of their regimen.

The highest impact of the physiologic changes in pregnancy on the pharmacokinetics of antiretrovirals is seen with the protease inhibitors class.[25–31] Several reports have shown that the AUCs for selective protease inhibitors during pregnancy in subjects taking standard adult dosage have been suboptimal[25,26,28–31] while boosted protease inhibitors or increase of the adult dose in the third trimester have been able to achieve adequate AUCs.[32–34] Most studies have also shown that the AUCs after delivery were compatible with those observed among nonpregnant adults. The likelihood of achieving adequate concentration during pregnancy is affected by the drug formulation and whether the drug or its active metabolite is measured.[27–29,35] At present most experts recommend the use of boosted protease regimens during pregnancy or an increase in the dose used for nonpregnant adults to ensure viral suppression and avert development of resistance.[32–35]

On the other hand, currently approved protease inhibitors do not readily cross the placenta in high amounts, which decrease the concern of fetal exposure and teratogenicity with this class.[13,25,26,31,36] Thus, women who receive these antiretrovirals for their own health could continue their use during the first trimester and avert viral rebound with its potential for in-utero transmission.[37] This approach could also protect the unborn child of women who undergo prenatal diagnosis[38] and could help ARV-experienced women who desire to conceive without putting at risk their own health. A recent analysis of a phase 1 study of Tenofovir used only during labor showed low transplacental passage of this nucleotide[39] but there is limited knowledge of the pharmacokinetics of newly approved entry inhibitors and integrase inhibitors during pregnancy.

Once the patient initiates antiretroviral therapy treatment, adherence should be evaluated at every visit at least by self-report and counseling provided if poor or inconsistent adherence is detected. Monitoring the patient's virologic response is essential to confirm adherence to treatment and determine optimal route of delivery. Although the goal is to attain viral load <50 copies/ml close to the patient's estimated date of confinement (EDC), achieving <1,000 copies/ml decreases risk of transmission to 2%. Women who have not reached that target by 36-weeks gestation should be offered operative delivery. Patients should also be educated regarding common and rare but severe toxicities of their regimen (as mentioned in Table 1).

Health care providers should not withhold therapy from pregnant women solely for fetal concerns since the best indicator of a good pregnancy outcome is a healthy mother. They should discuss with their patients the risks and benefits of a given treatment strategy and jointly select the most effective regimen that is less likely to adversely affect the unborn child if the woman conceives. Discussion of contraceptive options should also be addressed prior to treatment initiation given that most pregnancies are unplanned, any given women might initiate treatment with agents for which there is limited fetal safety data available, and there are known or potential drug interactions between antiretrovirals and some contraceptive modalities. Providers with limited HIV experience should consider referral or consultations with HIV experts in the field to maximize likelihood of success in decreasing MTCT while ensuring optimization of maternal health. The interested reader should also review updates to this topic at Public Health Service (PHS) guidelines for the management of HIV-infected adults and adolescents, or for the treatment of the HIV-infected pregnant women for their own health and to decrease MTCT (www.aidsinfo.nih.gov), as well as the APR (www.apregistry.com).

Some patients will be diagnosed late in pregnancy or during labor, so the immediate challenge for that population is to prevent MTCT. The initial approach in the U.S. to decrease MTCT consisted of ZDV monotherapy during pregnancy, intrapartum and to the neonate for asymptomatic women as used in the Pediatrics AIDS Clinical Trial Group (PACTG) protocol 076. The investigators observed a two-thirds decrease in transmission from 25% in the placebo arm to 8% in the treatment arm.[40] A significant reduction in HIV MTCT was also observed in the PACTG protocol 185, which enrolled women with more advanced HIV disease who also use the ZDV chemoprophylaxis.[41] Most of the patients enrolled in both studies (82–86%) were from racial ethnic minority groups. The mechanism for the MTCT reduction in both studies was a decrease in maternal HIV viral load as well as neonatal postexposure prophylaxis.[42, 43] The results of these studies lead to the development of the national guidelines for the management of the HIV-infected pregnant women, which recommended "the 076 regimen" or any of its components based on the time at which women enter into care or their HIV status was ascertain. The validity of this approach in routine care was confirmed by several investigators including Garcia et al. using clinical and laboratory information from the Women's and Infants

Transmission Study as well as the report by Wade and collaborators from the NY State Department of Health.[44,45] The majority of the women involved in these studies were also of underrepresented minority groups, which emphasizes the burden of the disease among this population and the potential for benefit if they have access to and utilize up-to-date treatment options. These investigators showed that the MTCT was lowest if the HIV viral load was <1,000 copies/ml and among women who received ZDV prophylaxis. Wade et al. also showed the systematic decrease in MTCT rates for women who received the complete PACTG 076 regimen versus those who only received a component of the regimen (intrapartum and neonatal therapy, or only the neonatal therapy) or no therapy at all.[45] The public impact and cost-effectiveness of implementing guidelines for HIV testing and MTCT prevention in the U.S. and other resource-rich countries has been published.[46,47] Over the years we have modified our approach to decrease maternal viral load and HIV MTCT with the use of highly active antiretroviral therapy (HAART) during pregnancy with intrapartum and neonatal postexposure prophylaxis as the preferred approach. This strategy has decreased MTCT to 1.5–2% among women delivering in clinical settings with access to HIV-experienced providers.[48,49] This algorithm is detailed in Fig. 2.

An alternative approach for those patients unable to achieve undetectable viral load by term, and for those with late diagnosis, limited or delayed access to care, or poor adherence to antiretroviral (ARV) therapy is to offer elective cesarean delivery (CD) without labor with intrapartum and neonatal ZDV. This approach also decreases MTCT rates to about 2%[50,51] and has been recommended by the American College of Obstetrics and Gynecology (ACOG) and the Perinatal HIV

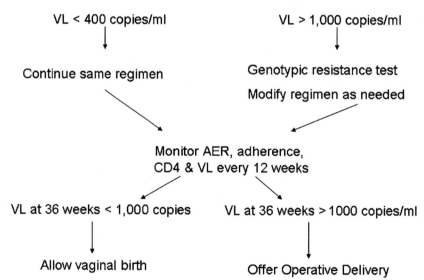

Fig. 2 Management for treatment experienced pregnant patients on HAART (nonteratogenic nor contraindicated during pregnancy)

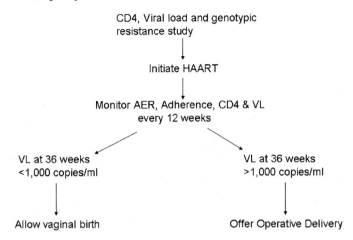

Fig. 3 Treatment naïve pregnant women or those who only received prior MTCT

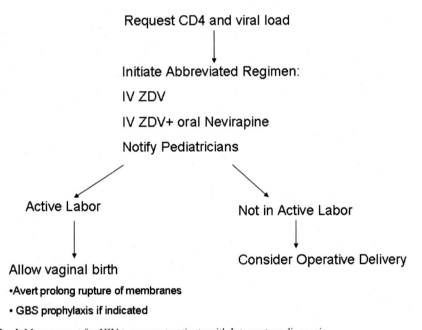

Fig. 4 Management for HIV+ pregnant patients with Intrapartum diagnosis

Guidelines Working Group of the Public Health Service Task Force.[13,52] Several concerns arise from the use of this strategy including an increased rate of maternal morbidity mostly due to infectious complications such as endometritis irrespective of antibiotic use, and the increased blood loss and length of hospital stay experienced by these patients.[53–57] Furthermore, the single most important factor for repeat CD in the U.S. is a prior CD, and studies have shown increased maternal morbidity and cesarean hysterectomy rates among patients with repeat cesarean section.[58–60] Thus, adequate education and counseling should be provided to HIV-positive women prior to and during pregnancy to decrease primary cesarean section due to HIV indications, in order to decrease the immediate and long-term complications of operative delivery and safeguard their future reproductive health.

Although some populations in the U.S. are disenfranchised from the health care system and receive limited or no prenatal care,[8,9,61] the study by Wade et al. showed that utilization of abbreviated regimen can reduce MTCT if at least intrapartum and neonatal ZDV or only neonatal ZDV is used instead of no treatment (10% vs. 26.6%, respectively).[45] These observations gave impetus to the use of rapid testing during labor with abbreviated ZDV or ZDV plus nevirapine regimen to curtail transmission among patients with late diagnosis and limited or no prior antiretroviral treatment, as detailed in Fig. 4.[13]

The feasibility and acceptance of rapid testing during labor for women with unknown HIV serostatus was evaluated in the Mother-Infant Rapid Intervention at Delivery Study (MYRIAD).[62,63] This multicenter study offered rapid HIV testing to 5,744 pregnant women with undocumented HIV status at the time of labor; 84% of them agreed to have the test (4,849) and 34 women had a positive test for an HIV prevalence of 7/1,000. The positive predictive value of the test was 90% and the results were available within an hour. Although this approach is inferior to early diagnosis and treatment during pregnancy it could still avail care to late presenters leading to significant reduction in MTCT rates.[3,13] Nonetheless, health care providers, pregnant women, and the community as a whole should be aware that early HIV diagnosis linked to care and treatment optimize maternal and fetal outcome as it allows time to modify other cofactors associated with increase in transmission, such as sexually transmitted infections (STIs), drug use, preterm birth, and prevention of chorioamnionitis among women with preterm or prolonged rupture of membranes.

A growing concern with the use of abbreviated MTCT regimens such as intrapartum nevirapine is that 20–69% of the women who use this strategy develop resistance, which could hinder future treatment options for maternal health.[64,65] Studies have shown that the observed genotypic resistance seen shortly after exposure to nevirapine (6–12 weeks) fades over time and its incidence varies with HIV clade, maternal viral load, CD4 count, and dose exposure.[13] The detrimental effect of this treatment on women's health is that for those who require initiation of HIV-related therapy for their own health shortly after their nevirapine exposure the risk of treatment failure is higher.[66,67] Several strategies had been evaluated to avert resistance development after exposure to nevirapine during labor including the use of additional antiretroviral drug for 7–10 days after nevirapine exposure, also known as using a "tail." Both Combivir and Tenofovir had been used for this purpose but poor adherence to a tail regimen consisting of ZDV and 3TC was associated with virologic failure due to 3TC resistance.[68]

Other algorithms are under evaluation including a tail with a protease inhibitor.[69,70] Because at the present time there is no consensus regarding which is the most cost-effective approach for women who required intrapartum antiretroviral to decrease MTCT the interested reader should refer the U.S. PHS guidelines for updates on this topic or request consultation with an HIV expert in this area.

Maternal, Fetal, and Neonatal Safety of Antiretroviral Therapy

Although many clinicians rely on the FDA class categories to ascertain the safety of drugs used during pregnancy, the available data are frequently insufficient to determine human teratogenic risk.[71] Pregnant women frequently find themselves using medications for which there is limited information regarding fetal toxicity and neonatal safety. A recent study showed that about 64% of pregnant women receive a drug other than a vitamin during pregnancy, primarily anti-infectives including antiretrovirals. Indeed, as many as 37.8–45% of the women received a category C or D while pregnant, and 21% of them had first trimester exposures, which is the vulnerable period for congenital fetal anomalies.[71,72]

Increased efforts have been made by the Centers for Disease Control and Prevention, national and state birth defects registries, academic centers, and other health-related societies to increase our knowledge of the potential teratogenicity of drug treatments in human pregnancy.[71] The APR represents one of these efforts for HIV-infected pregnant women.[24] It collects voluntary reports of antiretroviral exposures from the primary care provider. Each year they enroll approximately 1,000 pregnant women exposed to antiretrovirals, which represents 15% of the 6,000–7,000 HIV-positive women who give birth annually in the U.S. Their most recent report showed that the prevalence of birth defects by 100 live births among women with fist trimester exposure to any of the therapies included in the registry was 2.8 (95% CI: 2.2–3.5), which is not significantly different from the prevalence of defects among women exposed to these medications in the second or third trimester of pregnancy (2.6 per 100 live births) nor with the background rate of birth defects reported by CDC 2.72 per 100 live births (95% CI: 2.68, 2.76). Analysis of individual drugs with sufficient data to warrant separate analysis showed an increase in the frequency of defects only for didanosine although no specific pattern of defect was detected. The interested reader can seek more detailed information from the APR[24] (www.APRegistry.com). Other publications support the low overall risk of birth defects among HIV-infected women exposed to selective antiretrovirals in the first trimester.[73–77]

In 2005, Bristol-Myers Squibb (BMS) Company distributed a letter to Health Care providers alerting them of the change in the FDA classification of Sustiva (Efavirenz) from category C to D. This change was based on four retrospective reports of NTD (three meningomyelocele and one Dandy-Walker Syndrome) in infants born to women with first trimester exposure to this drug. Although these data were compatible with preclinical studies done in the cynomolgus monkeys, only seven defects/live births have been prospectively reported to the APR, which leads to a prevalence of 2.4% that is compatible with the background rate of birth defects reported by CDC.[24]

Most reports on maternal and fetal safety after exposure to antiretroviral monotherapy or combination had been encouraging with low rate of severe maternal or fetal toxicities. Sperling et al. reported mild hematologic toxicities among participants in the PACTG 076 study.[78] Bardeguez et al. showed that the discontinuation of antiretroviral therapy postpartum used solely for reducing MTCT did not alter HIV disease progression. This investigator also showed that only 9% of women initially exposed to ZDV monotherapy for MTCT had evidence of genotypic resistance when ZDV was subsequently used as part of a treatment regimen for maternal health.[79] The progression of HIV disease was not affected after MTCT treatment discontinuation in women with CD4 counts with more advanced disease, such as the participants in the PACTG 185 study.[80]

The increased use of HAART during pregnancy since late 1990s[81] has led to ongoing assessment of the maternal and fetal safety of such approach.[26,27,31,82–84] Most studies to date have shown good maternal outcomes, and few grade three or four toxicities among women receiving a protease-based regimen with saquinavir, indinavir, lopinavir, and nelfinavir.[26,27,31,82–84] The most commonly observed toxicities have been hematological, hepatic, and some amylase increases with infrequent need for treatment discontinuation.

In spite of these reassuring reports, unique life-threatening or lethal toxicities have been reported among pregnant women on antiretroviral therapy including hepatic failure and death.[13,85,86] The majority of these reports have been among women exposed to ddI/d4t combination or in women with CD4 counts greater than 250 cells who received nevirapine.[85,86] While some authors suggest that nevirapine hepatotoxicity is more frequent among pregnant women than among their nonpregnant counterparts, others suggest that the frequency of adverse events is higher among those initiating treatment late in pregnancy (third trimester) compared with those with early treatment initiation (first trimester).[87,88] Given that we do not have a good screening tool to ascertain individuals at risk for nevirapine hepatotoxicity and that other options are feasible for this population, this regimen should be avoided as initial antiretroviral therapy in women with high CD4 (CD4 count >250) and among those with higher predisposition for adverse hepatic events such as those coinfected with Hepatitis B or C.[13]

A rare but potentially lethal toxicity seen in newborns exposed to postnatal antiretroviral therapy is mitochondrial toxicity. Blanche et al. reported two deaths ascribed to mitochondrial dysfunction among HIV-uninfected children exposed to combination therapy with ZDV and 3TC (Combivir).[89] Systematic review in several U.S. longitudinal cohorts failed to find any occurrence of this event among infants exposed to either ZDV monotherapy or Combivir during pregnancy.[90] Likewise a report by the European Collaborative confirmed the lack of mitochondrial abnormalities among children whose mothers were exposed to antiretrovirals.[77] Thus, although patients should be aware of this potential complication they can be reassured that this event is extremely rare in the U.S. and these therapies should not be withheld from pregnant women when indicated.

The reported toxicities among infants whose mother received protease-based regimens had been low, with anemia or neutropenia being the most commonly reported. These toxicities have been rapidly resolved with minimal or no intervention.[27,83]

The long-term neonatal safety of ZDV in HIV-exposed uninfected children has been reported by several investigators. Culnane evaluated the growth, cognitive, and developmental function in children enrolled in PACTG 219, and observed no adverse effects among HIV-uninfected children with in utero exposure to ZDV who were followed-up to 5.6 years of age.[91] Hanson ascertain the risk of tumors in children enrolled in PACTG 219 and in the Women and Infants Transmission Study (WITS) and observed no tumors of any kind among children with a mean follow-up of 38.3 and 14.5 months, respectively, in these clinical cohorts.[92] While these data are extremely reassuring, as new treatment options are introduced to pregnant women the long-term outcomes of their exposed children should continue to be monitored.

Adherence to Antiretroviral Therapy During Pregnancy

Adherence is defined by the Webster Dictionary[93] as the "Act to stay attached, firm and in support to a plan or cause." So at its basic level it requires adequate health literacy, willingness to follow a plan of management, and resources to complete such a plan. We know that lack of adherence had been a problem with individuals with chronic illnesses such as diabetes and hypertension, which can jeopardize their long-term survival and quality of life.[94] But the unique importance of poor adherence for the HIV-infected individual is that (1) the number of treatment options for this disease is still comparatively fewer than for other chronic illnesses, (2) development of resistance can cause failure across a class of antivirals significantly reducing treatment options for a given individual, and (3) antiretroviral resistance can affect other individuals beyond the index person if that resistance is transmitted to a sexual partner or the unborn child.[91,92,95–97] Thus, in order to achieve and maintain viral suppression, which can translate to increased survival and quality of life, the HIV-infected individuals must remain adherent to their therapy.[98] Despite this, the rate of adherence for many groups afflicted by this epidemic including adolescents, substance users, depressed individuals, and pregnant women has been found to be less than optimal.[98–103]

It is therefore important that the selection of antiretroviral regimen to be used during pregnancy have a low likelihood of resistance development in order to protect future maternal treatment options and avoid transmission of drug-resistant strains to the newborn child. Adherence counseling and surveillance during pregnancy are also recommended as several studies have shown poor self-reported adherence rates in 20% or more of this population independent of whether they received monotherapy, combination therapy, or HAART.[102–105] Antiretroviral experience, drug use, and depression have been associated with poor adherence among pregnant women, and modification of these factors could lead to increased adherence.[102,103]

Pregnancy-Related Complications in the HIV-Infected Pregnant Women

Several medical and obstetrical complications have been reported among HIV-infected women prior to and during the HAART era. Anemia and thrombocytopenia are the most common hematological complications observed among HIV-infected pregnant women.[78,84,106] While for some patients anemia can be due to the physiologic changes of pregnancy, poor nutrition, HIV treatment (such as ZDV), and low erythropoietin levels can be observed in this population. Erythropoietin therapy can be used during pregnancy if this is deemed the etiologic factor.[107] HIV-related thrombocytopenia has also been described among HIV-infected women with diverse severity spectrum. Some patients respond favorably to use of antiretroviral therapy while others require treatment with steroids, gamma globulin, platelets transfusion, or even splenectomy. Because HIV infection is only one among many other etiologies for thrombocytopenia during pregnancy (which includes alloimmune thrombocytopenia, anticardiolipin syndrome, ITP, severe preeclampsia, HELLP syndrome) health care providers must first ascertain the etiology of this complication to effectively implement a treatment plan. This is particularly relevant for cases with platelets below 60,000 since adverse fetal outcome is more common with alloimmune thrombocytopenia than with ITP, and the treatment algorithm for these diseases also differ.[108–110]

Spontaneous rupture of membranes has also been frequently reported in cohorts of HIV-infected pregnant women. Indeed, when this event occurs in term or late preterm pregnancies it has been recommended that patients be offered induction of labor or operative delivery if a prolonged induction is anticipated to avert development of chorioamnionitis and to decrease the risk of HIV MTCT as documented in many pre-HAART cohorts and meta-analyses.[111–113] These patients should also receive Group B streptococcus (GBS) prophylaxis when indicated, and the frequency of vaginal exams during labor should be minimized.[114,115] Prophylaxis for genital herpes is also recommended for women with history or documented infection during pregnancy. Most experts will initiate prophylaxis in the third trimester but for women with history of frequent recurrences prophylaxis can be initiated earlier in pregnancy as this drug is well tolerated in pregnancy and its safety in the unborn child and neonate is known.[115–117]

Behavioral modifications to avert factors associated with increased risk of rupture of membranes such as smoking and cocaine abuse should also be implemented. Most experts agreed that patients with preterm premature rupture of membranes (PPROM) with a gestational age greater or equal to 34 weeks should delivered as the risk for in-utero infection of such infants outweighs the potential benefits of conservative treatment. On the other hand the optimal management for the women with PPROM at gestational age <34 weeks is controversial. On one hand, we know that the longer the interval between rupture of membranes and delivery, the higher the increase in HIV MTCT in the background of subclinical or overt infection such as chorioammnionitis.[111–113] However, delivery of a preterm or very preterm infant can also lead to significant short- and long-term neonatal morbidity and mortality.[115] A recent retrospective analysis by Alvarez et al. described the outcome of conservative management of such patients at a single institution.[118] The authors implemented conservative management in 18 HIV-infected pregnant patients who had PPROM prior to 34-weeks gestation. All patients received GBS prophylaxis and steroids for lung maturity, and they were monitored for evidence of chorioamnionitis and other complications of PPROM such as abnormal fetal heart rate tracing, vaginal bleeding, or labor. None of the newborns from women who were on HAART prior to rupture of membranes were HIV infected while two neonates born to women without prior prenatal care or antirerovirals were perinatally infected. Given the lack of consensus at present regarding management of these pregnancy complications, health care providers should (1) initiate antiretroviral therapy as soon as possible for those patients who have not received therapy prior to this event, (2) ensure that adequate prophylaxis is initiated promptly for GBS or any other suspected or documented STIs, (3) consider maternal transfer to a tertiary health care facility to ensure optimal management of the newborn if born preterm, (4) provide steroids for lung maturity if there are no contraindications, and (5) request consultation with HIV experts for such cases.

Another controversial topic is the effect of HAART on PTD first described by Lorenzi et al. in 1998.[119] In the U.S., small cohorts and retrospective data analysis dismissed the effect of HAART on preterm birth.[120] However, other studies continue to suggest an association between protease-based regimens and preterm birth including a recent report by Cotter et al.[121] The largest series to date regarding safety of antiretroviral therapy during pregnancy was reported by Tuomala et al. who analyzed data from 2,123 HIV infected women who delivered between 1990 and 1998, in seven large U.S. cohorts.[122] These authors found similar rates of premature delivery, low birth weight (LBW), and very low birth weight (VLBW) among patients who received antiretroviral therapy and those who did not, after controlling for CD4 cell count and use of tobacco, alcohol, or illicit drugs. Because of the conflicting observations reported in the literature regarding the effect of HAART on PTD and low birthweight infants,[123–128] women receiving HAART should at the very least be (1) educated of the early signs and symptoms of labor, (2) screened for STIs as needed, (3) counseled to avoid behaviors that increase the risk of preterm birth such as smoking or illicit drug use, and (4) encouraged to seek prompt evaluation if they suspect labor or have increased contractions.

The mechanisms for low birth weight among patients exposed to protease inhibitors are uncertain. However, Beitune et al.[129] reported lower umbilical cord insulin levels among infants born to mothers treated with protease-based regimen than among infants whose mother received only ZDV, and Chmait et al.[130] suggested that the impaired fetal growth could be due to the protease inhibition of GLUT4 glucose transport activity, which has been observed in vitro. These observations support the need for the long-term surveillance of the effect of PI-based regimens on the newborn birth weight and growth pattern.

Studies in HIV-infected nonpregnant women suggested that obesity, older age, and a protease inhibitor regimen increased the likelihood of developing type 2 diabetes.[131] Gestational diabetes, defined as carbohydrate intolerance first diagnosed during pregnancy, complicates 2–5% of pregnancies in the U.S.[132] Early, observational studies of pregnant women using protease-based antiretroviral therapy reported increased prevalence rates among this group (8%).[119] However, more recent reports from observational cohorts in the U.S. found no difference in gestational diabetes among HIV-infected pregnant women and their seronegative counterpart.[133] Dinsmoor et al. reported no differences in the rates of gestational diabetes among women receiving PI or non-PI regimens for a short interval during pregnancy, suggesting that this complication was infrequent when the ARV treatment was initiated and used only during pregnancy. Hitti et al. confirmed these observations in a prospective cohort study. These authors observed no difference in the rate of abnormal glucose challenge test (GCT), abnormal glucose tolerance test (GTT), or gestational diabetes among women who received protease-based versus protease-sparing regimens.[134] They also observed that women with a high body mass index (BMI) were more likely to have abnormal impaired glucose tolerance or gestational diabetes. These reports are compatible with the observations reported in nonpregnant women.[131] On the other hand, the rates of gestational diabetes and impaired glucose tolerance are higher among women who have received a PI-based regimen prior to pregnancy.[135] Thus, we recommend that early diabetic screening be done in all women who conceived on a protease-based regimen, in those with high BMI at entry to care, and in all HIV-infected women in the third trimester if the GCT early in pregnancy was normal (Table 1).

Pregnancy is characterized by dramatic changes in lipid metabolism geared toward supporting fetal growth and hormone development.[136–138] The effect of protease-based versus protease-sparing regimen by pregnant women on the lipid profile was recently evaluated by Livingston et al. using data from the ACTG protocol 5084.[139] These investigators observed higher cholesterol and triglycerides among women receiving protease-based regimen and an increased number of low birth weight infants among women with high triglycerides. Clearly more information is needed in this area to assess the short- and long-term implications of these observations for the woman and her child. However, clinicians should remember that lipid-lowering drugs are contraindicated in pregnancy but dietary changes can be implemented.

Prenatal Diagnosis for the HIV-Infected Women

Several obstetrical protocols have been used to screen for fetal anomalies during pregnancy both for women with low or high risk for structural or chromosomal anomalies in their unborn fetus.[140–144] Maternal characteristics and risk factors frequently included in such protocols are advanced maternal (those ≥35-years old) or paternal age, exposure to teratogenic drugs, hereditary illness such as sickle cell, and clinical diseases such as poorly controlled diabetes. Access to early prenatal diagnosis allows patients to seek reproductive services if they decide not to continue the pregnancy or transfer their care to a tertiary health care facility where early interventions by specialist can be rendered to improve long-term outcome and quality of life of such infants. Corrective factors have been used for certain populations, such as obese or diabetic patients to increase accuracy of noninvasive screening tests and avoid false-positive or false-negative results that could lead to unnecessary anxiety, invasive testing, or termination of a normal pregnancy. Indeed the success of a noninvasive approach for prenatal diagnosis relies on the accuracy and predictive value of the tools used among the populations who used them.[141–143]

The most frequently used second trimester screening tests for diagnosis of neural tube defect NTD, trisomy 13 or 18, are the triple or quad screen. This test is performed between weeks 14 and 21 of gestation and the levels of maternal serum alpha-feto protein (MSAFP), unconjugated estriol (uE3), and β-hCG are analyzed. The analysis provides a risk estimate for each patient, which is then used to counsel on the risk/benefit of using an invasive including amniocentesis to obtain a definite diagnosis. Women over 35 years of age are advised that amniocentesis is the gold standard but some opt for noninvasive approaches to decrease procedure-related complications including pregnancy loss.[142]

Several studies suggest that HIV-infected women are more likely to have an abnormal triple or quad screen than the general obstetrical population.[145, 146] Gross et al. showed that the abnormal screen was primarily due to elevations in hCG or in maternal serum alpha fetoprotein (MSAFP),[145] while Einstein et al. showed a correlation between the degree of maternal immune suppression and the likelihood of false-positive triple screen but no effect of the antiretroviral regimen used on this screening test.[147] These studies raised the concern that we could be offering invasive diagnosis to this population based on false-positive screening. As the field of prenatal diagnosis strives for first trimester detection of children with chromosomal or anatomical abnormalities with the combined use of nuchal translucency and other serum markers, the sensitivity and specificity in the HIV-infected women must be ascertained.

Target scan is a useful tool to identify fetus at risk of chromosomal anomalies based on the association of certain structural anomalies with an abnormal karyotype.[140, 142, 143] Detection of nuchal-fold thickness, absent nasal bone, renal anomalies, abnormal head anatomy, and short femur or humerus had been used as potential markers among other biometric parameters. For non-HIV-infected women with advanced maternal age the combination of sonogram with triple or quad screen test has increased the positive predictive value of the latter and provided more information to patients to decide if they want to opt out of invasive diagnosis.[141, 142]

For the HIV-infected women, the target scan can also be useful to rule out presence of fetal anomalies due to maternal or paternal age, or exposure to potential teratogenic drugs such as Sustiva or other teratogenic drugs. However, the false-positive rates of the triple and quad screen in the HIV-infected population could limit its utility to ascertain the risk of the infant to have a chromosomal anomaly. If the patients decide to proceed with invasive diagnosis they should be adequately counseled of its risk and benefits. We know that between 5 and 15% of perinatal HIV infections are in utero (prior to delivery), and studies have shown that events that increase maternal-fetal bleeding (such as amniocentesis, external cephalic version, or placental abruption) could increase the risk for in-utero MTCT.[13, 148] There is limited and conflicting information regarding the risk of HIV MTCT among women exposed to early invasive techniques during pregnancy. Pre-HAART reports describe MTCT rates of 40–55% among infants born to mothers exposed to amniocentesis, amnioscopies, and other needling procedures – who received mono or combination therapy,[148–150] while more recent publications observed rates as low as 0–3.3% for women receiving HAART.[68, 144] These low transmission rates in the HAART era are comparable with overall MTCT rates for HIV-infected women in developed countries and suggest that access to definite diagnosis by invasive procedures should be available and supported in this population. Adequate counseling of the risk and benefits must be provided prior to the procedure so that the HIV-infected women can make an informed decision given that most of our current knowledge is based on small retrospective case series.

Special Populations: Perinatally Infected Adolescents

Use of combination therapy including protease inhibitors has markedly reduced the mortality among children and adolescents infected with HIV-1 in developed countries.[151, 152] The benefits of HAART in this population include improved growth, better immune function, lower incidence of infectious complications, and decreased risk of death.[151–153] As the quality of life improves in this population many become sexually active around the same age as their seronegative counterparts.[153] However, limited health knowledge of sexually transmitted disease, contraception, reproductive choices, and common complications experienced by HIV-infected adolescents increase their risk for unplanned pregnancies and STD acquisition.[154, 155]

Adolescent pregnancies account for over 400,000 deliveries/year in the U.S. Frequent complications seen in this population during pregnancy include anemia, preterm labor, hypertensive disorders of pregnancy, low birth weight, and neonatal death.[156–158] For the perinatally infected adolescent the challenges are increased by their degree of antiretroviral experience and acquired resistance to prior antiretrovirals, which can limit drug selection,[159] the potential for glucose or lipid abnormalities, their adherence rates, and the need for treatment of other comorbid conditions such as pulmonary disease.[160] Other interrelated social issues include psychological adaptation, disclosure of HIV serostatus to the partner, and prevention of horizontal and perinatal transmission.

Some authors have shown that the rates of operative delivery for HIV indications, STIs, and preterm birth are high in this population.[155, 160, 161] Thus, although most HIV MTCT can be averted to the third generation it can come with a high price of increased operative deliveries to these young mothers due to treatment failure and poor adherence.[154, 160] Intense counseling and monitoring of such pregnancies, early surveillance and prevention of STIs, and management of abnormal cervical cytology must be a priority for heath care providers serving this unique population. It is also imperative that contraceptive counseling be provided.

Special Populations: HIV-Experienced Patients (Long-Term Survivors)

The widespread utilization of HAART among perinatally HIV-infected children and HIV-infected adults and adolescents has increased their survival rates and improved their quality of life. Parallel to those improved health outcomes and to the dramatic reduction of MTCT with the use of HAART[151] we have witnessed an increase in pregnancy rates in these populations and their acknowledgement of their desire to procreate.[154, 155, 162] The management of such cases is more complex as most of these patients are treatment experienced, often have prior treatment failures, or have experienced other HIV or treatment complications such as genital premalignant conditions, concomitant illnesses such as Hepatitis C, CMV, herpes infection, or lipodystrophy, all of which increase the complexity of their management. Some of them are also older,[162] which increases their risk of medical conditions that could adversely affect pregnancy outcomes and/or fetal survival such as hypertension, cervical premalignant lesions,[163] diabetes, and pulmonary or renal disease.

For the women over 35 years, their age, selective medical complications, or the treatment of comorbidities could increase the risk of fetal anomalies.[140, 144] Older women are also more likely to have experienced an abnormal Pap smear or diagnostic or treatment evaluations such as cone biopsies, which could increase their risk for cervical incompetence or preterm labor.[163, 164] But even perinatal survivors have increased rates of high-grade cervical squamous epithelial lesions and invasive cancer[165] or have experienced coinfections, which could lead to perinatal transmission of these pathogens, or have experienced chronic cardiac and pulmonary illness, which can lead to suboptimal pregnancy outcomes.[160] These conditions can also increase pill burden and daily demands in order to adhere with primary or secondary prophylaxis of opportunistic infections. Thus, not all pregnancies are the same and just because we can lower HIV viral load, it does not guarantee good pregnancy outcomes.

To optimize pregnancy outcomes it is crucial that these patients avail themselves of preconceptional counseling. During that session, the HIV expert should address issues such as appropriateness of current regimen to achieve viral load suppression, prevent teratogenicity to the unborn child, maintain therapeutic antiretroviral drug levels during pregnancy, and avert maternal toxicities. This encounter allows the woman and her partner to understand how their unique clinical history influences or deters attaining the best pregnancy outcome. It also provides them an opportunity for evaluation and management of such conditions prior to conception. For example, patients who have abnormal Papanicolao screening should undergo colposcopy and biopsy to rule out invasive disease. Some of the patients who were treated with cone biopsy to remove localized disease and who have no further recurrence in the past might require evaluation for incompetent cervix in early pregnancy and cerclage placement. Patients with genital herpes could either be offered suppression in the third trimester of pregnancy or through pregnancy if the patient experiences multiple recurrences. For those with hepatitis C infection, no treatment at present is safe in pregnancy, due to the high teratogenic nature of these agents, so conception should be deferred until completion of therapy, if feasible. Alternatively, patients should be informed of the potential risk of perinatal hepatitis C transmission, and studies conducted in the pre-HAART era suggest that coinfection with Hepatitis C could increase the risk of perinatal HIV transmission. Option for operative delivery for such cases should also be considered, as some observational studies showed that this approach could reduce transmission of both pathogens. These coinfected patients could also be at increased risk of hepatotoxicity upon initiation of antiretroviral therapy and should be closely monitored.[166, 167] For patients coinfected with hepatitis B, their prenatal care is not modified other than close surveillance for liver toxicities and assurance that infants receive both immunoglobulin and Hepatitis vaccine at birth.[166] Consideration has been recently given to the selection of NRTI regimen for these pregnancies but limited data have impeded evidence-based recommendations at present for pregnant women. Those interested in this topic should monitor new reported data incorporated to the PHS treatment guidelines.

Patients with a history of CMV infection need to know that if reactivation occurs the fetus could be affected in utero, and deafness, blindness, and other congenital anomalies can be seen among those infants. Other patients who have prolonged antiretroviral exposure have developed metabolic changes with or without lipodystrophy prior to conception. For such cases, we recommend discontinuation of cholesterol-reducing drugs and diet modification during pregnancy. For those showing evidence of hyperglycemia or overt diabetes adequate glucose control should be achieved prior to conception. Long-term survivors could also have other illnesses that adversely affect pregnancy outcomes such as hypertension, asthma, or hematologic complications such as thrombocytopenia and anemia. Again, given the complexity of these cases management by a maternal fetal medicine expert is highly recommended.

Finally, we should address during the preconceptional counseling the status of the partner and how we can achieve conception while reducing acquisition risk to a uninfected partner. This could be achieved by using intrauterine insemination, obtaining lavage sperm samples or using intracytoplasmic sperm injection. More detailed information of these options is provided in a later section of this review.

A Glimpse to the Future: Assisted Reproductive Technologies for HIV-Infected/Affected Couples

Irrespective of age, race, or mode of HIV-1 acquisition, many infected patients and their partners have expressed a desire to have children.[168–170] Indeed, the clinical milestone achieved during the last decade regarding long-term survival, improved quality of life, and reduction of MTCT challenge the validity of our former advice to this population to defer pregnancy. Although most of the pregnancies occur among asymptomatic, nondrug users, younger patients with increased number of pregnancies have also been seen among women between the ages of 35 and 44.[171,172] Uninfected partners of long-term survivors frequently expect to have children of their own instead of choosing adoption.[170] Use of reproductive technologies for HIV-infected couples has been advocated by some clinicians and investigators in the last 15 years. Assisted reproductive technology (ART) is defined as the use of artificial insemination, in vitro fertilization (IVF), or intracytoplasmic sperm injection (ICSI).[173] Who should benefit from access to these technologies is still controversial and some clinicians have proposed a systematic criteria for patient selection. The ethics, challenges, and controversies of assisted reproduction in this population have also been previously discussed.[174,175] It is possible that in addition to assisting the couple to conceive, the society as a whole could benefit by the use of these technologies by decreasing unprotected encounters and therefore transmission among discordant partners. The extent of the benefit will depend on the balance between the desire or urgency to conceive, alternative approach to decrease horizontal transmission among discordant couples, cost of the intervention, and access to the intervention by all society groups independent of their income.

Clearly, it is also important to monitor the outcomes of elective medical intervention for the patient, the couple, the unborn child, and the society. Several reports have shown that the use of intrauterine insemination and ICSI has been successful in achieving pregnancies without documented seroconversion of neither the uninfected partner nor the newborn. On the other hand, it is well known that a complication of ICI and induction ovulation is the higher rates of multiple gestations with its underlying risk of preterm birth and operative delivery. It is also recognized that this approach limits access due to its increased cost. Thus, as the HIV/AIDS epidemic matures, novel, cheaper approaches must be sought to meet the needs of this growing population globally.

In summary, we have provided a comprehensive overview of the most salient topics related to HIV screening and the management of pregnant women with emphasis on common complications and age-specific issues. We understand that this is a dynamic field and while some of the basic concepts will remain, such as the need for comprehensive history, thorough physical exam, and knowledge of patients' desires and plans for conception, our understanding of the optimal management of HIV and its complications will evolve over time. It is thus essential that clinicians view this chapter as a basic overview, but still seek updated information from experts in the field as well as national guidelines.

References

1. Centers for Disease Control and Prevention. HIV/AIDS surveillance report 2006;18:1–56.
2. UNAIDS. 2006 report on the global AIDS epidemic. A UNAIDS 10th anniversary special edition.
3. Centers for Disease Control and Prevention. Revised recommendations for HIV testing of adults, adolescents, and pregnant women in health care settings. MMWR 2006;55(No RR-14):1–16.
4. Jamieson DJ, Clark J, Kourtis AP, et al. Recommendations for human immunodeficiency virus screening, prophylaxis, and treatment for pregnant women in the United States. Am J Obstet Gynecol 2007;197(Suppl 3):S26–32.
5. Centers for Disease Control and Prevention. Enhanced Perinatal Surveillance-United States, 1999–2001. Atlanta: U.S. Department of Health and Human Services, Centers for Disease Control and prevention 2004:1–22. Special surveillance report 4.
6. Brooke Steele C, Lehida M-M, Campoluci R, DeLuca N, Dean H.D. *Health Disparities in HIV/AIDS, Viral Hepatitis, Sexually Transmitted Diseases, and Tuberculosis: Issues, Burden, and Response, A Retrospective Review, 2000–2004.* Atlanta, GA: Department of Health and Human Services, Centers for Disease Control and Prevention, November 2007. Available at: http://www.cdc.gov/nchhstp/healthdisparities/.
7. Donegan SP, Steger KA, Lakambini R, et al. Seroprevalence of human immunodeficiency virus in parturients at Boston City Hospital: Implications for public health and obstetric practice. Am J Obstet Gynecol 1992;167:622–9.
8. Wiznia AA, Crane M, Lambert G, et al. Zidovudine use to reduce perinatal HIV type 1 transmission in an urban center. JAMA 1996;275:1504–6.
9. Sambamoorthi U, Akincigil A, McSpiritt E, et al. Zidovudine use during pregnancy among HIV-infected women on Medicaid. J Acquir Immune Defic Syndr 2002;30(4):429–39.
10. Anderson JE, Ebrahim SH, Sansom S. Women's Knowledge about treatment to prevent mother to child human immunodeficiency virus transmission. Obstet Gynecol 2004;103:165–8.
11. ACOG Committee Opinion Health Literacy. Number 391, December 2007. Obstet Gynecol 2007;110(6):1489–91.
12. Panel on Antiretroviral Guidelines for Adults and Adolescents. Guidelines for the use of antitretroviral agents in HIV-1 infected adult and adolescents. Department of Health and Human Services. January 29, 2008;1–128. Available at http://www.aidsinfo.nih.gov.
13. Public Health Service Task Force recommendations for use of antiretroviral drugs in pregnant HIV-1-infected women for maternal health and interventions to reduce perinatal HIV-1 transmission in the United States. July 8, 2008. AIDSinfo Web site (http://AIDSinfo.nih.gov).
14. Little BB. Pharmacokinetics during pregnancy: Evidence-Based maternal dose formulation. Obstet Gynecol 1999;93:858–68.
15. Tracy TS, Venkataramanan R, Glover DD, Caritis SN, for the NICHD Network of MFM units. Temporal changes in drug metabolism (CY1A2, CYP2D6 and CYP 3A activity) during pregnancy. Am J Obstet Gynecol 2005;192:633–9.
16. O'Sullivan MJ, Boyer PJ, Scott GB, Parks WP, Weller S, Blum MR, et al. The pharmacokinetics and safety of zidovudine in the third trimester of pregnancy for women infected with human immunodeficiency virus and their infants: Phase I acquired immunodeficiency syndrome Clinical Trials Group Study (protocol 082). Am J Obstet Gynecol 1993;168(5):1510–16.
17. Mandelbrot L, Peytavin G, Firtion G, Farinotti R. Maternal-fetal transfer and amniotic fluid accumulation of lamivudine in human immunodeficiency virus-infected pregnant women. Am J Obstet Gynecol 2001;184:153–8.
18. Wang Y, Livingston E, Patil S, McKinney RE, Bardeguez A, et al. Pharmacokinetics of didanosine in antepartum and postpartum human immunodeficiency virus-infected pregnant women and their neonates: An AIDS Clinical Trials Group Study. JID 1999;180:1536–41.

19. Wade NA, Unadkat JD, Huang S, Shapiro DE, Mathias A, et al. Pharmacokinetics and safety of stavudine in HIV infected pregnant women and their infants: Pediatrics AIDS Clinical Trials Group protocol 332. The Journal of Infectious Diseases 2004;190:2167–74.

20. Brokie BM, Mirochnick M, Caparelli EV, et al., for the PACTG 1026s Study Team. Impact of pregnancy on abacavir pharmacokinetics. AIDS 2006;20(4):553–60.

21. Mirochnick M, Fenton T, Gagnier P, et al., for the Pediatric AIDS Clinical Trials Group Protocol 250 Team. Pharmacokinetics of nevirapine in human imunodeficiency virus type 1 infected pregnant women and their neonates. J Infect Dis 1998;178(2):368–74.

22. Fundaro C, Genovese O, Rendeli C, et al. Myelomeningocele in a child with intrauterine exposure to efavirenz. AIDS 2002;16(2):299–300.

23. Dear Health Care Provider. Re: Important change in Sustiva (Efavienz) package insert-Change from Pregnancy Category C to D Bristol Myers Squibb Company. March 2005.

24. Antiretroviral Pregnancy Registry Steering Committee. Antiretroviral Pregnancy Registry International Interim Report for 1 January 1989 through 31 July 2007. Wilmington, NC: Registry Coordinating Center; 2007. Available at www.APRegistry.com.

25. Acosta EP, Zorrilla C, Van Dyke R, Bardeguez A, Smith E, et al. Pharmacokinetics of saquinavir SGC in HIV Infected pregnant women. HIV Clin. Trials 2001;2(6):460–5.

26. Stek A, Mirochnick M, Capparelli E, et al., for the Pediatric AIDS Clinical Trials Group (PACTG) 1026 Team. Reduced lopinavir exposure during pregnancy. AIDS 2006;20: 1931–9.

27. Bryson Y, Mirochnick M, Stek A, Mofenson L, et al. Pharmacokinetics and safety of nelfinavir when used in combination with zidovudine and lamidivine in HIV-infected pregnant women: Pediatrics AIDS Clinical Trials Group (PACTG) protocol 353. HIV Clin Trials 2008;9(2):115–25.

28. Nellen JF, Schillevoort I, Ferdinand WN, Bergshoeff AS, Godfried MH, et al. Nelfinavir plasma concentrations are low during pregnancy. CID 2004;39:736–40.

29. Van Heeswijk RP, Khaliq Y, Gallicano KE, Bourbeau M, Seguin I, et al. The pharmacokinetics of nelfinavir and M8 during pregnancy and postpartum. Clin Pharmacol Ther 2004;76:588–97.

30. Hayashi S, Beckerman K, Homma M, et al. Pharmacokinetics of indinavir in HIV-positive pregnant women. AIDS 2000;14(8):1061–2.

31. Unadkat JD, Wara DW, Hughes MD, Mathias AA, et al. Pharmacokinetics and safety of indinavir in human immunodeficiency virus-infected pregnant women. Antimicrob Agents Chemother 2007;51(2):783–6.

32. Acosta EP, Bardeguez A, Zorrilla CD, Van Dyke R, et al., for the Pediatrics AIDS Clinical Trials Group 386 Protocol Team. Pharmacokinetics of saquinavir plus low dose ritonavir in human immunodeficiency virus-infected pregnant women. Antimicrob Agents Chemother 2004;48(2):430–6.

33. Ripamonti D, Cattaneo D, Maggiolo F, et al. Atazanavir plus low-dose ritonavir in pregnancy: Pharmacokinetics and placental transfer. AIDS 2007;21:2409–15.

34. Mirochnick M, Best B, Stek A, Capparelli E, et al., for the PACTG 1026s Protocol Team. Lopinavir exposure with an increased dose during pregnancy. J Acquir Immune Defic Syndr 2008;49:485–91.

35. Best B, Stek A, Hu C, et al. High dose lopinavir and standard-dose emtricitabine pharamacokinetics during pregnancy and postpartum. Abstract 629. 15th Conference on Retroviruses and Opportunistic Infections, Boston, U.S., 2008.

36. Marzolini C, Rudin C, Decosterd LA, Telenti A, et al. Transplacental passage of protease inhibitors at delivery. AIDS 2002;16:889–93.

37. Bucceri AM, Somigliana E, Matrone R, Uberti-Foppa C, Vigano P, et al. Discontinuing combination antiretroviral therapy during the first trimester of pregnancy: Insights from plasma human immunodefiency virus-1 RNA viral load and CD4 cell count. Am J Obstet Gynecol 2003;189:545–51.

38. Somigliana E, Bucceri AM, Tibaldi C, Alberico S, et al. Early invasive diagnostic techniques in pregnant women who are infected with HIV: A multicenter cases series. Am J Obstet Gynecol 2005;193:437–42.

39. Rodman J, Flynn P, Shapiro D, Bardeguez A, et al., for te PACTG 394 Study Team. Pharmacokinetics and safety of tenofovir disoproxil fumarate in HIV infected pregnant women and their infants. Abstarct 708; 13th Conference on Retroviruses and Opportunistic Infections, Denver, U.S., 2006.

40. Connor EM, Sperling RS, Gelber R, et al. Reduction of maternal-infant transmission of human immunodeficiency virus type 1 with zidovudine treatment. N Engl J Med 1994;331(18):1173–80.

41. Stiehm ER, Lambert JS, Mofenson LM, et al. Efficacy of zidovudine and human immunodeficiency virus (HIV) hyperimmne immunoglobulin for reducing perinatal HIV transmission from HIV-infected women with advanced disease: Results of Pediatrics AIDS Clinical Trials Group protocol 185. J Infect Dis 1999;179:567–75.

42. Sperling R, Shapiro D, Coombs R, et al. Maternal viral load, zidovudine treatment, and the risk of transmission of human immunodeficiency virus type 1 from mother to infant. N Engl J Med 1996;335(22):1621–9.

43. Mofenson LM, Lambert JS, Stiehm ER, et al. Risk factors for perinatal transmission of human immunodeficiency virus type 1 in women treated with zidovudine. N Engl J Med 1999;341:385–93.

44. Garcia PM. Maternal levels of plasma human immunodeficiency virus type 1 RNA and the risk of perinatal transmission. N Engl J Med 1999;341(6):394–402.

45. Wade NA, Birkhead GS, Warren BL, et al. Abbreviated regimens of zidovudine prophylaxis and perinatal transmission of the human immunodeficiency virus. N Engl J Med 1998;339:1409–14.

46. Fiscus SA, Adimora AA, Schoenback VJ, et al. Trends in human immunodeficiency virus(HIV) counseling, testing and antiretroviral treatment of HIV infected women and perinatal transmission in North Carolina. J Infect 1999;180:99–105.

47. Mayaux MJ, Teglas JP, Mandelbrot L, et al. Acceptability and impact of zidovudine prevention on mother-to-child HIV-1 transmission in France. J Pediatr 1997;131:857–62.

48. Dorenbaum A, Cunningham CK, Gelber RD, et al. Two-dose intrapartum/newborn nevirapine and standard antiretroviral therapy to reduce perinatal HIV transmission. JAMA 2002;288(2):189–98.

49. Cooper ER, Charurat M, Mofenson, L et al. Combination antiretroviral strategies for the treatment of pregnant HIV-1-infected women and prevention of perinatal HIV-1 transmission. J Acquir Immune Defic Syndr 2002;29(5):484–94.

50. The European Mode of Delivery Collaboration. Elective cesarean-section versus vaginal delivery in prevention of vertical HIV-1 transmission: a randomized clinical trial. Lancet 1999;353(9158):1035–9.

51. The International Perinatal HIV Group. The mode of delivery and the risk of vertical transmission of human immunodeficiency virus type 1 – A meta-analysis of 15 prospective cohort studies. N Engl J Med 1999;340(13):977–87.

52. ACOG Committee Opinion. Scheduled cesarean delivery and the prevention of vertical transmission of HIV infection. May 2000; Number 234 (219).

53. Read JS, Tuomala R, Kpamegan E, et al. Mode of delivery and postpartum morbidity among HIV-infected women: The Women and Infants Transmission Study. J Acquir Immune Defic Syndr 2001;26:236–45.

54. Marcollet A, Goffinet F, Firtion G, et al. Differences in postpartum morbidity in women who are infected with the human immunodeficiency virus after elective cesarean delivery, emergency cesarean delivery, or vaginal delivery. Am J Obstet Gynecol 2002;186:784–9.

55. Duarte G, Read JS, Gonin R, et al. Mode of delivery and postpartum morbidity in Latin America and Caribbean countries among women who are infected with human immunodeficiency virus-1: The NICHD International Site Development Initiative (NISDI) Perinatal study. Am J Obstet Gynecol 2006;195:215–29.

56. Louis J, Landon MB, Gersnoviez RJ, et al. Perioperative morbidity and mortality among human immunodeficiency virus-infected women undergoing cesarean delivery. Obstet Gynecol 2007;110:385–90.

57. Sebitloane HM, Modly J, Esterhuinzen TM. Prophylactic antibiotics for the prevention of postpartum infectious morbidity in women infected with human immunodeficiency virus: A randomized controlled trial. Am J Obstet Gynecol 2008;198:189–90.

58. Menacker F. Trends in cesarean rates for first births and repeat cesarean rates for low risk women, United States, 1990–2003. National Vital Statistics Report, Center for Disease Control and Prevention.

59. Silver RM, Landon MB, Rouse DJ, et al. Maternal morbidity associated with multiple repeat cesarean deliveries, Obstet Gynecol 2006;107:1226–32.

60. Knight M, Kurinczuk JJ, Spark P, Brocklehurst, P., for the United Kingdom Obstetrics Surveillance System Steering Committee. Cesarean delivery and peripartum hysterectomy. Obstet Gynecol 2008;111:97–105.

61. CDC. Success in implementing PHS guidelines to reduce perinatal transmission of HIV-Louisiana, Michigan, New Jersey, and South Carolina, 1993, 1995 and 1996. MMWR 1998;47:688–91.

62. Bulterys M, Jamieson DJ, O'Sullivan MJ, et al. Rapid HIV-testing during labor: A multicenter study. JAMA 2004;292:219–23.

63. Jamieson DJ, Cohen MH, Maupin R, et al. Rapid human immunodeficiency virus-1 testing on labor and delivery in 17 U.S. hospitals: the MIRIAD experience. Am J Obstet Gynecol 2007;197(Suppl 3):S72–82.

64. Eshleman SH, Mracna M, Guay LA, et al. Selection and fading of resistence mutations in women and infants receiving nevirapine to prevent HIV-1 vertical transmission (HIVNET 012). AIDS 2001;15(15):1951–7.

65. Cunningham CK, Chaix M, Rekaccwicz C, et al. Development of resistance mutations in women receiving standard antiretroviral therapy who received intrapartum nevirapine to prevent perinatal human immunodeficiency virus type 1 transmission: A substudy of Pediatric AIDS Clinical Trials Group Protocol 316. J Infect Dis 2002;186:181–8.

66. Jourdain G, Ngo-Giang-Huong N, Le Coeur S, et al. Intrapartum exposure to nevirapine and subsequent maternal responses to nevirapine-based antiretroviral therapy. N Engl J Med. 2004;315(3):229–39.

67. Lockman S, Shapiro RL, Smeaton LM, et al. Response to antiretroviral therapy after a single, peripartum dose of nevirapine. N Engl J Med 2007;356:135–47.

68. Coffie PA, Ekouevi DK, Chaix M, et al. Maternal 12 month response to antiretroviral therapy following prevention of mother-to -child transmission of HIV type1, Ivory Coast, 2003–2006. Clin Infect Dis 2006;46:611–2.

69. Chaix M, Ekouevi DK, Rouet F, et al. Low risk of nevirapine resistance mutations in the prevention of mother to child transmission of HIV: Agence Nationale de Recherches sur le SIDa Ditrame Plus, Abidjan, Cote d'Ivorie. J Infect Dis 2006;193:482–7.

70. Chi B, Sinkala M, Mbewe F, et al. Single-dose tenofovir and emtricitabine for reduction of viral resistance to non-nucleoside reverse transcriptase inhibitor drugs in women given intrapartum nevirapine foe perinatal HIV prevention: An open-label randomized trial. Lancet 2007;370:1698–705.

71. Lo WY, Friedman JM. Teratogenicity of recently introduced medications in human pregnancy. Obstet Gynecol 2002;100:465–73.

72. Andrade SE, Gurwitz JH, Davis RL, Chan KA, Finkelstein JA, et al. Prescription use in pregnancy. Am J Obstet Gynecol 2004;191:398–407.

73. Newschaffer CJ, Cocroft J, Anderson CE, et al. Prenatal zidovudine use and congenital anomalies in a Medicaid population. J Acquir Immune Defic Syndr 2000;24:249–56.

74. Watts HD, Covington DL, Beckerman K, Garcia P, Scheuerle A, et al. Asssesing the risk of birth defects associated with antiretroviral exposure during pregnancy. Am J Obstet Gynecol 2004;191:985–92.

75. Watts HD, Li D, Handlelsman E, et al. Assessment of birth defects according to maternal therapy among infants in the women and Infants transmission study. J Acquir Immune Defic Syndr 2007;44(3):299–305.

76. Covington DL, Conner SD, Doi PA, Swinson J, Daniels EM. Risk of birth defects associated with nelfinavir exposure during pregnancy. Obstet Gynecol 2004;103:1181–9.

77. European Collaborative study. Exposure to antiretroviral therapy in utero or early life: The health of uninfected children born to HIV-infected women. J Acquir Immune Defic Syndr 2003;32:380–7.
78. Sperling RS, Shapiro DE, McSherry GD, et al. Safety of the maternal-infant zidovudine regimen utilized in the Pediatric AIDS Clinical Trial Group 076 Study. AIDS 1998;12:1805–13.
79. Bardeguez A, Shapiro D, Mofenson LM, et al. Effect of cessation of zidovudine prophylaxis to reduce vertical transmission on maternal disease progression and survival. J Acquir Immune Defic Syndr 2003;32:170–81.
80. Watts DH, Lambert JS, Stiehm ER, Harrris R, et al., for the Pediatric AIDS Clinical Trials Group 185 Study Team. Progression of HIV disease among women following delivery. J Acquir Immune Defic Syndr 2003;33:585–93.
81. Minkoff H, Ahdieh L, Watts H, Greenblatt RM, et al. The relationship of pregnancy to the use of highly active antiretroviral therapy. Am J Obstet Gynecol 2001;184:1221–7.
82. Watts DH, Rajalakshmi B, Maupin R, Delke I, et al. Maternal toxicity and pregnancy complications in human immunodeficiency virus-infected women receiving antiretroviral therapy: PACTG 316. Am J Obstet Gynecol 204;190:506–16.
83. Zorrilla CD, Van Dyke R, Bardeguez A, Acosta E, et al., for the Pediatrics AIDS Clinical Trials Group 386 Protocol Team. Clinical response, safety and tolerability to saquinavir with low-dose ritonavir in HIV-1 infected mothers and their infants. Antimicrob Agents Chemother 2007:2208–10.
84. Tuomala RE, Watts H, Li D, et al. Improved obstetrics outcomes and few maternal toxicities are associated with antiretroviral therapy, including highly active antiretroviral therapy during pregnancy. J Acquir Immune Defic Syndr 2005;38:449–73.
85. Bristol-Myers Squibb Company. Healthcare provider important drug warning letter. January 5, 2001.
86. Hitti J, Frenkel LM, Stek AM, et al. Maternal toxicity with continuous nevirapine in pregnancy results from PACTG 1022. J Acquir Immune Defic Syndr 2004;36:772–6.
87. Timmermans S, Templlman C, Godfried MH, et al. Nelfinavir and nevirapine side effects during pregnancy. AIDS 2005;19:795–9.
88. Joy S, Poi M, Hughes L, et al. Third trimester maternal toxicity with nevirapine use in pregnancy. Obstet Gynecol 2005;106:1032–8.
89. Blanche S, Tardieu M, Rustin P, et al. Persistent mitochondrial dysfunction and perinatal exposure to antiretroviral nucleoside analogues. Lancet 1999;354:1084–9.
90. The Perinatal Safety Review Working Group. Nucleoside exposure in the children of HIV-infected women receiving antiretroviral drugs: Absence of clear evidence for mitochondrial disease in children who died before 5 years of age in five United States cohorts. JAIDS 2000;25(3):261–8.
91. Culnane M, Fowler M, Lee SS, et al. Lack of long-term effects of in utero exposure to zidovudine among uninfected children born to HIV-infected women. JAMA 1999;281:151–7.
92. Hanson IC, Antonelli TA, Sperling RS, et al. Lack of tumors in infants with perinatal HIV-1 exposure and fetal/neonatal exposure to zidovudine. J Acquir Immune Defic Syndr 1999;20(5):463–7.
93. Webster Dictionary, 3rd College Edition.
94. Osterberg L, Blaschke T. Adherence to medications. N Eng J Med 2005;353:487–97.
95. Bangsberg DR, Hecht FM, Charlebois ED, et al. Adherence to protease inhibitors, HIV-1 viral load, and development of drug resistance in an indigent population. AIDS 2000;14(4):357–66.
96. Ross L, Lim ML, Liao Q, et al. Prevalence of antiretrovirak drug resistance and resistance associated mutations in antiretroviral naïve HIV infected individuals from 40 United States cities. HIV Clin Trials 2007;8:1–8.
97. Johnson VA, Petropoulos CJ, Woods CR, et al. Vertical transmission of multidrug-resistant human immunodeficiency virus type 1 (HIV-1) and continued evolution of drug resistance in an HIV-1-infected infant. J Infect Dis 2001;183:1688–93.

98. Paterson DL, Swindells S, Mohr JA, et al. Adherence to protease inhibitor therapy and outcomes in patients with HIV infection. Ann Intern Med 2000;133:21–30.

99. Murphy DA, Wilson CM, Durako SJ, et al. Antiretroviral medication adherence among the REACH HIV-infected adolescent cohort in the U.S. AIDS Care 2001;13:27–40.

100. Lucas GM, Cheever LW, Chaison RE, et al. Detrimental effects of continued illicit drug use on the treatment of HIV-1 infection. J Acquir Immune Defic Syndr 2001;71:251–9.

101. Starace F, Ammassari A, Trotta MP, et al. Depression is a risk factor for suboptimal adherence to highly active antiretroviral therapy. J Acquir Immune Defic Syndr 2002;3(Suppl 3):S136–9.

102. Cohn SE, Umbleja T, Mrus J, Bardeguez AD, Anderson J, Chesney MA. Prior illicit drug use and missed prenatal vitamins predict non-adherence to antiretroviral therapy in pregnancy: Adherence analysis A5084. AIDS Patient Care STDs 2008;22(1):29–40.

103. Bardeguez A, Lindsey JC, Shannon M, et al. Adherence to antiretrovirals (arvs) in U.S. women during and after pregnancy. J Acquir Immune Defic Syndr 2008;48(4):408–17.

104. Wilson T, Ickovics JR, Fernandez MI, et al., for the Perinatal Guidelines Evaluation Project. Self-reported zidovudine adherence among pregnant women with human immunodeficiency virus infection in four U.S. states. Am J Obstet Gynecol. 2001;184(6):1235–40.

105. Ickovics JR, Wilson TE, Royce RA, et al. Prenatal and postpartum zidovudine adherence among pregnant women with HIV: Results of a MEMS sub-study from the perinatal guidelines evaluation project. J Acquir Immune Defic Syndr 2002;30(3):311–5.

106. van den Broek NR, White SA, Neilson JP. The relationship between asymptomatic human immunodeficiency virus infection and the prevalence and severity of anemia in pregnant Malawian women. Am J Trop Med Hyg 1998;59:1004–7.

107. Henry DH, Volberding PA, Leitz G. Epoetin alfa for the treatment of anemia in HIV-infected patients. J Acquir Immune Defic Syndr 2004;37:1221–7.

108. Sullivan PS, Hanson D, Chu SY, et al. Surveillance for thrombocytopenia in persons infected with HIV: Results from the multistate adult and adolescent spectrum of disease project. J Acquir Immune Defic Syndr 1997;14:374–9.

109. Miguez-Burbano MJ, Jackson J, Hadrigan S. Thrombocytopenia in HIV disease: Clinical relevance, pathophysiology and management. Curr Med Chem–Cardiovasc Hematol Agents 2005;3:365–76.

110. Thrombocytopenia in Pregnancy. ACOG practice bulletin. Clinical management guidelines for obstetrician-gynecologist. Number 6, September 1999. In ACOG 2008 Compendium of Selected Publications. Volume 2: Practice Bulletins, pp. 581–91.

111. Duration of rupture membranes and vertical transmission of HIV-1: A meta-analysis from 15 prospective cohort studies. The International Perinatal group. AIDS 2001;15:357–68.

112. Minkoff H, Burns DN, Landesman S, et al. The relationship of the duration of ruptured membranes to vertical transmission of human immunodeficiency virus type. Am J Obstet Gynecol 1995;173:585–9.

113. Landesman SH, Kalish LA, Burns DN, et al. Obstetrical factors and the transmission of human immunodeficiency virus type 1 from mother to child. N Engl J Med 1996;34:1617–23.

114. ACOG Committee Opinion Prevention of Early Onset Group B Streptococcal Disease in Newborns. Number 279. December 2002. In ACOG 2008 compendium of selected publications. Volume 1: Committee opinions and policy statements, pp. 425–32.

115. Premature Rupture of Membranes. ACOG practice bulletin. Clinical management guidelines for obstetrician-gynecologists. Number 80, April 2007. In ACOG 2008 compendium of selected publications. Volume 2: Practice Bulletin, pp. 940–52.

116. Major CA, Towers CV, Lewis DF, and Garite TJ. Expectant management of preterm premature rupture of membranes complicated by active recurrent genital herpes. Am J Obstet Gynecol 2003;188:1551–5.

117. Drake AL, John-Steward GC, Wald A, et al. Herpes Simplex virus type 2 and Risk of intrapartum human immunodeficiency virus transmission. Obstet Gynecol 2007;109:403–9.

118. Alvarez JR, Bardeguez A, Iffy L, Apuzzio J. Preterm premature rupture of membraines in pregnancies complicated by human immunodeficiency virus infection: A single center's five-year experience. J Matern-Fetal Neonat Med 2007;20:853–7.

119. Lorenzi P, Spicher VM, Laubereau B, et al. Antiretroviral therapies in pregnancy: Maternal, fetal, and neonatal effects. Swiss HIV Cohort Study, The Swiss Collaborative HIV and Pregnancy Study, and The Swiss Neonatal HIV Study. AIDS 1998;12(18):F241–7.

120. Morris AB, Cu-Uvin S, Harwell JI, et al. Multicenter review of protease inhibitors in 89 pregnancies. J Acquir Immune Defic Syndr 2000;25:306–11.

121. Cotter AM, Gonzalez A, Duthely LM, et al. Is antiretroviral therapy during pregnancy associated with increased risk of preterm delivery, low birth weight, or stillbirth? J Infect Dis 2006;193:1195–201.

122. Tuomala RE, Shapiro DE, Mofenson LM, et al. Antiretroviral therapy during pregnancy and the risk of an adverse outcome. N Engl J Med 2002;346(24):1863–70.

123. Grosch-Woerner I, Puck K, Maier RF, et al. Increased rate of prematurity associated with antenatal antiretroviral therapy in a German/Austrian cohort of HIV-1-infected women. HIV Med 2008;9:6–13.

124. Schulte J, Dominguez K, Sukalac T, et al. Declines in low birth weight and preterm among infants who were born to HIV-infected women duringan era of increased use of maternal antiretrovital drugs: Pediatric spectrum of HIV disease, 1989–2004. Pediatrics 2007;119:e 900–6.

125. Martin F, Taylor GP. Increased rates of preterm delivery are associated with the initiation of highly active antiretroviral therapy during pregnancy: A single center cohort study. JID 2007;196:558–61.

126. Ravizza M, Martinelli P, Bucceri A, et al. Treatmment with protease inhibitors and co-infection with hepatitis C virus are independent predictors of preterm delivery in HIV-1 infectedpregnant women. JID 2007;195:913–4.

127. Kourtis AP, Schmid CH, Jamieson DJ, Lau J. Use of antiretroviraltherapy in pregnant HIV-infected women and the risk of premature delivery: A meta analysi. AIDS 2007;21:607–15.

128. Szyld EG, Warley EM, Freimanis L, et al. Maternal antiretroviral drugs during pregnancy and infant lowbirthweight and preterm birth. AIDS 2006;20:2345–53.

129. Beitune PA, Duarte G, Foss M, Montenegro RM, et al. Effect of maternal use of antiretroviral agents on serum insulin levels of the newborn infant. Diabetes Care 2005;28:856–9.

130. Chamait R, franklin P, Spector SA, Hull AD. Protease inhibitors and decreased birth weight in HIV infected pregnant women with impaired glucose tolerance. J Perinatol 2002;22:370–3.

131. Justman JE, Benning L, Danoff A, Minkoff H, et al. Protease inhibitor use and the incidence of diabetes mellitus in a large cohort of HIV-infected women. JAIDS 2003;32:298–302.

132. Gestational Diabetes. ACOG Practice Bulletin. Clinical management guidelines for obstetrician-gynecologists. Number 30, September 2001. In ACOG 2008 compendium of selected publications. Volume 2: Practice Bulletin, pp. 695–708.

133. Dinsmoor MJ, Forrest ST. Lack of an effect of protease inhibitor use on glucose tolerance during pregnancy. Infect Dis Obstet Gynecol 2002;10:187–91.

134. Hitti J, Anderson J, McComsey G, et al., for the AIDS Clinical Trials Group 5084 Study Team. Protease inhibitor-based antiretroviral therapy and glucose tolerance in pregnancy: AIDS Clinical Trials Group A5084. Am J Obstet Gynecol 2007;196:331.e1–7.

135. Watts DH, Balasubraman R, Maupin ET, et al. Maternal toxicity and pregnancy complications in HIV-infected women receiving antiretroviral therapy: PACTG 316. Am J Obstet Gynecol 2004;190:506–16.

136. Hollingsworth DR, Moore TR. Diabetes and pregnancy Chapter 46. In *Maternal Fetal Medicine: Principles and Practice.* Creasy RK, Resnick R, editors, 1989, 2nd ed., p. 835.

137. Brizzi P, Tonolo G, Esposito F, et al. lipoprotein metabolism during normal pregnancy. Am J Obstet Gynecol 1999;181:430–4.

138. Fahraeus L, Larsson-Cohn U, Wallentin L, et al. Plasma lipo-proteins including high density lipoproteins sub-fractions during normal pregnancy. Obstet Gynecol 1985;66:468–72.

139. Livingston E, Cohn SE, Yang Y, et al., for the AIDS Clinical Trials Group A5084 Study team. Lipids & lactate in HIV-1 infected pregnancies with/without protease inhibitor-based therapy. Obstet Gynecol 2007;110:391–7.

140. DeVore GR, Romero R. Genetic sonography: An option for women of advanced maternal age with negative triple-marker maternal serum screening results. J Ultrasound Med 2003;22:1191–9.

141. Pinette MG, Egan JFX, Wax JR, et al. Combined sonographic and biochemical markers for down syndrome screening. J Ultrasound Med 2003;22:1185–90.

142. Biggio JR, Morris C, Owen J, Stringer JS. An outcome analysis of five prenatal screening strategies for trisomy 21 in women younger than 35 years. Am J Obstet Gynecol 2004;190:721–9.

143. Hobbins JC, Lezotte DC, Persutte WH, et al. An 8-center study to evaluate the utility of midterm genetic sonograms among high risk pregnancies. J Ultrasound Med 2003;22:33–8.

144. (a) Coll O, Suy A, Hernandez S, et al. Prenatal diagnosis in human immunodeficiency virus-infected women: A new screening program for chromosomal anomalies. Am J Obstet Gynecol 2006;194:192–8.
    (b) Mandelbrot L, Jasseron C, Ekoukou D, et al., for the ANRS French Perinatal Cohort. Ammniocentesis and mother to child human immunodeficiency virus transmission in the Agence Nationale de Reserches sur le Sida et les Hepatites Virales French Perinatal Cohort. Am J Obstet Gynecol 2009;200:160.e1–9.

145. Gross S, Castillo W, Crane M, et al. Maternal serum alpha fetoprotein and human chorionic gonadotropin levels in women with HIV. Am J Obstet Gynecol 2003;188:1052–6.

146. Yudin MH, Prosen TL, Landers DV. Multiple marker screening in HIV positive pregnant women: Screen positivity rates with the triple and quad screen. Am J Obstet Gynecol 2003;189:973–6.

147. Einstein FH, Wright RL, Trentacoste S, et al. The impact of protease inhibitors on maternal serum screening analyte levels in pregnant women who are HIV positive. Am J Obstet Gynecol 2004;191:1004–8.

148. Shapiro DE, Sperling RS, Mandelbrot L, et al. Risk factors for perinatal human immunodeficiency transmission in patients receiving zidovudine prophylaxis. PACTG Protocol 076 Study Group. Obstet Gynecol 1999;94:897–908.

149. Mandelbrot L, Mayaux MJ, Bongain A, et al. Obstetrics factors and mother-to-child transmission of human immunodeficiency virus type1: The French Perinatal Cohorts. Am J Obstet Gynecol 1996;175:661–7.

150. Bucceri AM, Somigliana E, Vignali M. Early invasive diagnostic techniques during pregnancy in HIV-infected women. Acta Obstet Gynecol Scan 2001;80:82–3.

151. The European Collaborative Study. Fluctuations in symptoms in human immunodeficiency virus-infected children: The first 10 years of life. Pediatrics 2001;108:116–22.

152. Gortmaker SL, Hughes M, Cervia J, et al. Effect of combination therapy including protease inhibitors on mortality among children and adolescents infected with HIV-1. N Engl J Med 2001;345:1522–28.

153. Resino S, Bellon JM, Resino R, Navarro L, et al. Extensive implementation of highly active antiretroviral therapy shows great effect on survival and surrogate markers in vertically HIV-infected children. CID 2004;38:1605–12.

154. Zorrilla C, Febo I, Ortiz I, et al. Pregnancy in perinatally HIV-infected adolescents and young adults – Puerto Rico, 2002. MMWR Weekly 2003;52:149–51.

155. Brogly SB, Watts DH, Ylitalo N, et al. Reproductive health of adolescent girls perinatally infected with HIV. Am J Public Health 2007;97:1047–52.

156. Fraser AM, Brockert JE, Ward RH. Association of young maternal age with adverse reproductive outcomes. N Engl J Med 1995;332:1113–7.

157. Jolly MC, Sebire N, Harris J, Robinson S, Regan L. Obstetric risks of pregnancy in women less than 18 years old. Obstet Gynecol 2000;96:962–6.

158. Chen XK, Wen SW, Fleming N, Demissie K, Rhoads GG, Walker M. Teenage pregnancy and adverse birth outcomes: A large population based retrospective cohort study. Int J Epidemiol 2007;36:368–73.

159. Williams S, Keane M, Bettica L, Dieudonne A, Bardeguez A. Adeherence issues and viral suppression in perinatally-infected pregnant adolescents. Infectious Disease Society for Obstetrics and Gynecology. 34th Annual Scientific Meeting, Boston, MA, August 9, 2007.

160. Williams S, Keane M, Bettica L, Dieudonne A, Bardeguez A. Pregnancy outcomes in young women with perinatally acquired human immunodeficiency virus-1. Am J Obstet Gynecol 2009;200:149.e1–5.

161. McConnell M, Clark H, Zorrilla C, et al. Pregnancy in perinatally HIV-infected youth. 3rd IAS Conference on HIV Pathogenesis and Treatment, Rio de Janeiro, Brazil, July 24–27, 2005. Abstract number: MoPeLB9.5C01.

162. Sharma A, Feldman JG, Golub ET, et al. Live birth patterns among human immunodeficiency virus-infected women before and after the availability of highly active antiretroviral therapy. Am J Obstet Gynecol 2007;196:541.e1–6.

163. Hawes SE, Critchlow CW, Faye MA, et al. Increased risk of high grade cervical squamous intraepithelial lesions and invasive cancer among African women with human immunodeficiency virus type 1 and 2 infections. J Infect Dis 2003;188:55–63.

164. Jakobson M, Gissler M, Sainio S, et al. Preterm delivery after surgical treatment for cervical intraepithelial neoplasia. Obstet Gynecol 2007;109:309–13.

165. Moscicki A, Ellenberg JH, Crowley-Nowick P, et al. Risk of high-grade squamous intraepithelial lesion in HIV infected adolescents. JID 2004;190:1413–21.

166. Viral Hepatitis in Pregnancy. ACOG Practice Bulletin. Clinical management guidelines for obstetrician-gynecologists. Number 86, October 2007. Obstet Gynecol 2007;110(4):941–55.

167. Santiago-Munoz P, Scott R, Sheffield J, et al. Prevalence of hepatitis B and C in pregnant women who are infected with human immunodeficiency virus. Am J Obstet Gynecol 2005;193:1270–3.

168. Chen JL, Phillips KA, Kanouse DE, Collins RL, Miu A. Fertility desires and intentions of HIV-positive men and women. Family Planning Perspect 2001;33(4):144–52.

169. Bedimo-Rung AL, Clark RA, Dumestre J Rice J, Kissinger P. Reproductive decision-making among HIV-infected women. J Nat Med Assoc 2005;97:1403–10.

170. Klein J, Pena JE, Thornton II MH, Sauer MV. Understanding the motivations, concerns and desires of human immunodefiviency virus 1 serodiscordant couples wishing to have children through assisted reproduction. Obstet Gynecol 2003;101:987–94.

171. Massad LS, Springer G, Jacobson L, et al. Pregnancy rates and predictors on conception. Miscarriage and abortion in U.S. women with HIV. AIDS 2004;18:281–6.

172. Blair JM, Hanson DL, Jones JL, Dworkin MS. Trends in pregnancy rates among women with human immunodeficiency virus. Obstet Gynecol 2004;103:663–8.

173. Goldman-Clery J, Pena JE, Thornton MH, et al. Obstetrics outcomes of human immunodeficiency virus 1 serodiscordant couples following in vitro fertilization with intracytoplasmic sperm injection. Am J Perinatol 2003;29:305–11.

174. Al-Khan A, Colon J, Palta V, Bardeguez A. Assisted Reproductive technology for men and women infected with human immunodeficiency virus type 1. CID 2003;36:195–200.

175. Lyerly AD, Anderson J. Human immunodeficiency virus and assisted reproduction: reconsidering evidence, reframing ethics. Fertil Steril 2001;75:843–58.

The Dermatological Manifestations of HIV Infection in Ethnic Skin

Dina D. Strachan

Introduction

It is well known that HIV infection is associated with an increased burden of dermatologic disease.[1,2] Some studies show that greater than 90% of HIV-positive people have skin-related complaints.[1,2] Taking into account that the scope of dermatology includes the skin, hair, nails, and mucosa, approximately a quarter of the conditions listed as AIDS-defining illnesses are dermatologic in nature (Table 1).[3] Historically, dermatologists were among some of the first doctors to recognize AIDS as a distinct condition.

Dermatologic conditions may be the presenting manifestation of HIV infection, prompting testing,[2] or a marker for disease progression (Table 2).[4] Patients may have unusual, more severe, or recalcitrant cases of common conditions (e.g., warts, seborrheic dermatitis) or present with diseases relatively unique to HIV infection (e.g., eosinophilic folliculitis, Kaposi's sarcoma). In untreated patients, the type of dermatologic disease seen tends to have a pattern that correlates with CD4 count; however, the introduction of HAART in the mid-1990s changed the pattern of the conditions seen.[5] Complications from HAART and other medicines used to treat HIV infection, such as lipodystrophy, added to the list of the many HIV-related cutaneous manifestations.

In the U.S., ethnic minorities, particularly African Americans and Latinos, bear a disproportionately high burden of HIV/AIDS infection.[6] Within the subpopulation of people infected with HIV, ethnic minorities may also have a greater incidence of skin disease. In 2001, Mirmirani et al. reported African American race as an independent risk factor for skin disease in a study of 2,018 HIV-infected women.[7] Recent recognition of the differences in the diagnosis and treatment of ethnic skin adds to the complexity of treating skin disease in this population.

D.D. Strachan
161 Sixth Avenue, 13th floor, New York, NY 10013, U.S.
E-mail: drstrachan@yahoo.com

V. Stone et al. (eds.), *HIV/AIDS in U.S. Communities of Color*.
DOI: 10.1007/978-0-387-98152-9_8, © Springer Science + Business Media, LLC 2009

Table 1 Conditions included in the 1993 AIDS surveillance case definition (Adapted from 1993 Revised Classification System for HIV Infection and Expanded Surveillance Case Definition for AIDS Among Adolescents and Adults)

Candidiasis of bronchi, trachea, or lungs
Candidiasis, esophageal
Cervical cancer, invasive[a]
Coccidioidomycosis, disseminated or extrapulmonary
Cryptococcosis, extrapulmonary
Cryptosporidiosis, chronic intestinal (greater than 1 month's duration)
Cytomegalovirus disease (other than liver, spleen, or nodes)
Cytomegalovirus retinitis (with loss of vision)
Encephalopathy, HIV-related
Herpes simplex: chronic ulcer(s) (greater than 1 month's duration); or bronchitis, pneumonitis, or
    esophagitis
Histoplasmosis, disseminated or extrapulmonary
Isosporiasis, chronic intestinal (greater than 1 month's duration)
Kaposi's sarcoma
Lymphoma, Burkitt's (or equivalent term)
Lymphoma, immunoblastic (or equivalent term)
Lymphoma, primary, of brain
Mycobacterium avium complex or M. kansasii, disseminated or extrapulmonary
Mycobacterium tuberculosis, any site (pulmonary[a] or extrapulmonary)
Mycobacterium, other species or unidentified species, disseminated or extrapulmonary
Pneumocystis carinii pneumonia
Pneumonia, recurrent[a]
Progressive multifocal leukoencephalopathy
Salmonella septicemia, recurrent
Toxoplasmosis of brain
Wasting syndrome due to HIV

[a] Added in the 1993 expansion of the AIDS surveillance case definition

Just as there may be distinct clinical manifestations and incidence of skin disease in an HIV-infected population, ethnicity may also impact epidemiology, clinical presentation, prognosis, and management. Demographic differences in the cutaneous manifestations of HIV may reflect genetic differences, comorbidities, differences in HIV risk factors, and environment. In 2006, Zancanaro et al. reported no reduction in the prevalence of some conditions, such as seborrheic dermatitis, among HAART users in their study of the spectrum of skin disease in a largely urban, majority African American HIV-infected population.[5] This contradicted previous reports of variations in the prevalence of seborrheic dermatitis in studies with different ethnic demographic compositions. Zancaro et al. also found that folliculitis was the most common skin disease identified, seen in 18% of patients, followed by condyloma acuminatum in 11.5%, seborrheic dermatitis in 10.6%, xerosis cutis in 9.7%, and dermatophyte infection in 7.1%.[5]

To further complicate the picture, the spectrum of skin disease in HIV also varies with respect to gender. In 1999, Barton and Bushness reported the appearance of molluscum contagiosum at a higher CD4 count and a lower prevalence of Kaposi's sarcoma, oral hairy leukoplakia, and onychomycosis in women.[8]

In light of the high dermatologic morbidity in HIV-infected patients, any practitioner who provides primary medical care to this population should have a partnership with a dermatologist. Although a comprehensive review of the dermatologic

Table 2 Chronology of skin disease in HIV infection[8] (Adapted from Wong 1996)

Seroconversion
Mononucleosis-like syndrome with exanthema and enanthem
CD4 count < 500
Dermatophyte infection
Psoriasis
Seborrheic deramatitis
CD4 count 500–200
Bacterial folliculitis
Pityriasis versicolor
Verruca vulgaris
Molluscum contagiosum
Herpes zoster
CD4 < 200
Acquired ichthyosis
Herpes simplex
Kaposi's sarcoma
Crusted scabies
Oral candidiasis
Oral hairy leukoplakia
Other opportunistic infections
Papular/follicular eruptions
Pruritus

manifestations of HIV is beyond the scope of this chapter, to follow is a discussion of some of the common conditions seen in HIV-infected patients in the ambulatory setting with particular attention to how these present and may differ in ethnic minorities.

Infection

Bacterial

Staphylococcus aureus

Staphylococcus aureus is a Gram-positive bacterial pathogen responsible for a wide variety of skin infections including cellulitis, impetigo, folliculitis, and abscesses. Patients may present with erythematous, indurated, tender papules, plaques, pustules, furuncles, and abscesses. A honey-colored crust may also be present. Patients with underlying skin conditions that compromise barrier function, such as atopic dermatitis, are at increased risk of infection and colonization. Recently there has been concern about the growing prevalence of the highly virulent community-acquired methicillin-resistant *Staphlococcus aureus* (MRSA) infection. HIV infection acquired through male homosexual activity and through injection drug use are independent risk factors for MRSA infection.[9] Patients infected with HIV, particularly those with clinical AIDS, have a high rate of nasal colonization with MRSA and are at increased risk of serious systemic infection such as pneumonia, bacteremia, endocarditis, and death (Nyguen et al.[10] and Miller et al.[11]). Patients with severe or resistant infections may require hospitalization.

Liberal use of antibiotics is believed to be the cause of the increased incidence of resistant strains, such as MRSA, even in community settings, in both HIV-infected and uninfected populations.[9, 12] MRSA infections involve the skin in 85% of cases most commonly as abscesses or folliculitis.[9] Patients colonized by resistant strains may experience recurrent infection and may require more aggressive management strategies, including efforts to eradicate MRSA colonization.

Sending pus or crust for culture and antibiotic sensitivity testing is recommended when *Staphylococcus* infection is suspected. Pus-filled lesions should be incised and drained. Elston recommends using a sulfa or tetracycline first-line for pus-filled lesions as there is currently less resistance to these antibiotics. In other types of uncomplicated skin infections, a cephalosporin, a penicillinase-resistant penicillin, or a beta-lactam/beta-lactamase inhibitor combination (such as amoxicillin/clavulanic acid) is recommended.[9]

Use of antimicrobial cleansers, such as chlorhexidine, and topical mupirocin in the nares, axilla, and groin is useful in the treatment of patients suspected of being colonized. Various oral antibiotic treatment protocols, using combinations of rifampin and other antibiotics including tetracyclines, may be required; rifampin monotherapy may lead to resistance. Close contacts of infected patients have a high risk of colonization and may require at least a topical decolonization protocol.

Syphilis

Syphilis is an ancient, ubiquitous infection caused by the spirochete *Treponema pallidum*. Infection generally occurs through the skin or mucous membranes and is usually the result of sexual contact. Hematogenous and congenital transmissions also occur. It is characterized by primary, secondary, latent, and tertiary stages, each with its own distinct clinical characteristics. Syphilis can also be passed congenitally resulting in visual and auditory impairment, as well as tooth deformities. Although often recognized only for its genitoulcerative lesions, syphilis has a variety of presentations, thus its moniker, *the great imitator*. The many cutaneous manifestations of syphilis, particularly in the secondary stage, resulted in dermatologists being the experts in identifying and managing this disease in the preantibiotic era. In fact, many professional societies and journals were named for "dermatology and syphiliology" in the nineteenth and early twentieth centuries.

The primary stage of syphilis is characterized by a "chancre," which is a painless, cutaneous ulcer at the point of entry, usually the genitals. Patients may have more than one chancre and a chancre may be painful if it becomes superinfected. The average time from incubation to primary syphilis is 21 days but can range from 10 to 90 days. Untreated, the chancre may resolve in 1–6 weeks; however, the infection remains. The differential diagnosis includes other genital ulcers such as ulcers due to herpes simplex, and chancroid.

Secondary syphilis is characterized by a variety of mucocutaneous and constitutional signs and symptoms. It generally presents 3–6 weeks after the appearance of the chancre, which may still be present in the secondary phase. Cutaneous signs of secondary syphilis include patchy hair loss, maculopapular eruption, psoriasiform eruptions (Figs. 1 and 2), verrucous papules known as condylomata lata on the genital or perianal region (Fig. 3), silvery papules on the oral mucosa (mucous patches), and scaly red-brown papules on the palms and soles (copper penny lesions) (Figs. 4 and 5). Palmar and plantar involvement of an eruption of unknown etiology should raise suspicion for secondary syphilis; however, be aware that in patients with dark skin, nonscaly macular hyperpigmentation of the palms and soles is common

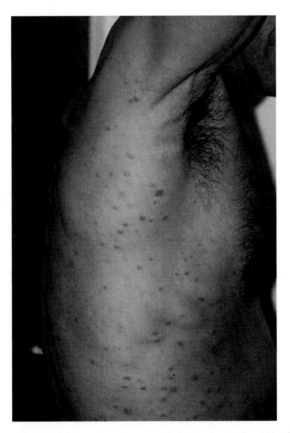

Fig. 1 An eruption of well-demarcated erythematous scaly papules on the trunk of a Hispanic man with HIV and syphilis. The patient presented with pharyngitis and was initially thought to have guttate psoriasis

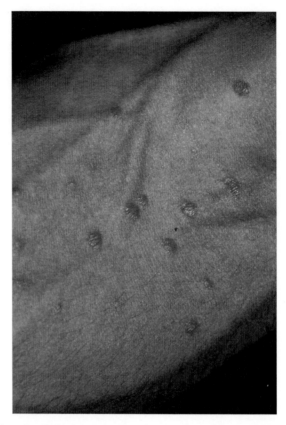

Fig. 2 An eruption of well-demarcated erythematous scaly papules on the forearm of a Hispanic man with HIV and syphilis. The patient presented with pharyngitis and was initially thought to have guttate psoriasis

(Fig. 6). If the lesions have been present for years they are unlikely to be a sign of syphilis.

The differential diagnosis of the lesions of secondary syphilis includes pityriasis rosea, sarcoidosis, psoriasis, lichen planus, viral examthem, drug eruption, and herpetic seroconversion. Additionally, emtricitabine (FTC) has also been reported to cause hyperpigmentation of the palms and soles almost exclusively in patients of African descent, thus drug reaction should be on the differential of these types of lesions in patients on FTC.[13] Cutaneous findings may be accompanied by lymphadenopathy and constitutional symptoms such as fever, pharyngitis, and conjunctival injection. In order to not miss a diagnosis of syphilis, it is important to include it appropriately in the differential diagnosis of a variety of cutaneous eruptions.

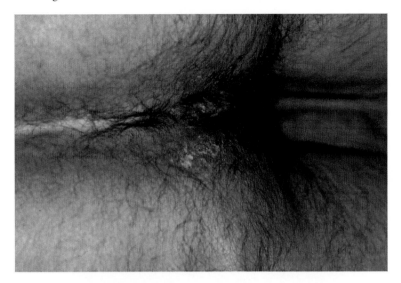

Fig. 3 Condylomata lata in the perianal area

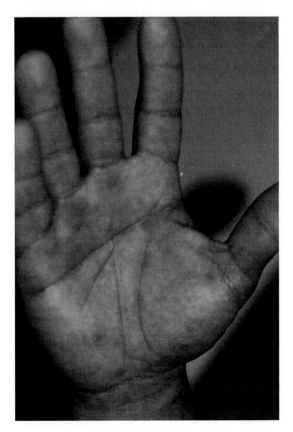

Fig. 4 Syphilis on the palm in a patient with HIV

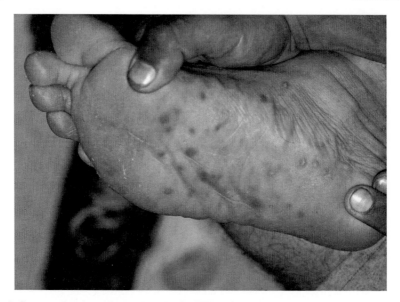

Fig. 5 Copper-colored papules on the sole of a HIV-positive Hispanic man

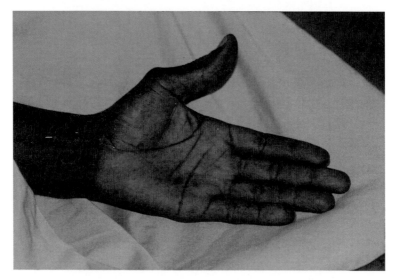

Fig. 6 Palmoplantar hyperpigmentation on a 53-year-old African American man. The lesions were present for years. The patient was referred to the dermatology clinic with an unreactive RPR

Syphilis and HIV

It is no surprise that being HIV-infected increases the likelihood of acquiring syphilis given its similar mode of transmission. Furthermore, as a genital ulcer disease, syphilis likely increases the risk of both acquiring and transmitting HIV infection.[11,12] Coinfection of syphilis and HIV can create diagnostic challenges both clinically and serologically. Coinfection may change the presentation and progression of syphilis.[14] Cutaneous lesions may be more exuberant or appear at uncharacteristic times. Chancres may persist into the secondary stage. Gutierrez-Galhardo et al. reported in 2005 an increased frequency of multiple genital ulcers in secondary and latent syphilis in the setting of HIV infection.[15] The prozone phenomenon, a false-negative nontreponemal test with a reactive treponeme-specific test in the setting of excessive antibody, occurs more commonly in HIV, which may make serologic diagnosis less reliable. Accurate diagnosis of a suspicious eruption may require a skin biopsy. Timely diagnosis of syphilis is especially important in the setting of HIV, as patients have been reported to progress to neurosyphilis earlier despite appropriate treatment.[16]

Fungal

Dermatophytes

Superficial fungal infection of the skin is most commonly caused by the dermatophytes, a group of fungi that only penetrate a few millimeters into the skin. The dermatophytes include the genera Epidermophyton, Microsporum, and Trichophyton. Conditions caused by dermatophytes are usually named for the affected region, e.g., Tinea corporis (body), Tinea capitis (scalp), Tinea cruris (inguinal), Tinea pedis (feet), and Tinea ungium (nails). Infection is opportunistic. It is usually contracted from the environment and depends on host immune factors. Reinfection and recurrence are common. Although a common diagnosis in HIV-infected patients, dermatophyte infection is common in the general population and is not considered a specific marker for HIV infection except in the setting of noninflammatory, widespread infection.[17]

The classic presentation of dermatophyte infection on the skin is an erythematous, annular (thus its name "ringworm"), scaly plaque. Lesions are typically pruritic but may be asymptomatic in HIV.[17] It may present with scale, hair loss, pustules, and itch with lymphadenopathy on the scalp. Folliculitis may lead to cellulitis and abscess formation. Maceration and vesicles are common on the feet. Nail involvement typically presents with hyperkeratosis, and white, yellow, or black discoloration. In HIV infection, toenail involvement may occur in the absence of T. pedis and may involve both palms (usually only one palm is involved in immunocompetent patients[17]). Proximal subungual thickening is almost exclusively seen in the setting of HIV infection. Although dermatophyte infection does not penetrate deeper than the skin or nail, it compromises the skin barrier function, especially if patients excoriate the skin, thus increasing the risk of potentially dangerous bacterial superinfection.

It may be difficult to distinguish dermatophyte infections from seborrheic dermatitis, psoriaisis, or crusted scabies (all more common in HIV-infected patients). Although scalp infection is far more common in children, particularly African American children, it has been identified as a growing problem in adults, particularly African American women.[18] This increase seems to be unrelated to HIV infection but rather exposure to the high-risk group (i.e., children).

If clinical diagnosis or pathogen identification is required, there are a number of options. Sampling technique is dependent on the location of interest. Diagnosis of dermatophyte infection can be achieved with a KOH (potassium hydroxide) preparation, fungal culture, or staining of the fungi on tissue biopsy. Although fungal culture tends to have a low yield, which may be a result of poor sampling technique, it may be required for species identification. This tool may be particularly useful in distinguishing Tinea from other scaly scalp conditions. Although many clinicians are skilled at making a clinical diagnosis, laboratory support is recommended particularly with scalp or nail disease, as many weeks of systemic therapy may be required.

When Tinea is suspected, a thorough history of previous treatments, particularly topical steroids, should be obtained to rule out Tinea incognito, which is described and identified as follows. When treated with topical steroids, a dermatophyte infection may react in a variety of ways. It may appear to improve as a result of a masked inflammatory response, followed by a flare with the withdrawal of treatment. Topical steroids may also cause clinical worsening or result in a change in morphology steering the observer from the correct diagnosis of dermatophytosis.

Candida

Mucocutaneous candidiasis may present as thrush, oral erosions, intertrigo, atrophic glossitis (Fig. 7), esophagitis, vulvovaginitis, paronychia, and rarely onychomycosis. Candida nail infection usually represents secondary invasion of a primary dermatophytosis.[17]

Deep Fungal

Cryptococcus neoformans

The cutaneous lesions of cryptococcosis are umbilicated papules (Fig. 8) usually less than 5 mm in diameter that may be confused with mollusca contagiosa (Table 3). Skin lesions are a sign of disseminated infection, most commonly meningitis. If identified, a search for systemic involvement should follow. Skin biopsy or culture can establish diagnosis.

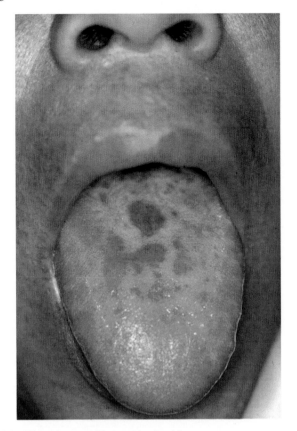

Fig. 7 HIV-positive Hispanic man with atrophic glossitis

Table 3 Differential diagnosis of umbilicated lesion in HIV

Molluscum contagiosum
Penecillium marnefii
Basal cell carcinoma
Cryptococcus neoformans
Pneumocyctis carinii pneumonia
Sebaceous hyperplasia

Viral

Acute Retroviral Syndrome (ARS)

Acute HIV infection may present with a mononucleosis-like condition commonly associated with dermatological findings. Fever is the most common symptom followed by oral and skin lesions.[19] The cutaneous lesions of ARS are usually asymptomatic macules and papules on the face and trunk.[20] Lymphadenopathy,

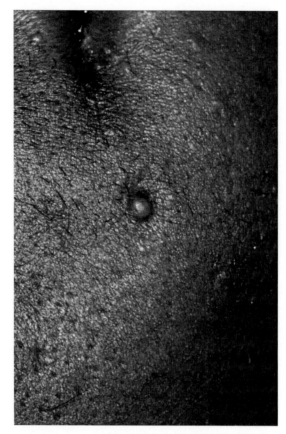

Fig. 8 Cutaneous cryptococcosus on the cheek of an HIV-positive African American woman admitted for headache and neurological complaints. Diagnosis was confirmed on skin biopsy

pharyngitis, myalgias, weight loss, and aseptic meningitis may also occur. The condition starts 2–4 weeks after exposure and resolves in 2–3 weeks.[20] Consider HIV testing in any individual presenting with fever and a rash especially if there is a history of high-risk behaviors associated with HIV infection.

Human Papilloma Virus Infection (Warts)

Common warts (verruca vulgaris), flat warts (verruca plana), and genital warts (condyloma acuminate) all represent infection with the human papilloma virus (HPV). There are numerous HPV serotypes each of which has a penchant for certain anatomical sites. The virus intercalates into the DNA of the host epithelial cell inducing hyperplasia. The result is the characteristic lesions. Common warts of the hands and feet, associated with HPV serotypes 2 and 4, typically present as verrucous, brush-like, papules on nonmucosal skin. Serotypes 6 and 11 are most

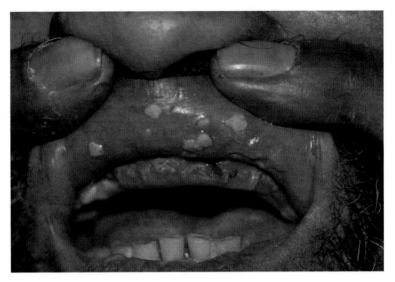

Fig. 9 Oral warts in an HIV-infected Hispanic man

commonly associated with genital warts. Other serotypes, such as 16 and 18 are well known for their oncogenic potential in cervical cancer. Common warts may have visible black specks that represent superficial, thrombosed capillaries, which may bleed with paring. Flat warts are flat-topped papules that are usually under 5 mm in diameter. Autoinnoculation is common in areas where people commonly shave such as the face, genitals, and legs. Warts on the genital, perianal, and oral areas, condyloma accuminata, may be white, brown, pink macerated papules or confluent plaques. They may or may not be clinically verrucous. Oral warts (Fig. 9) are uncommon outside of HIV infection. Given the similar clinical appearance of the condyloma lata, it is important to rule out syphilis when considering a diagnosis of oral or genital warts. This can be done with either serologies or skin biopsy.

HPV is ubiquitous. Warts are difficult to treat, even in immunocompetent individuals. Although warts tend to thrive in the setting of depressed immunity, they may not improve with immune reconstitution. In fact, warts tend to be seen early in HIV infection with no increased incidence with disease progression.[21]

In the anogenital area, nail, and oral cavity, HPV is commonly associated with squamous cell carcinoma (SCC) in patients with HIV infection.[22] There should be a low threshold for tissue biopsy of lesions in these areas.

Mollusca Contagiosa

Mollusca contagiosa is caused by cutaneous infection with a pox virus. Much like the HPV, the molluscum virus infects the skin inducing the growth of the

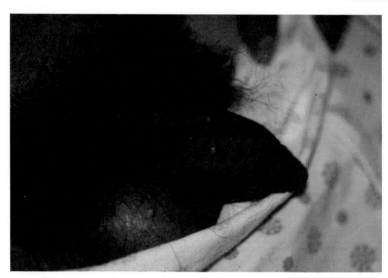

Fig. 10 Mollusca contagiosa on the genitals

characteristic umbilicated papules. Transmission is usually secondary to wet skin-to-skin contact. This highly contagious opportunistic infection is common in healthy children. In adults molluscum infection is typically the result of sexual transmission (Fig. 10).

Even in the immunocompetent, treatment can be challenging. Most modalities are destructive (cryosurgery, electrodessication, curettage, chemodestruction) and often painful and scarring. Liquid nitrogen therapy (cryosurgery) should be used with caution in patients with dark skin as it can be toxic to melanocytes resulting in permanent depigmentation. Use of the immune response modifier, imiquimod, may be a helpful adjunctive therapy as may be the chemotherapeutic agent 5-fluorouracil.

In the pre-HAART era, molluscum infection was the scourge of the dermatology clinic. HIV-infected patients were often disfigured with dozens, if not hundreds, of lesions that responded poorly to painful treatment. Fortunately, immune reconstitution is very effective in clearing this infection.

Diagnosis of molluscum contagiosum lesions is usually clinical. Diagnostic aids include KOH prep on which molluscum bodies may be visualized. In HIV infection, it is important to consider the differential diagnosis of umbilicated lesions (Table 3) particularly in patients who present with systemic symptoms. The presentation of deep fungal infection, such as that caused by *Cryptococcus* and *Penicillium marnefii*, may include molluscum-like cutaneous lesions. Verrucous or giant lesions (>1 cm) may also occur in the setting of HIV infection.

Herpes Simplex Infection

Classic herpes simplex virus infection presents as grouped vesicles on the oral mucosa (usually associated with HISV-1) and on the anogenital area (associated with HSV-2). In recent years, increased oral-genital sexual practice has resulted in more genital infection with HSV-1. Herpes simplex virus coinfection in HIV can have a number of atypical clinical presentations including verrucous lesions, chronic lesions, and paronychia (paronychia in HIV should be cultured for HSV-2). Foscarnet-resistant HSV is also more common in HIV. Diagnosis can be established through either Tzanck smear, viral culture, or direct fluorescent antibody stain (DFA). Skin biopsy can suggest a diagnosis of herpes simplex and rule in an alternative cause, such as syphilis; however, like the Tzanck smear, it will not establish herpes simplex type. It is important to culture ulcers for other types of infection.

In addition to its own altered clinical presentation, HSV also appears to affect the transmission and progression of HIV disease. In 1993, Hook et al. reported that HSV-2 (but not HSV-1) infection was an independent risk factor for HIV infection.[23] It is no surprise that HSV-2, a genital ulcer disease, is more common in HIV-positive people. In a study of pregnant women delivering at a Seattle hospital, 75% of the HIV-infected mothers versus 32% of the controls were found to be seropositive for HSV-2.[24] Active HSV-2 has been shown to cause an increase in HIV-1 RNA viral load.[25] Both genital and plasma levels of HIV-1 RNA have been shown to decrease when women were treated with valacyclovir.[26]

Race and poverty are independent risk factors for herpes simplex infection (HSV). The 1999–2002 NHANES data of the HSV-1 seroprevalence in children of age 6–13 years showed the rates for non-Hispanic white, black, and Mexican American children to be 24.7, 47.8, and 42.1, respectively.[27] The rates were 51.8% for children below poverty level and only 24.0% for children at or above poverty level.[27] McQuillan et al. reported in 2004 that the increased prevalence in HSV-2 in non-Hispanic blacks and Mexican Americans was not changed when controlled for high- and low-risk populations.[28] Given the greater burden of HSV infection in ethnic minority populations, regardless of risk factors, and the impact of HSV on both transmission and progression of HIV disease, prevention strategies aimed at minority groups regardless of risk status may play a greater role in reducing the disease burden in both cases.

Herpes Zoster Infection

Herpes Zoster is a viral infection, which represents recrudescence of latent infection with Varicella Zoster virus (VZV). Primary infection ("chicken pox") is characterized by a centrifugal vesicular eruption, lesions being described as "dew drops on a rose petal." Pruritus is a common symptom. The infection resolves in 3 weeks, at which time the virus rests in the dorsal root ganglia. With recrudescence the virus travels down the nerve resulting in pain and the eruption of lesions in a dermatomal pattern.

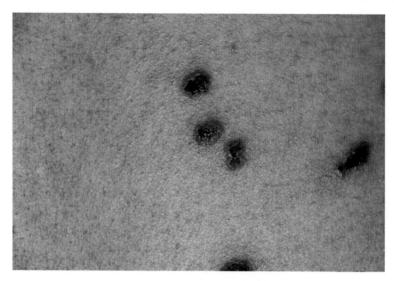

Fig. 11 Verrucous zoster lesions on the back of a HIV-positive Hispanic man

The primary lesion of herpes zoster is a vesicle; however, in HIV-infected people, the lesions may be more chronic and become verrucous or crusted (Fig. 11). It is thought that the cause of these lesions is an altered pattern of VZV gene expression, specifically diminished gE or gB expression.[29] Blacks have been documented to have a later onset of primary varicella infection and a lower risk of developing zoster in general when compared with whites.[30] Although there is an increased incidence of Zoster with HAART initiation, this diagnosis is excluded as part of the defining criteria of immune reconstitution syndrome (IRS) because rates of zoster remain constant irrespective of the host's ability to mount an immune response.[31] Herpes zoster may be recurrent and followed by postherpetic neuralgia, even in young patients.

Infestations

Scabies (Crusted Scabies)

Scabies, also described as the "7-year itch," is an infestation by the female mite *Sarcoptes scabei* var *hominis*. Although there are different animal species of scabies, cross-species infestation usually does not occur.[32] Transmission most commonly occurs as a result of prolonged, direct skin-to-skin contact, such as sharing a bed. Infestation results in generalized pruritus and a variety of clinical lesions including papules, scale, erythema, and burrows, which are typically found in the body folds. The number of mites present, typically 12, is small given the extent of anatomic involvement. Mites tend to burrow in specific areas, such as the web spaces, axilla,

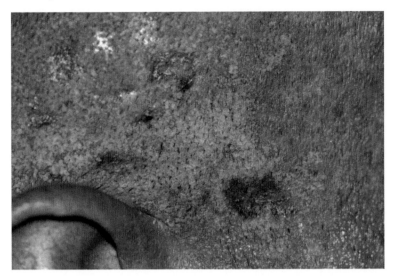

Fig. 12 "Sand on egg white" scale of crusted scabies on the scalp of patient with AIDS

genitals, and folds. The general dermatologic symptoms represent a hypersensitivity reaction to the mite and its byproducts.

Crusted or Norwegian scabies is a condition in which the patient is infested with thousands of mites, much like sarcoptic mange in animals. It is associated with declining immune status, especially HIV, and neurological disorders. A type of scale that develops on the skin in crusted scabies has been described as "sand on egg white" (Fig. 12). Diagnosis is much easier than in a conventional infestation as parasites, eggs, and feces are easily visualized on KOH preparation. Given the greatly increased number of mites, a patient with crusted scabies is much more contagious.

The differential diagnosis of crusted scabies includes seborrheic dermatitis, psoriasis, and eczema. The identification of "pruritic penile papules" in males should greatly increase confidence in a diagnosis of scabies.

Inflammatory

Xerosis

Xerosis (dry skin) is a diagnosis of exclusion in which the skin feels and appears scaly. It is distinguished from ichthyosis in that the scales tend to be finer. Xerosis can be a primary problem, a sign of an underlying condition such as atopic dermatitis, HIV, thyroid, or renal disease, or the side effect of a drug. People with darker skin may be more concerned about this condition because the light skin scales are more prominent against their darker skin. Cosmetic issues aside, xerosis is not a petty concern. The skin is one of our largest organs. It functions as a barrier between us and the outside world. Xerosis results in a compromise in the skin's barrier function and can result in a number of problems. Dry skin is the most common cause of itch, especially in the winter months. Dry cold outside, dry heat inside, and a tendency to want to take long, hot showers or baths to cut the chill contribute to the problem. Xerosis can progress to eczema (Figs. 13 and 14), which can become

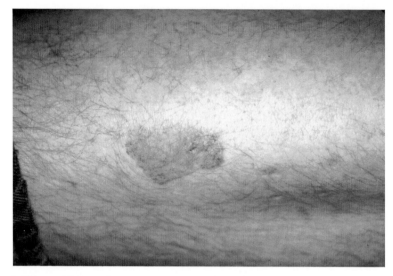

Fig. 13 This pruritic plaque of nummular eczema had been present on this HIV-positive patient's leg for over 3 months

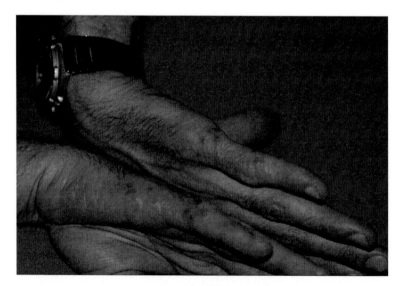

Fig. 14 Dyshidrotic eczema on the hands of an HIV-positive man

superinfected with bacteria from scratching. Xerosis should be managed with a regimen of gentle skin care as follows: Minimize bathing or showering; once a day is adequate. If a second cleaning is required (e.g., after exercise) consider just rinsing off the sweat. Use a gentle, soapless cleanser. Most people do not have dirty jobs that require use of soap over their whole bodies. Use of cleanser on the hairy areas of the body daily (e.g., armpits, groin, buttocks) is usually adequate. Bathing should be followed by an application of a moisturizer. Petroleum jelly is popular among African Americans and it does provide an excellent barrier. However, it should be applied to wet skin only, because when it is applied to dry skin it seals water out.

Seborrheic Dermatitis

Seborrheic dermatitis (SD) is a chronic, inflammatory skin condition characterized by erythema and greasy scaling on the scalp, glabella, ears, alar creases, and melolabial folds. Other areas sometimes affected include the bearded areas in men, the upper chest and back (particularly on hairy individuals), axilla, and groin. Patients may refer to it scalp involvement as "dry scalp." Rather than merely dry, however, the area is scaly and inflamed. Affected areas may itch or burn. In people with dark skin SD may present as hyperpigmented (dark) or hypopigmented (light) areas.

Although the cause of SD is unclear, it is thought to be a hypersensitivity reaction to normal yeast on the skin. Malassezia species (Pityrosprum) is a yeast that is an inhabitant of normal skin usually found on the scalp, face, neck, chest, and back, which are rich in the fatty acids it survives on. SD tends to flare with season change and in the cold, winter months. It is one of the most common skin conditions in the HIV-infected population. SD may be more severe and treatment resistant in the setting of HIV infection.

There are a variety of effective treatments for seborrheic dermatitis. These include topical steroids, ketoconazole cream or gel, and zinc pyrothione or selenium sulfide shampoo or lotion. Sulfacetamide creams, lotions, or washes are also effective. Patients with scalp involvement should shampoo at least once in a week. Although many antidandruff shampoos are labeled to be used multiple times a week, suggesting daily shampooing to many African American patients may result in noncompliance. Curly kinky hair is more susceptible to becoming dry and brittle with too frequent washing. Many dandruff shampoos are particularly drying. Furthermore, many African Americans have hair-grooming practices that require less frequent washing to maintain. Shampooing at least once in a week should be encouraged however, as without debulking the yeast and the scale on the skin, the condition can be difficult to control.

Conditions that can be confused with seborrheic dermatitis include psoriasis, xerosis, atopic dermatitis, and crusted scabies.

Neoplastic

Kaposi's Sarcoma

Kaposi's sarcoma (KS) is a malignancy caused by the virus Human Herpes Virus 8. It was rare in the U.S. before the start of the AIDS epidemic in the 1980s. Prior to this time, KS was primarily a disease of middle-aged men of Mediterranan and Eastern European descent. Although endemic in part of Africa, KS is unusual in African Americans. In the HIV-infected population, KS is much more common among men who have sex with men. Women also have a much lower incidence of KS. It is now less prevalent in the post-HAART era.

On the skin Kaposi's sarcoma is characterized by violaceous papules, plaques, tumors, and nodules, which may present early in HIV infection. Lesions may also be verrucous. The violaceous color may be challenging for some observers to appreciate on patients with dark skin.

Disorders of Hair

Acquired Trichomegaly

Acquired trichomegaly of the eyelashes has been reported in patients with advanced HIV infection. In 1991, Kaplan et al. reported a case in which the trichomegaly reversed with successful treatment of the HIV infection.[33] A survey of 204 patients in Spain by Almagro et al. in 2003, however, found no correlation between eyelash length and CD4 count.[34]

Hair Straightening

Hair loss associated with a straightening of the hair texture has been reported in black patients with HIV infection. In 1996, Smith et al. looked at ten HIV-infected patients, eight of whom were black, who reported hair loss, straightening not associated with heat styling or chemical processing. Histology was consistent with telogen effluvium associated with inflammation, necrotic keratinocytes, and hair dystrophy.[35]

Disorders of Nails

AZT-Induced Melanonychia

AZT therapy is a well-known cause of longitudinal hyperpigmented bands of the nails. Melanonychia striata, dark longitudinal bands of the nails, are common in people with dark skin. In the setting of treatment with AZT they have also been reported in Caucasians.[36]

HIV-Associated Lipodystrophy Syndrome

Lipoatrophy of the face and peripheral areas and/or lipohypertrophy in other areas of the body can be a side effect of HAART therapy. This may be accompanied by dyslipidemias and insulin resistance (the metabolic syndrome) resulting in increased cardiovascular risk. Lipohypertrophy usually manifests as fat accumulation in the dorsocervical area, breasts, and abdominal viscera. Facial lipoatrophy, or fat loss, can be a normal part of the aging process.

HAART therapy can result in a syndrome of fat wasting, particularly on the face, resulting in a sickly, prematurely aged appearance of patients with restored immune status. Although primarily a cosmetic problem, lipoatrophy can be a cause of great psychological distress, social stigma, delayed entry into HIV treatment, and poor adherence to treatment. The result is a hollow appearance of the face, with sunken cheeks, deep melolabial folding, and wasting in the temporal area. Interestingly, central facial aging with deepening of the melolabial folds is characteristic of aging in African Americans who happen to be less frequently affected by HIV-associated lipodystrophy than whites are. Men are also affected more than women.

Peripheral lipoatrophy commonly involves the limbs and buttocks. In 2005, Dube et al. found that regimens containing nelfinavir and didanosine/stavudine resulted in greater rates of limb atrophy.[37] All but one of the 20 patients treated in a Norwegian study had been on stavudine.[38] Risk for development of this syndrome is likely multifactorial[39] as white race is an increased risk factor. On the face the wasting involves the nasolabial folds, the cheeks, and the periorbital areas.

Switching of the treatment regimen may reverse the signs and symptoms of lipodystrophy.[40,41] For example, in the SWEET Study, switching from Combivir with efavirenz to TDF/FTC with efavirenz preserved limb fat while maintaining virologic control.[41] Consistent with these findings, there is now a general consensus that NRTIs contribute the most to the development of lipoatrophy, and lipoatrophy varies substantially depending on which NRTI is used. The thymdine analogues, d4T and AZT, have been found to have the greatest association with lipoatrophy.

The explosion in cosmetic dermatology has resulted in the availability of a variety of injectable, volume replacement fillers. Both temporary (e.g., collagen, hyaluronic acid) and permanent (e.g., silicone, autologous fat) options exist. Given the hypersensitivity and infection concerns with injectable collagen, which is derived from cows, hyaluronic acid leads in popularity. Bugge et al. found that injection of Restylane SubQ, a large particle hyaluronic acid, in patients with HIV-associated lipoatrophy was safe, effective, and resulted in a statistically significant improvement in skin thickness and self-esteem; the clinical and psychological benefits lasted up to 12 months.[38] Hyaluronic acid gel dermal fillers also appear to be safe in patients with dark skin. A study presented by Taylor et al. reported no adverse reactions outside of the expected routine side effects in 150 patients treated with Fitzpatrick Skin Types IV–VI.[42] Injectable-L-poly-lactic acid (Sculptra[TM]) is an FDA-approved treatment for correction of facial lipoatrophy in people with HIV. Results may last up to 2 years. Side effects include formation of subcutaneous nodules. Although Sculptra is the FDA-approved treatment, it has the disadvantage of delayed gratification as it may require months and multiple sessions to see clinical results. It is also more technique-dependent than some of the other fillers and has a greater risk of hypersensitivity/nodule formation.

Immune Reconstitution Syndrome

IRS is an inflammatory reaction characterized by a paradoxical worsening of symptoms of a variety of conditions within days to months of initiating HAART. IRS affects a variety of organs systems and includes both infectious and noninfectious diseases. Skin conditions reported as part of IRS include Mycobacterium Avium intracellulare, Mycobacterium leprae, chronic ulcers of HSV, Zoster, HPV, mollusca contagiosa, balanitis circinata (*Chlamydia trachomatis*), and sarcoidosis.[40] Although there is an increased incidence of Zoster with HAART initiation this diagnosis is excluded as part of the defining criteria of IRS because rates of zoster remain constant irrespective of the host's ability to mount an immune response.[31]

For most dermatologic manifestations, antiretroviral therapy can be continued and the condition treated with a secondary modality.[43]

Postinflammatory Pigmentary Alteration

Deeply pigmented skin characteristically responds with a change in the degree of pigmentation in response to trauma. People of color may primarily complain of hyperpigmentation (most common), or even hypo- and depigmentation when affected by conditions such as acne vulgaris,[44] eczema, or dermatophytosis. It is important to encourage the patient to treat the underlying condition in addition to addressing the discoloration. In many cases, the pigmentary alteration will resolve once the primary problem has resolved. This, however, may take many months to years. Sun protection and the use of hydroquinone products can speed up the fading.

Patients should be cautioned not to abuse hydroquinone as chronic use can result in permanent skin darkening and thickening, a condition called ochronosis.

Summary

The vast majority of people with HIV/AIDS will require some type of dermatological care. Identifying and managing the dermatologic manifestations of HIV infection has evolved with the changing nature and demographics of the epidemic. Populations of color have different risk factors and comorbidities, which may impact the type and diagnosis of skin, hair, or nail pathology seen.

References

1. Valle SL. Dermatologic findings related to human immunodeficiency virus infection in high-risk individuals. J Am Acad Dermatol. 1987 Dec; 17(6): 951–61.
2. McGrath E, Evans A, Masenga J, Fuller C. Skin diagnoses prompting serological testing for HIV: an 8-year retrospective analysis of HIV testing in a regional dermatology centre, Tanzania. J Am Acad Dermatol. 2005 Mar; 52: 107.
3. MMWR December 18, 1992/41(RR-17) 1993 Revised classification system for HIV infection and expanded surveillance case definition for AIDS among adolescents and adults.
4. Wong D and Shumack S. HIV and skin disease. MJA 1996; 164: 352.
5. Zancanaro PCQ, McGirt LY, Mamelak AJ, Nguyen RHN, Martins C. Cutaneous manifestations of HIV in the ear of highly active antiretroviral therapy: An institutional urban clinic experience. J Am Acad Dermatol. 2006; 54: 581–8.
6. HIV Infection in the United States Household Population Aged 18–49 Years: Results from 1999–2006. hppt://cdc.gov/NCHS/data/databriefs/db04.htm. (Accessed April 13, 2008)
7. Mirmirani P, Hessol NA, Mauer TA, Berger TG, Nguyen P, Khalsa A, Gurtman A, Micci S, Young M, Holman S, Gange SJ, Greenblatt R. Prevalence and predictors of skin disease in the Women's Interagency HIV Study (WIHS). J Am Acad Dermatol. 2001; 44: 785–8.
8. Barton JC, Buchness MR. Nongenital dermatologic diseases in HIV-infected women. J Am Acad Dermatol. 1999; 40: 938–948.
9. Elston D. Community-acquired methicillin-resistant *Staphylococcus areus*. J Am Acad Dermatol. 2007; 56: 1–16.
10. Nguyen MH, Kauffman CA, Goodman RP, Squier C, Arbeit RD, Singh N, Wagener MM, Yu VL. Nasal carriage of and infection with Staphylococcus aureus in HIV-infected patients annals of internal medicine. Ann Int Med. 1999 Feb; 130(3): 221–225.
11. Miller M, Cespedes C, Vavagiakis P, Klein RS, Lowy FD. *Staphylococcus aureus* colonization in a community sample of HIV-infected and HIV-uninfected drug users. Staphylococcus aureus colonization in a community sample of HIV-infected and HIV-uninfected drug users. Eur J Clin Microbiol. Infect Dis. 2003 Aug; 22(8): 463–9. Epub 2003 Jul 18.
12. Crum-Cianflone NF, Burgi AA, Hale BR. Increasing rates of community-acquired methicillin-resistant *Staphylococcus aureus* infections among HIV-infected persons. Int J STD AIDS. 2007 Aug; 18(8): 521–6.
13. Nelson M, Schiavone M. Emtricitabine (FTC) for the treatment of HIV infection. Int J Clinic Pract. 2004 May; 58(5): 504–10.
14. Bari MM et al. Ulcerative syphilis in acquired immunodeficiency syndrome: a case of precocious tertiary syphilis in a patient infected with human immunodeficiency virus. J Am Acad Dermatol. 1989; 21(6): 1310.

15. Gutierrez-Galhardho MC, do Valle GF, de Silva FC, Schumbach AO, do Valle ACF. Clinical characteristics and evolution of syphilis in 24 HIV + individuals in Rio de Janeiro, Brazil. Rev Inst Med Trop S Paulo. 2005 May–Jun; 47(3): 153–157.
16. Cherneskie T. Update and Review of the Diagnosis and Management of Syphilis, Region II STD/HIV Prevention Training Center; New York City Department of Health and Mental Hygiene, New York: 2006.
17. Johnson, RA. Dermatophyte infection in human immune deficiency virus (HIV) disease. J Am Acad Dermatol. 2000 Nov; 43: S135–42.
18. Silverberg N, Weinberg J, DeLeo V. Tinea capitis: Focus on African American women. J Am Acad Dermatol. 2002; 46(2): S120–S124.
19. Kinloch-de Loës S, de Saussure P, Saurat JH, Stalder H, Hirschel B, Perrin LH. Symptomatic primary infection due to human immunodeficiency virus type 1: review of 31 cases. Clin Infect Dis – 01-JUL-1993; 17(1): 59–65.
20. MacNeil RJ, Dinulos JGH. Acute retroviral syndrome. Dermatol Clin. 2006 Oct; 24(4): 431–8.
21. Smith KJ, Skelton HG, Yeager J, Ledsky R, McCarthy W, Baxter D, et al. Cutaneous findings in HIV-1-positive patients: a 42 month prospective study. Military Medical Consortium for he Advancement of Retroviral Research (MMCARR). J Am Acad Dermatol. Nov 1994; 31(5 pt 1): 746–54.
22. Wilkins K, Turner R, Doley J, LeBoit P, Berger T, Maurer T. Cutaneous malignancy and human immunodeficiency virus disease. J Am Acad Dermatol. 2006; 54(2): 189–206.
23. Hook EW III, Cannon RO, Nahmias AJ, Lee FF, Campbell CH Jr, glasser D, Quinn TC. Herpes simplex virus infection as a risk factor for human immunodeficiency virus infection in heterosexual. J Infect Dis. 1992 Feb; 165(2): 251–5.
24. Hitti J, Watts DH, Burchett SK, Schacker T, Selke S, Brown ZA, Lawrence C. Herpes simplex virus seropositivity and reactivation at delivery among pregnant women infected with human immunodeficiency virus-1. Am J Obstet Gynecol. 1997 Aug; 177(2): 450–4.
25. Reynolds SJ. Developments in STD/HIV Interactions: The Intertwining Epidemics of HIV and HSV-2. Infect Dis Clin North Am. Jun 2005; 19(2): 415–25.
26. Wilkinson E. Herpes treatment may limit HIV transmission and progression. Lancet Infect Dis. Apr 2007; 7(4): 249.
27. Xu F, Lee FK, Marrow RA, Sternberg MR, Luther KE, Dubin G, Markowitz LE. Seroprevalence of Herpes Simplex Virus Type 1 in children in the United States. J Pediatr. 2007 Oct; 151(40): 374–7.
28. McQuillan GM, Kruszon-Moran D, Kottiri BJ, Curtin LR, Lucas JW, Kington RS. Racial and ethnic differences in the seroprevalence of 6 infectious diseases in the United States: Data from NHANES III, 1988–1994. Am J Public Health. 2004 Nov; 94(11): 1952–1958.
29. Nikkels AF, Rentier B, Pierard GE. Chronic varicella-zoster virus skin lesions in patients with human immunodeficiency virus are related to decreased expression of gE and gB. J Infect Dis. 1997 Jul; 176(1): 261–4.
30. Schmader K, George LK, Burchett BM, Hamilton JD, Pieper CF. Race and stress in the incidence of herpes zoster in older adults J Am Geriatr Soc.1998 Aug; 46(8): 973–7.
31. Robertson J, Meier M, Wall J, Ying J, Fichtenbaum CJ. Immune reconstitution syndrome in HIV: Validating a case definition and identifying clinical predictors in persons initiating antiretroviral therapy. Clin Infect Dis. 2006; 42: 1639–1646.
32. Mellanby K. Scabies. 2nd ed. Hampton, Middlesex, UK: E.W. Ltd; 1972: 1–81.
33. Kaplan MH, Sadick NS, Talmor M. Acquired trichomegaly of the eyelashes: a cutaneous marker of acquired immunodeficiency syndrome. J Am Acad Dermatol. 1991 Nov; 25 (5 pt 1): 801–4.
34. Almagro M, del Pozo J, Garcia-Silva J, Martinez W, Castro A, Fonseca E. Eyelash length in HIV-infected patients. AIDS. 2003 Jul 25; 17(11): 1695–6.
35. Smith KJ, Skelton HG, DeRusso D, Sperling L, Yeager J, Wagner KF, Angritt P. Clinical and histopathologic features of hair loss in patients with HIV-1 infection. J Am Acad Dermatol. 1996 Jan; 34(1): 63–8.
36. Tosti A, Gaddoni G, Fanti PA, D'Antuono A, Albertini F. Longitudinal melanonychia induced by 3′-azidodeoxythymidine. Report of 9 cases. Dermatologica. 1990; 180(4): 217–20.

37. Dube M, Parker R, Tebas P, Grinspoon S, Zackin R, Robbins G, Roubenoff R, Shafer R, Wininger D, Meyer W, Snyder S, Mulligan K. Glucose metabolism, lipid, and body fat changes in antiretroviral-naïve subjects randomized to nelfinavir or efavirenz plus dual nucleosides. AIDS. 19(16): 1807–1818, November 4, 2005.
38. Bugge H, Negaard A, Skeie L, Bergersen B. Hyaluronic acid Treatment of facial fat atrophy in HIV-positive Patients. HIV Med. 2007; 8(8): 475–482.
39. Balasubramanyam A. "HIV-associated lipodystrophy syndrome: an accelerated form of the metabolic syndrome of insulin resistance due to altered fat distribution". Research Initiative/Treatment Action!. Fall 2006. Find Articles.com. 24 May, 2008.
40. Lafeuillade A, Clumeck N, Mallolas J, Jaeger H, Livrozet J-M, Ferreira M, Johnson M, Cheret A, Antoun Z. Comparison of metabolic abnormalities and clinical lipodystrophy 48 weeks after switching from HAART to Trizivir TM versus continued HAART: The Trizal study. HIV Clin Trials. 2003; 4(1): 37–43.
41. Fisher AM, Moyle G, Ebrahimi R, and others (SWEET Study Group). Switching from Combivir (CBV, AZT/3TC) to Truvada (TVD, TDF/FTC) Maintains Viral Suppression, Prevents and Reverses Limb Fat Loss, and Improves Biochemical Parameters: Results of a 48 Week Randomised Study. 11th European AIDS Conference (EACS). Madrid, Spain. October 24–27, 2007. Abstract PS5/7.
42. Taylor SC, Callendar VD, Burgess CM. Assessment of Adverse Experiences, keloid formation, and pigmentary changes in subjects with Fitzpatrick skin types IV, V or VI injected with hyaluronic acid gel dermal fillers. Presented November 11, 2007 at the LOreal 4th International Symposium, Ethnic Hair & Skin: Defining the Research Agenda in Miami, Fl.
43. Hirsch H, Kaufmann G, Sendi P, Battegay M. Immune reconstitution in HIV-infected patients. Clini Infect Dis. 2004; 38: 1159–1166.
44. Taylor SC, Cook-Bolden F, Rahman Z, Strachan D. Acne vulgaris in skin of color. J Am Acad Dermatol. 2002 Feb; 46(2): S98–S106.

Comorbidities in Black Patients with HIV/AIDS

M. Keith Rawlings and Oluwatoyin Adeyemi

Chronic diseases account for three-quarters of the U.S. health care expenditures and a majority of early deaths and loss of productive years of life. Health disparities exist among the common chronic diseases, such as hypertension, diabetes mellitus, HIV/AIDS, cardiovascular disease, renal disease, and obesity, with ethnic minorities and the poor having higher incidence or worse outcomes.[1]

Hepatitis C in Minorities: Focus on African Americans

Chronic hepatitis C virus (HCV) infection affects up to 170 million people worldwide, and in the U.S. it is estimated that 3.9 million individuals have a positive HCV antibody test. Approximately 60–85% and 10–15% of patients develop chronic infection and cirrhosis of the liver, respectively.[2,3] These patients are at risk of hepatic failure and hepatocellular carcinoma (HCC) (up to 3% per year once cirrhosis is present), and in the U.S. and many parts of the world chronic HCV infection is a leading cause of liver transplantation. Annually, at least 8,000–12,000 deaths are attributed to complications from chronic HCV infection.

In the U.S. and Europe, up to 30% of the 900,000 HIV-infected people are also infected with HCV. The rate of coinfection is as high as 90% among people who contracted HIV infection through injection drug use (IDU).[4–6] With the advent of highly active antiretroviral therapy (HAART) and improved survival in HIV-infected patients, HCV-related end-stage liver disease (ESLD) has become a significant cause of morbidity and mortality in coinfected patients. In many published series, HCV-related deaths are increasing in HIV-infected patients in the era of HAART.[7–9]

The advances in the last decade in the understanding of hepatitis C virus (HCV) infection have led to significant improvements in treatment responses. However, it

O. Adeyemi (✉)
Cook County Hospital and Rush University medical College, Chicago, IL, U.S.
E-mail: oluwatoyin_adeyemi@rush.edu

V. Stone et al. (eds.), *HIV/AIDS in U.S. Communities of Color*.
DOI: 10.1007/978-0-387-98152-9_9, © Springer Science + Business Media, LLC 2009

is now known that HCV behaves differently in African Americans, even though African Americans were underrepresented in many of the initial treatment trials. It is important to note that there are even fewer studies in HIV-coinfected patients, so most of the information is extrapolated from HIV-negative populations.

Natural History of Hepatitis C Infection

There are disparities in the prevalence of hepatitis C in the U.S. HCV infection is more prevalent in the African American population than in any other racial group. The mode of transmission of HCV appears to be similar for white and black African American individuals, and IDU has been identified as the primary transmission route among both whites and African Americans in many series. A report using the NHANES III survey data estimated that 1.8% (3.9 million) of the US population had a positive HCV antibody test but found that this rate was higher in blacks than in whites (3.2% vs. 1.5%). The study also found that 74% of these people had chronic infection, and the rate of viremia was higher in blacks than in whites (86% vs. 68%). Black men had higher rates of infection, with the highest prevalence rate (9.8%) observed among black males of age 40–49 years.[10]

African Americans represent only 12% of the US population, yet account for 22% of those with chronic HCV infection.[11] Although 70% of overall HCV isolates in the U.S. are of genotype 1, there is a difference among racial groups with a higher prevalence of genotype 1 among African Americans than among any other racial group.[12–14] The explanation for this disparity is currently unknown. Despite the higher prevalence, natural history data has suggested a more favorable outcome for African Americans. HCV RNA levels were similar, but liver enzymes (ALT) were lower in African Americans. African Americans had less inflammation and fibrosis in their liver biopsies, and there was a trend toward less cirrhosis than non-blacks (22% vs. 30%). In another study the results were similar with African Americans having lower ALT levels and more genotype 1 virus (94% vs. 67%). In this study also, African Americans had less necrosis and lower fibrosis scores independent of age and ALT compared with Caucasians.[15]

Although fibrosis may evolve more slowly in African Americans, the rate of HCC is increasing more quickly in this population. The rates of HCC and liver cancer-related mortality are 2–3 times higher among African American persons than among white persons.[16, 17]

HIV–HCV Coinfection

There are no data on the natural history of HCV disease in HIV-coinfected patients stratified by ethnicity, but it is reasonable to extrapolate from the data in HIV-negative patients. HCV-associated liver damage appears to be more likely to develop in HIV/HCV-coinfected people than in those with HCV infection only. Coinfected people with <200 CD4 cells/mL are at greatest risk for ESLD. One study evaluated paired liver biopsies from 61 coinfected patients and found that liver disease progressed by two stages or more in 28% (17 of 61 participants) over an interval of less than 3 years.[18] A similar study in people with HCV mono infection reported that only 11% (23 of 210 participants) progressed by two stages or more in a similar time period (median of 2.5 years). A meta-analysis of eight studies reported that coinfected patients were twice more likely to develop cirrhosis than patients with HCV alone and had a sixfold greater risk for hepatic decompensation.[11] In the HIV-infected population, recent data have shown that compared with the HIV-negative population fewer patients are listed for orthotopic liver transplantation (OLT) and more die while waiting for OLT.[19] In addition, HIV–HCV-coinfected patients are more likely to develop HCC at a younger age.[20]

The mechanism for the possible discrepancies in the natural history of hepatitis C is unknown; however, the answer may lie in disparate HCV-specific CD4 T cell responses between African Americans and Caucasians. Various aberrations in the immune response and differences in the HLA alleles are also present in African Americans as in Caucasians. The strength and sustenance of HCV-specific T-cell responses have been identified as critical determinants of viral clearance during acute HCV infection, which requires a potent IFN-g response. In African American patients, HCV-specific CD4 T-cell proliferative responses were not accompanied by IFN-g production, suggesting a dysregulated, virus-specific T-cell function in cases of chronic infection in this population.[21,22] Other mechanisms invoked to explain the disparities in the natural history among different races include the stronger association of certain human leukocyte antigen class II alleles with HCV clearance and the lack of immune system recognition of the virus in African Americans.[23] In a recent study, variants of the immunomodulatory *IL-10* and *IL-19/20* genes seemed to play a role in the spontaneous clearance of HCV in African American patients; no such relationship was found in white patients.[24]

Eligibility for Treatment

The first studies showing limitations of eligibility and barriers to treatment were published in 2002 and 2003. One from the Cleveland Clinic reported that only 28% of 327 HCV-positive patients referred were eligible for treatment.[25] Similarly in a study from Boston only 30% of coinfected patients were deemed eligible for treatment.[26] In both studies, the top reasons for ineligibility were nonadherence with evaluation follow-up, psychiatric issues, active substance abuse, and comorbidities. In a study comparing HCV-monoinfected patients to HIV-coinfected patients, there was no difference in treatment eligibility by HIV-coinfection status.[27] In this referral cohort of mostly ethnic minorities (75% of the 131 HIV–HCV-coinfected patients were African American), only 33% of the patients were eligible for treatment and reasons for nontreatment were similar to those previously mentioned. Interestingly, HIV-coinfected patients were less likely to be lost to follow-up during treatment evaluation. Patients with well-controlled HIV, who understand the need for adherence and follow-up, may actually be better treatment candidates compared with HIV-negative persons. It is important to note that in all the studies discussed earlier, not all eligible patients received treatment and in some cases patients refuses to initiate treatment even when deemed eligible.

In the Veterans Administration (VA) system, two large studies on HCV treatment were both published in 2006. Findings of one study analyzing over 120,000 HCV-positive veterans (of whom 6,500 were HIV-positive) found that independent predictors of nontreatment for HCV were older age, being African American, or being HIV-positive. Only 7% of the coinfected patients were treated and among coinfected patients, non-white ethnicity remained an independent predictor of nontreatment.[28] In the other study that compared coinfected patients who received HCV treatment to those who did not, investigators found that independent predictors of starting treatment included being white and having well-controlled HIV as determined by use of HAART, higher CD4 counts, and undetectable HIV viral loads.[29]

Even in the absence of HCV treatment, the importance of adequate control of HIV infection by HAART cannot be overstated. A recently published large retrospective analysis showed that HIV–HCV-coinfected patients with undetectable HIV RNA as a result of HAART had slower fibrosis progression rate (FPR) than those with detectable virus and a FPR similar to HCV-monoinfected patients. Factors independently correlated to FPR in the coinfected patients were HIV RNA level, necroinflammation on biopsy, and age at HCV infection.[30]

Treatment and Outcomes

The ultimate goal of treatment is to prevent complications of HCV infection such as decompensated cirrhosis, HCC, liver transplantation, and death. This is primarily achieved by eradication of infection. Accordingly, treatment responses are frequently characterized by the results of HCV RNA testing. Infection is considered eradicated when there is a *sustained virologic response* (SVR), defined as the absence of HCV RNA in serum by a sensitive test at the end of treatment and 6 months later. Persons who achieve an SVR almost always have a dramatic earlier reduction in the HCV RNA level defined in some studies as a 2-log drop or loss of HCV RNA 12 weeks into therapy, referred to as an *early virologic response* (EVR). Continued absence of detectable virus at termination of treatment is referred to as *end of treatment response* (ETR). A patient is considered to have relapsed when HCV RNA becomes undetectable on treatment but is detected again after discontinuation of treatment. Persons in whom HCV RNA levels remain stable on treatment are considered *nonresponders*, while those whose HCV RNA levels decline (e.g., by 2 logs) but never become undetectable are referred to as *partial responders*. Improvement in liver histology, including improvement in fibrosis, has been observed in patients receiving interferon or pegylated interferon (peg interferon) in combination with ribavirin, particularly in those with an SVR to therapy.

Although the improvements in response rates with current therapeutic regimens have been encouraging, reports have also emerged during the last several years that the response rate is lower in African Americans. African American subjects represent only 5–10% of participants in clinical trials involving HCV infection. As a group, African Americans respond less well to interferon therapy than persons of other races. In an early study of patients treated with unmodified interferon alfa-2b and interferon alfacon-1 (also known as consensus interferon), it was found that only 1 of 40 black patients (2%) had a SVR.[31] One study challenged these findings and reported the experience of treatment with unmodified interferon alfa-2b and ribavirin. In this analysis the overall response rate was lower among black patients, at 11%. However, a higher observed they also proportion of genotype 1 infection in the black patients (genotype 1 is known to be less responsive to treatment). In the subset analysis of genotype 1 patients who received unmodified interferon alfa-2b and ribavirin, the SVR rates were similar: 22% and 23% for whites and blacks, respectively. These data suggested that genotype and not race was the critical predictor of a response.[32] Several other reports then followed with similarly dismal response rates.[33–35] In the registration trials of treatment with pegylated IFN and ribavirin, too few African American subjects were enrolled to make outcome assessments.[36–39]

More recently three controlled clinical trials have examined the effect of pegylated IFN treatment in a large number of African Americans. These trials have clearly documented that the SVR rate in African Americans with genotype 1 is approximately 40–50% lower than that observed in Caucasians. The first trial compared a group of 100 African American patients with a control group of 100 non-Hispanic white patients, both of which were treated with pegylated IFN and ribavirin for 48 weeks. Both groups were equally matched with regard to age, HCV viral load, genotype, and other attributes. Treatment was well tolerated in both groups; 81% of African Americans and 79% of white patients completed therapy. Rates of adherence to treatment and of adverse events were also similar in both groups, and depression was the most common reason for discontinuation of therapy, regardless of ethnicity. Compared with non-Hispanic white subjects, African American subjects had substantially poorer rates of SVR (19% vs. 52%) The only predictor of SVR in multivariate analysis was race. Also analyzed was the predictive value of an EVR, defined as a ≥ 2 $\log_{10}$ reduction in HCV RNA level at week 12 of therapy. None of the subjects who failed to achieve an EVR at week 12 reached a SVR, irrespective of ethnicity. Thus, the negative predictive value of EVR was 100%. This was the first time the EVR was validated in African Americans.[40]

The second study enrolled 78 African American subjects and 28 white subjects who were infected with HCV genotype 1 and were HCV treatment-naive. All subjects received pegylated IFN and ribavirin for 48 weeks. Rates of adverse events were higher among white patients. Thirty-nine percent of white subjects discontinued therapy, compared with 23% of African American subjects. At week 72, in the African American group, the rate of SVR was 26%, significantly lower than the

39% rate for the white group. Interestingly, of the 36 African American patients who did not achieve SVR and who underwent both liver biopsies, 22% achieved fibrosis improvement. These data may support the concept that some patients may achieve reversal in fibrosis, irrespective of whether they achieve a SVR.[41] These two studies clearly show that after controlling for many variables and with similar or even better adherence rates in African Americans, response rates among African Americans with HCV are still much lower.

To further explore the differences in response, the National Institute of Diabetes and Digestive and Kidney Diseases (NIDDK) launched the VIRAHEP-C Study (Viral Resistance to Antiviral Therapy of Chronic Hepatitis C). This study was conducted at eight medical centers in the U.S. and was designed to examine the treatment responses of African Americans, along with the immune response, virologic kinetics, and genetic factors to better understand the reason for any disparity in treatment. In this multicenter study, 196 African American and 205 Caucasian patients with HCV genotype 1 were treated with pegylated IFN and ribavirin. The SVR rate was much lower in African Americans (28% vs. 52%), and differences in response by ethnicity were clear early in the treatment course. Relapse rates, rates of treatment discontinuations, modifications, and side effects were similar in both groups.[42]

Another important study conducted recently was the WIN-R trial. Findings from the weight-based dosing of Peg-Intron and Rebetrol (WIN-R) trial demonstrate that weight-based dosing of ribavirin confers a significant advantage in the treatment of African American persons infected with genotype 1, compared with fixed dosing of ribavirin. Three-hundred eighty-seven genotype 1 infected African American patients were among the 5,000 patients treated. Of the 362 African American subjects who weighed $\geq$65 kg, those who received weight-based ribavirin dosing had better end-of-treatment and SVR rates than did those who received flat dosing. VR rates were more than doubled (SVR rate, 21% vs. 10%; $P = 0.004$). However, even though African American patients achieved higher response rates with weight-based doses of ribavirin, rates of SVR were still inferior to the rates for white patients.[43] Of the three large trials focusing on HCV treatment in HIV/HCV-coinfected subjects, only two enrolled a significant percentage of African American subjects. The overall SVR rates in these studies were 14–29%; however, race was not predictive for sustained response.[44–46] Many other studies have been published from centers across the world; however, African Americans remain a minority of the study population and therefore the studies are not powered to detect differences in response based on ethnicity.

A multitude of hypotheses have been promulgated to explain the dissimilar treatment responses among ethnic groups. In all these studies, the lower SVR rates observed in African Americans were due to both a decrease in the rate of virologic response and an increase in the rate of relapse. The reasons include host factors and HCV virus factors. Host factors may include a higher body-mass index in African Americans, a higher rate of dose lowering, or treatment discontinuation due to side effects. However, in studies adjusting for these factors, African Americans still had a lower SVR leading investigators to explore viral factors. Viral factors implicated include higher HCV RNA in African Americans and intrinsic interferon resistance in African Americans. It also seems that African Americans have a global defect in the ability to respond to interferon and eradicate HCV. Other possibilities include discrepant viral kinetics, cytokine production, and iron stores. An initial decrease in the HCV RNA level, referred to as "phase 1," occurs hours after the administration of IFN; it represents blocking of viral replication. The subsequent, slower decrease in the viral level (phase 2) represents the clearance of HCV-infected hepatocytes and usually occurs days to months after IFN therapy is initiated. The phase 2 decrease is the better predictor of ultimate HCV RNA clearance. Ethnicity may influence these phases. In a kinetics study that compared African American and white subjects who received combination therapy, a significant difference was found between African American and white subjects with regard to inhibition of viral production on the first day of treatment. The findings for phase 2 decrease in the viral load were also discordant; the rate of loss of infected cells was lower in African American subjects.[47] In a recent small study addressing the issue of early viral kinetics, as measured by HCV RNA, decline was slower in African Americans in both first and second phases, which may explain the lower SVR rates, but first and second phase decline was similar in both HIV-positive and -negative patients.[48]

Ethnicity-associated cytokine production may also explain dissimilar treatment responses. A study compared cytokine production in phytohemaglutinin-stimulated PBMCs obtained from infected and control participants, both African American and white. Relative to healthy white control subjects, African American subjects produced higher levels of proinflammatory(TH1) cytokines IL-2 and TNF-a and lower levels of downregulatory (TH2) cytokine IL-10.[49] Elevated hepatic iron stores have also been invoked to explain resistance to IFN-based therapy in African Americans because the response to standard IFN monotherapy may be influenced by hepatic iron content.[50–53] While the earlier hypotheses are interesting and are being explored, it is likely that the reasons for the disparity in treatment response are multifactorial.

Newer Agents for HCV Treatment

Significant research is ongoing among African Americans with HCV infection. Nevertheless, many clinicians are aware of the literature suggesting a lower response for African Americans. As more patients are identified as ineligible for treatment or as treatment nonresponders both clinicians and patients await the development of new agents. This is especially pertinent in African Americans and HIV-coinfected patients who have much lower treatment response rates. If we find that African Americans in particular respond well to one of these new therapies, this may provide even greater breakthroughs in the understanding of the pathogenesis of HCV. These new agents, specifically targeted antiviral therapies for HCV (STAT-C), are being studied in conjunction with current standard therapies and may allow shorter dosing durations or an induction-maintenance approach while improving SVR rates. While there are numerous agents in different stages of development, a few of the most promising agents include VX-950 (Telaprevir), Boceprevir, and Albuferon. Another agent that has shown promise is Nitazoxanide, an antiparasitic agent that is used commonly in the pre-HAART era for the treatment of cryptosporidiosis. These agents in addition to PegIFN and ribavirin increase SVR rates to 61–67% – a rate higher than that of standard of care.

Cardiovascular Disease in HIV-Infected Black Patients

For HIV-infected persons, the risk factors for cardiovascular disease are mostly similar to what we expect in the general population. A previous or family history of cardiovascular disease, male gender, aging, smoking, lipid abnormalities, hypertension, and diabetes are the traditional risk factors seen in all adults. Additionally, data suggest that both HIV infection and antiretroviral (ARV) therapy may also contribute to cardiovascular risk. However, the overall rate of myocardial infarction in the HIV-infected population is relatively low and is greatly overshadowed by the morbidity and mortality related to untreated HIV disease. Thus, while cardiovascular risk must be accounted for in the comprehensive treatment of individuals living with HIV, the initiation and choice of ARV therapy should be made to maximize viral suppression and reduce toxicities.

Cardiovascular disease is another of the conditions that disproportionately impacts the African American community. According to CDC data, African Americans were 30% more likely to die from heart disease, yet less likely to be diagnosed than whites.[54,55] As a group, blacks are 40% more likely to have hypertension, and 10% less likely to have it under control. This greater risk in the general population is also seen in higher rates of obesity and diabetes in black adults. The higher burden of cardiovascular risk in the black community thus raises concerns about the identification and management of these comorbid conditions in the population of blacks living with HIV/AIDS.

A recent study suggests that better cardiovascular outcomes are achieved when HIV-infected persons receive continuous ARV therapy without interruption, rather than CD4 cell count-driven interrupted therapy. The Strategies for the Management of Antiretroviral Therapy (SMART) study showed an increase in the relative hazards for clinical or silent MI, coronary artery disease requiring surgery or medication, cardiovascular death, peripheral vascular disease, or congestive heart failure in individuals who discontinue ARV compared with those who are on continuous therapy.[56] Furthermore, there does not appear to be a significant difference in pre-clinical markers of CVD in patients well controlled on HAART versus those who are not on ARV.[57] There is tremendous controversy and rapidly evolving data regarding the contribution that ARV therapy makes to cardiovascular risks and outcomes. The D:A:D Study confirmed that the cardiovascular risk factors in HIV-infected individuals consist mostly of behavioral or lipid abnormalities that are modifiable. Smoking had the highest prevalence, followed by elevated triglycerides. 203 mg/dL, HDL-C <35 mg/dL, lipodystrophy, elevated total cholesterol >239 mg/dL, hypertension,

BMI $>30\,kg/mm^2$, diabetes and previous cardiovascular disease.[1] In a separate population based cohort of causes of non-HIV related deaths among people with AIDS, cardiovascular disease was leading contributor across all racial groups.[2]

However, there have been changes in risk factors for cardiovascular disease and use of lipid-lowering drugs over time in HIV-infected individuals.[59] While there is little specific data some older studies do suggest a higher rate of atherosclerosis, cardiomegaly, and earlier age of CAD in blacks who are HIV-infected than in those who are not.[60]

Currently the assessment of cardiovascular risk in HIV-infected individuals is done using the Framingham risk score to determine 10-year risk in individuals with two or more cardiovascular risk factors.[61] However, recent studies have suggested that a more precise instrument may be needed to assess cardiovascular risk in HIV-infected individuals.[62–64] All patients should undergo metabolic assessment at the time of initiation of ARV and when switching regimens. There should be reevaluation at 3 and 6 months after initiation or switching and annually in patients on stable therapy. In addition to monitoring blood pressure and blood glucose, levels of total cholesterol, low-density lipoprotein (LDL) cholesterol, HDL cholesterol, and triglycerides should be measured. Consider oral glucose tolerance testing in patients at high risk for developing diabetes and hemoglobin A1C monitoring in those with diagnosed disease.

Present guidelines recommend treating cardiovascular disease in HIV-infected individuals in the same way as the general population is treated. Particular attention should be placed on smoking cessation, diet, exercise, treating dyslipidemia, and other concomitant conditions, which have established coronary artery risk (e.g., hypertension, diabetes).

Anemia in HIV and the Black Patients

For several years clinicians have known that anemia is associated with morbidity and mortality in individuals living with HIV. There are numerous causes of anemia including HIV disease,[65,66] infections or cancers of the bone marrow, nutritional substances such as vitamin B12 or folate,[67,68] and drug induced. Several of the medications used in the overall management of patients living with HIV have been shown to cause hemolytic anemia (e.g., dapsone and ribavirin) or marrow suppression (e.g., zidovudine, ganciclovir, trimethoprim sulfamethoxazole).

Analyses of race/ethnicity and prevalence of anemia related to HAART show that African American women and men are significantly more likely to have anemia than their white counterparts.[69] According to the Anemia Study Prevalence Group, highest prevalence of anemia was in patients with lower CD4 strata (CD4 counts

---

[1] Frlls-Moller N et al. Cardiovascular disease risk factors in HIV patients–associated with antiretroviral therapy. Results from the DAD study. *AIDS*. 2003;17:1179–1193

[2] Sackoff JE, Hanna DB, Pfeiffer MR, Torian LV. Causes of death among persons with AIDS in the era of highly active antiretroviral therapy: New York City. *Ann Intern Med*. 2006;145:397–406

<200). African American women had a relative risk of 1.5 vs. Caucasian women, and African American men had a relative risk of 2.5 vs. Caucasian men. The relative risk was 3.6 amongst patients with CD4 count <200 and 1.6 amongst patients with CD4 counts >200.[70]

To address anemia particularly in black patients, we would suggest strategies for monitoring hemoglobin, physical functioning, and quality of life routinely, rule out and correct treatable causes of low hemoglobin or symptomatic anemia, initiate HAART therapy as warranted, use erythropoietin or other therapies in anemic patients without correctable causes, and continue therapy until symptoms resolve.[71]

Lipodystrophy in HIV-Infected Black Patients

Lipodystrophy is a clinical manifestation comprising several conditions that may occur singularly or in combination. These include lipoatrophy, lipohypertrophy, and insulin resistance. Lipoatrophy clinically has consist of fat loss in the face (buccal fat pads), extremities, buttocks, and subcutaneous abdominal fat. Lipohypertrophy may include one or more of the following: visceral abdominal fat accumulation, dorsal cervical fat pad, parotid area fat accumulation, development of lipomata, or enlargement of breasts in women.[72,73] Several studies have shown that both lipoatrophy and lipohypertropthy can regularly manifest at the same time and in the same individual.[74–77]

The clinical implications of lipoatrophy appear to differ from those of lipohypertrophy. In one study coronary heart disease (CHD) risk estimates were greater in HIV-infected patients who had lipoatrophy than in those who had either lipohypertrophy or mixed fat redistribution.[78] While CHD risk is increased in HIV-infected patients with fat redistribution, the pattern of fat distribution appears to be an important component in determining the risk.

There are several contributors to the development of HIV lipodystrophy. Studies have suggested an associated relation to individual factors such as increasing age, white race, and low body fat and disease factors such as low CD4 cell count or an AIDS diagnosis.[79,80] In addition, several studies have demonstrated a contribution of ARV medications to both lipodystrophy and insulin resistance.[81,82] Within the African American population women appear to be the group that is most impacted.

There are some differences in the management of lipoatrophy and lipohypertrophy. While clinicians regularly recommend diet and exercise for weight reduction, lowering lipids, and reducing blood pressure, there is very little controlled data evaluating how diet, exercise, or both impacts HIV-infected patients with lipodystrophy.[83] For example exercise may reduce central fat while worsening lipoatrophy. Similarly, changing of ARV agents has shown mixed results with some minimal improvement in lipoatrophy, but limited to no impact on lipids, insulin resistance, or trunk fat when switching from a thymidine analog nucleoside agent.[84] While switching between protease inhibitors has not had an effect on lipoatrophy, there have been improvements in triglyceride and total cholesterol, on change in HDL-C, and variable impact on insulin resistance.[84]

To prevent fat loss it appears that the best approach is to select nucleoside reverse transcriptase inhibitors that have lower risk for producing lipoatrophy (either initially or by switching) and treating the fat lost prior to the development of advanced HIV.[85] Some treatments, such as rosiglitazone, have not been shown to have a significant benefit on HIV lipoatrophy.[86] With regard to surgical interventions such as polylactic acid injections, autologous fat transfer, and liposuction, there are advantages and disadvantages to each.[87–89]

Obesity in HIV-Infected Black Patients

Among black adults in the US, age 20 and above, 62.9% of men and 77.2% of women are overweight or obese [defined as a body mass index (BMI) of 25.0kg/m^2 or higher]. And 27.9% of black men and 49.0% of black women are obese (defined as a BMI of 30kg/m^2 or higher). Given the high rates of obesity in the general population of black adults it is not hard to speculate that this baseline level of obesity might be a significant contributor to the metabolic abnormalities associated with HIV or its treatment described in this group of patients living with HIV disease.[90]

Obesity in HIV-infected black patients is a much more common problem than HIV-associated wasting in the era of current therapy. Women, particularly those of color, are at high risk. As patients with HIV live longer, obesity-related complications may contribute to morbidity.[91] Current treatment recommendations should include diet and exercise. Appropriate use of insulin sensitizing agents such as metformin has been shown to improve visceral fat deposition in short-term trials, and surgical options may also be considered. Resection of abdominal fat distribution may be indicated especially in those causing pain or respiratory compromise. While issues of fat redistribution (lipoatrophy, lipohypertrophy) are separate from obesity, the combination of factors should be considered in all patients. Particular attention needs to be given to assess both lipoatrophy and lipohypertrophy within the context of obesity.

Diabetes and Metabolic Syndrome in HIV-Infected Black Patients

Metabolic syndrome is a constellation of abnormalities that include elevated waist circumference, elevated triglycerides, low HDL cholesterol, hypertension, and glucose intolerance.[92,93] Up to 40% of patients treated for HIV-1 infection have abnormal glucose metabolism with evidence of insulin resistance. Obesity and hypertension are frequently seen in black patients as part of the metabolic syndrome.

Diabetes is particularly common amongst the black population. According to the Centers for Disease Control, in 2004 of the total population of age 20 and above,

7.2% of men and 6.3% of women had physician-diagnosed diabetes. Amongst non-Hispanic blacks, the prevalence was 10.3% and 12.7%, respectively. In 2002, the overall death rate from diabetes mellitus was 25.4 per 100,000. However, the death rates for blacks were 49.4 per 100,000 for males and 48.6 per 100,000 for females.

The treatment of HIV, and the disease itself, may add to the risk for the development of metabolic and glucose metabolism problems. Long-term changes in glucose metabolism may be due to both the direct effects in vitro and in vivo of the disease. The role of HIV and disease stage is not as clear, but there is evidence that increasing fasting glucose concentrations over time have been associated with classes of ARV therapy. Increased risk for diabetes, hyperglycemia, and exacerbation of preexisting diabetes have also been demonstrated, and there are clear genetic predispositions within the black community at risk for metabolic syndrome and diabetes.[94–97] Thus, black patients living with HIV should be routinely screened for diabetes.

Recommendations currently indicate that patients who develop diabetes should have standard treatment initiated including obtaining fasting glucose and lipids (including total cholesterol, HDL cholesterol, and triglycerides), perform baseline measures before starting therapy, and repeat every 2–3 months after therapy has started or to evaluate change. Fasting insulin levels are not necessarily routine at this time. However, patients should be evaluated for both body fat changes and for abnormal fasting glucose levels. In addition, patients should have urinalysis checked as standard of care.[98]

Renal Disease in HIV-Infected Black Patients

With improved survival and increasing age, HIV-infected patients are increasingly likely to experience comorbidities that affect the general population, including renal disease. There are two aspects of renal disease of individuals in the black community with HIV infection. The first are patients who develop renal disease for the more common reasons – primarily diabetes and hypertension. In addition to these common risk factors for kidney disease, HIV-infected individuals have a high prevalence of other risk factors, including hepatitis C, cigarette smoking, and IDU. Furthermore, they have exposures unique to this population, including exposure to ARVs and other medications. In those with chronic kidney disease, interventions, such as aggressive blood pressure control with the use of ACE inhibitors or angiotensin receptor antagonists where tolerated, tight blood glucose control in those with diabetes, and avoidance of potentially nephrotoxic medications, can slow progression and prevent end-stage renal disease. In one study, mathematical modeling suggested that despite the potential benefit of HAART, the prevalence of HIV+ ESRD in the U.S. is expected to rise in the future as a result of the expansion of the AIDS population among black individuals.[99] HIV-infected African Americans are at increased risk of end-stage renal disease. Nearly 1% require renal replacement therapy (RRT) annually, a rate that was similar in the HAART and pre-HAART eras. While new cases of CKD decreased, the prevalence of CKD increased in the HAART era, primarily because survival in those with HIV-associated CKD has improved.[100] Among women, race is an independent predictor of renal disease along with age, high BMI, prior AIDS defining infection and hypertension.[101]

The second form of renal disease that is found in the population of black patients living with HIV is HIV-associated nephropathy (HIVAN), which is a focal segmental glomerulosclerosis that can lead to rapid deterioration of renal function. HIVAN is the most common HIV-specific cause of chronic renal disease in patients and is the third leading cause of end stage renal disease for African Americans between the ages of 20 and 64 years of age. Amongst those who develop end stage renal disease secondary to HIV, 88.4% of them are black compared with 7.7% being white. HIVAN is believed to be caused by a direct effect of infection on renal cells by HIV with the virus actively replicating within the renal cells. In addition, a history of familial clustering of end stage renal disease among blacks with HIV disease has been demonstrated.[102–104]

HIVAN occurs almost exclusively in blacks and Hispanics in the U.S. Blacks have been shown to be 12.2 times more likely to develop HIVAN than non-African Americans. This racial discordance has been demonstrated through multiple communities in France, London, and even Switzerland.[105, 106] The incidence of HIVAN increased consistently between 1990 and 1995, peaking in that year amongst African Americans, and has remained relatively consistent for the remaining decade.[107]

Several cohort studies have shown little cumulative association of progression of renal disease related to specific ARV therapy. Progression appears more related to the degree of immune destruction, age, and years of infection.[108, 109] The impact of race can be seen in other studies. Several studies have shown a correlation between black race and proteinuria.[110, 111] It is important to remember that the causes of renal disease in HIV-infected patients are complex and often multifactorial. As a result it is often recommended that a nephrologist be consulted and kidney biopsy be considered to assess the specific etiology of CKD.[112]

When indicated, corticosteroids, angiotensin-converting enzyme inhibitors, and HAART have been used for the treatment of HIVAN. HAART, in particular, generally produces dramatic improvement in both the pathologic changes and clinical course of HIVAN. It should be noted that many HIV-positive patients who go on to present with end stage renal disease may not have a single etiology, and the clinician should be mindful to look for varying causes of renal failure. Often, this requires a renal biopsy to determine other problems that may contribute to the development of chronic kidney disease.

Summary

It is clear that there are differences in the prevalence, natural history, and treatment response rates to various comorbid diseases between African Americans and non-Hispanic whites. While there has been some ongoing research focused on African Americans, however, the reasons for these differences are not yet clear and are still being explored. HIV–HCV-coinfected patients, regardless of ethnicity are less likely to receive HCV treatment when compared with HCV-monoinfected patients and have lower treatment response rates. Diabetes and renal disease occur at high rates in blacks than in other ethnic groups and have been shown to be exacerbated by increasing age and advanced HIV disease.

HIV–HCV-coinfected patients should be evaluated for HCV treatment as soon as HIV disease is well controlled and stable. HAART should be optimized and in some cases medications may need to be replaced prior to HCV treatment (e.g., didanosine and probably zidovudine). All coinfected patients, who initiate HCV treatment, should have HCV RNA levels measured at weeks 4 and 12 and treatment should be discontinued in those who do not achieve EVR. In the subset of patients who achieve EVR but did not have a RVR, some experts recommend treating for 18 months, depending on severity of liver disease at baseline and the ability to tolerate treatment. Treatment is for 48 weeks in coinfected patients with genotypes 2 and 3 and in those with genotype 1 who achieve RVR. While there is progress in the development of new agents active against HCV, there is currently only one STAT-C drug in phase III trials and none in coinfected patients. This means that providers need to focus on counseling for abstinence from alcohol, adequate control of HIV with suppression of viremia, and optimizing current treatment options for patients with significant liver disease. Also providers who care for African American patients need to encourage them to participate in HCV treatment clinical trials once available.

Overall, the management of HIV disease is complicated by the impact of the virus on other disease states, and those conditions on HIV. It is imperative that clinicians of all specialties be aware of the impact of the disease and its treatment on other medical conditions and their management.

References

1. Crook ED, Peters M. Health disparities in chronic diseases: where the money is. Am J Med Sci. 2008 Apr;335(4):266–70
2. Alter MJ, Kruszon-Moran D, Nainan OV, et al. The prevalence of hepatitis C virus infection in the United States, 1988 through 1994. New Engl J Med 1999;341:556–62
3. National Institutes of Health Consensus Development Conference Statement Management of Hepatitis C: Hepatology 2002;36:5 suppl 1:S3–20
4. Sulkowski MS, et al. Hepatitis C virus infection as an opportunistic disease in persons infected with human immunodeficiency virus. Clin Infect Dis 2000;suppl 1:s77–84
5. Broers B, et al. Prevalence and incidence rate of HIV, hepatitis B and C among drug users on methadone maintenance treatment in Geneva between 1988 and 1995. AIDS 1998;12:2059–66
6. Sherman KE, et al. Comparison of methodologies for quantification of hepatitis C virus (HCV) RNA in patients coinfected with HCV and human immunodeficiency virus. Clin Infect Dis. 2002 Aug 15;35(4):482–7. Epub 2002 Jul 22
7. Bica I, McGovern B, Dhar R, et al. Increasing mortality due to end-stage liver disease in patients with human immunodeficiency virus infection. Clin Infect Dis. 2001 Feb 1;32(3):492–7. Epub 2001 Jan 23

8. Monga HK, Rodriguez-Barradas MC, Breaux K, et al. Hepatitis C virus infection-related morbidity and mortality among patients with human immunodeficiency virus infection. 2001 Jul 15;33(2):240–7. Epub 2001 Jun 15

9. Rosenthal E, Pialoux G, Bernard N, et al. Liver-related mortality in human-immunodeficiency-virus-infected patients between 1995 and 2003 in the French GERMIVIC Joint Study Group Network (MORTAVIC 2003 Study). J Viral Hepat 2007 Mar;14(3):183–8

10. Hobbs F, Stoops N; 2002. Available at http://www.census.gov/prod/2002pubs/censr-4.pdf

11. Pearlman BL. Hepatitis C virus infection in African Americans. Clin Infect Dis. 2006 Jan 1;42(1):82–91. Epub 2005 Nov 29. Review

12. Lau JY, Davis GL, Prescott LE, et al. Distribution of hepatitis C virus genotypes determined by line probe assay in patients with chronic hepatitis C seen at tertiary referral centers in the United States. Hepatitis Interventional Therapy Group. Ann Intern Med. 1996 May 15;124(10):868–76

13. Howell C, Jeffers L, Hoofnagle JH. Hepatitis C in African Americans: summary of a workshop. Gastroenterology. 2000 Nov;119(5):1385–96

14. Bonacini M, Groshen MD, Yu MC, Govindarajan S, Lindsay KL. Chronic hepatitis C in ethnic minority patients evaluated in Los Angeles County. Am J Gastroenterol. 2001 Aug;96(8):2438–41

15. Sterling RK, Stravitz RT, Luketic VA, et al. A comparison of the spectrum of chronic hepatitis C virus between Caucasians and African Americans. Clin Gastroenterol Hepatol. 2004 Jun;2(6):469–73

16. El-Serag HB. Hepatocellular carcinoma: recent trends in the United States. Gastroenterology. 2004 Nov;127(5 Suppl 1):S27–34

17. Nguyen MH, Whittemore AS, Garcia RT, et al. Role of ethnicity in risk for hepatocellular carcinoma in patients with chronic hepatitis C and cirrhosis. Clin Gastroenterol Hepatol. 2004 Sep;2(9):820–4

18. Sulkowski MS, Mehta SH, Torbenson MS, et al. Rapid fibrosis progression among HIV/hepatitis C virus-co-infected adults. AIDS 2007 Oct 18;21(16):2209–16

19. Maida I, Nunez M, Gonzalez-lahoz J. Liver transplantation in HIV–HCV coinfected candidates: what is the most appropriate time for evaluation? AIDS Res Hum Retroviruses. 2005 Jul;21(7):599–601

20. Bräu N, Fox RK, Xiao P, et al. Presentation and outcome of hepatocellular carcinoma in HIV-infected patients: a U.S.-Canadian multicenter study. J Hepatol. 2007 Oct;47(4):527–37. Epub 2007 Jul 19

21. Lechner F, Wong DK, Dunbar PR, et al. Analysis of successful immune responses in persons infected with hepatitis C virus. J Exp Med. 2000 May 1;191(9):1499–512

22. Sugimoto K, Stadanlick J, Ikeda F, et al. Influence of ethnicity in the outcome of hepatitis C virus infection and cellular immune response. Hepatology. 2003 Mar;37(3):590–9

23. Thio CL, Thomas DL, Goedert JJ, et al. Racial differences in HLA class II associations with hepatitis C virus outcomes. J Infect Dis 2001 Jul 1;184(1):16–21. Epub 2001 May 30

24. Oleksyk TK, Thio CL, Truelove AL, et al. Single nucleotide polymorphisms and haplotypes in the IL10 region associated with HCV clearance. Genes Immun. 2005 Jun;6(4):347–57

25. Falck-Ytter Y, Kale H, Mullen KD, et al. Surprisingly small effect of antiviral treatment in patients with hepatitis C. Ann Intern Med. 2002 Feb 19;136(4):288–92

26. Fleming CA, Craven DE, Thorton D, et al. Hepatitis C virus and human immunodeficiency virus coinfection in an urban population: low eligibility for interferon treatment. Clin Infect Dis. 2003 Jan 1;36(1):97–100. Epub 2002 Dec 11

27. Adeyemi OM, Jensen D, Attar B, et al. Hepatitis C treatment eligibility in an urban population with and without HIV coinfection. AIDS Patient Care STDS. 2004 Apr;18(4):239–45

28. Butt AA, Justice AC, Skanderson M, et al. Rates and predictors of hepatitis C virus treatment in HCV-HIV-coinfected subjects. Aliment Pharmacol Ther. 2006 Aug 15;24(4):585–91

29. Backus LI, Boothroyd DB, Phillips BR, et al. Pretreatment assessment and predictors of hepatitis C virus treatment in US veterans coinfected with HIV and hepatitis C virus. J Viral Hepat. 2006 Dec;13(12):799–810

30. Bräu N, Salvatore M, Ríos-Bedoya CF, et al. J Hepatol. 2006 Jan;44(1):47–55. Epub 2005 Jul 27
31. Reddy KR, Hoofnagle JH, Tong MJ, et al. Racial differences in responses to therapy with interferon in chronic hepatitis C. Consensus Interferon Study Group. Hepatology 1999 Sep;30(3):787–93
32. McHutchison JG, Poynard T, Pianko S, et al. The impact of interferon plus ribavirin on response to therapy in black patients with chronic hepatitis C. The International Hepatitis Interventional Therapy Group. Gastroenterology. 2000 Nov;119(5):1317–23
33. De Maria N, Colantoni A, Idilman R, et al. Impaired response to high-dose interferon treatment in African Americans with chronic hepatitis C. Hepatogastroenterology. 2002 May–Jun;49(45):788–92
34. Kinzie JL, Naylor PH, Nathani MG, et al. African Americans with genotype 1 treated with interferon for chronic hepatitis C have a lower end of treatment response than Caucasians. J Viral Hepat. 2001 Jul;8(4):264–9
35. Theodore D, Shiffman ML, Sterling RK, et al. Intensive interferon therapy does not increase virological response rates in African Americans with chronic hepatitis C. Dig Dis Sci. 2003 Jan;48(1):140–5
36. Zeuzem S, Feinman SV, Rasenack J, et al. Peginterferon alfa-2a in patients with chronic hepatitis C. N Engl J Med. 2000 Dec 7;343(23):1666–72
37. Linday KL, Trepo C, Heintges T, et al. Hepatology. 2001 Aug;34(2):395–403
38. Manns MP, McHutchison JG, Gordon SC, et al. Lancet. 2001 Sep 22;358(9286):958–65
39. Fried MW, Shifmman ML, Reddy KR, et al. Peginterferon alfa-2b plus ribavirin compared with interferon alfa-2b plus ribavirin for initial treatment of chronic hepatitis C: a randomised trial. N Engl J Med. 2002;347:975–82
40. Jeffers L, Cassidy W, Howell CD, Hu S, Reddy KR. Peginterferon alfa-2a (40 kd) and ribavirin for black American patients with chronic HCV genotype 1. Hepatology. 2004 Jun;39(6):1702–8
41. Muir AJ, Bornstein JD, Killenberg PG, et al. Peginterferon alfa-2b and ribavirin for the treatment of chronic hepatitis C in blacks and non-Hispanic whites. N Engl J Med. 2004 May 27;350(22):2265–71
42. Conjeevaram HS, Fried MW, Jeffers LJ, et al. Peginterferon and ribavirin treatment in African American and Caucasian American patients with hepatitis C genotype 1. Gastroenterology. 2006 Aug;131(2):470–7
43. Jacobson IM, Brown RS, et al. Impact of weight-based ribavirin with peginterferon alfa-2b in African Americans with hepatitis C virus genotype 1. Hepatology. 2007 Oct;46(4):982–90
44. Carrat F, Bani-Sadr F, Pol S, et al. Pegylated interferon alfa-2b vs standard interferon alfa-2b, plus ribavirin, for chronic hepatitis C in HIV-infected patients: a randomized controlled trial. JAMA. 2004 Dec 15;292(23):2839–48
45. Toriani FJ, Rodriguez-Torres M, Rockstroh JK, et al. Peginterferon Alfa-2a plus ribavirin for chronic hepatitis C virus infection in HIV-infected patients. N Engl J Med. 2004 Jul 29;351(5):438–50
46. Chung RY, Andersen J, Volberding P, Robbins GK, et al. Peginterferon Alfa-2a plus ribavirin versus interferon alfa-2a plus ribavirin for chronic hepatitis C in HIV-coinfected persons. N Engl J Med. 2004 Jul 29;351(5):451–9
47. Layden-Almer JE, Ribeiro RM, Wiley T, et al. Viral dynamics and response differences in HCV-infected African American and white patients treated with IFN and ribavirin. Hepatology. 2003 Jun;37(6):1343–50
48. Jain M, Shelton J, Liston N, et al. 15th Conference on Retroviruses and Opportunistic Infections (CROI 2008). Boston, MA. February 3–6, 2008. Abstract 1077
49. Kimball P, Elswick RK, Shiffman M. Ethnicity and cytokine production gauge response of patients with hepatitis C to interferon-alpha therapy. J Med Virol. 2001 Nov;65(3):510–6
50. Ikura Y, Morimoto H, Hohmura H, et al. Relationship between hepatic iron deposits and response to interferon in chronic hepatitis C. Am J Gastroenterol. 1996;91:1367–73

51. Barton Al, Banner BF, Cable EE, et al. Distribution of iron in the liver predicts the response of chronic hepatitis C infection to interferon therapy. Am J Clin Pathol. 1995 Apr;103(4):419–24

52. Van Thiel DH, Friedlander L, Fagiuoli S, et al. Response to interferon alpha therapy is influenced by the iron content of the liver. J Hepatol. 1994 Mar;20(3):410–5

53. Ioannou GN, Dominitz JA, Weiss NS, et al. Racial differences in the relationship between hepatitis C infection and iron stores. Hepatology. 2003 Apr;37(4):795–801

54. CDC 2007. Summary Heath Statistic for US Adults: 2006. Table 2. http://www.cdc.gov/nchs/data/series/sr_10/sr10_235.pdf

55. CDC 2007. Heath United States, 2007. Table 35. http://www.cdc.gov/nchs/data/hus/hus07.pdf

56. Phillips A, Carr A, Visnegwala F, et al. Interruption of ART and risk of cardiovascular disease: findings from SMART. 14th Conference on retroviruses and opportunistic infections, 2007.

57. Mondy KE, de las Fuentes L, Waggoner A, et al. Insulin resistance predicts endothelial dysfunction and cardiovascular risk in HIV-infected persons on long-term highly active antiretroviral therapy. AIDS. 2008 Apr 23;22(7):849–56

58. D:A:D Study Group. Use of nucleoside transcriptase inhibitors and risk of myocardial infarction in HIV-infected patients enrolled in the D:A:D study: a multi-cohort collaboration. Lancet 2008; Published Online April 2, 2008

59. Sabin CA, d'Arminio Monforte A, Friis-Moller N, et al. Changes over time in risk factors for cardiovascular disease and use of lipid-lowering drugs in HIV-infected individuals and impact on myocardial infarction. Clin Infect Dis. 2008 Apr 1;46(7):1101–10

60. Choudhary SA, et al. 43rd ICAAC. Chicago, 2003. H-1937

61. Law MG, Friis-Møller N, El-Sadr WM, et al. The use of the Framingham equation to predict myocardial infarctions in HIV-infected patients: comparison with observed events in the D:A:D Study. HIV Med. 2006 May;7(4):218–30

62. Garcia-Lazaro M, et al. Variability in coronary risk assessment in HIV-infected patients. Med Clin (Barc). 2007 Oct 20;129(14):521–4

63. Kaplan RC, et al. Ten-year predicted coronary heart disease risk in HIV-infected men and women. Clin Infect Dis. 2007 Oct 15;45(8):1074–81. Epub 2007 Sep 12

64. May M, et al. A coronary heart disease risk model for predicting the effect of potent antiretroviral therapy in HIV-1 infected men. Int J Epidemiol. 2007 Dec;36(6):1309–18. Epub 2007 Jul 25

65. Huang SS, et al. Reversal of human immunodeficiency virus type 1-associated hematosuppression by effective antiretroviral therapy. Clin Infect Dis. 2000 Mar;30(3):504–10

66. Sullivan PS, et al. Epidemiology of anemia in human immunodeficiency virus (HIV)-infected persons: results from the multistate adult and adolescent spectrum of HIV disease surveillance project. Blood. 1998 Jan 1;91(1):301–8

67. Aalto-Setälä K, et al. Folic acid absorption in patients infected with the human immunodeficiency virus. J Intern Med. 1991 Sep;230(3):227–31

68. Guyatt GH, et al. Laboratory diagnosis of iron-deficiency anemia: an overview. J Gen Intern Med. 1992 Mar–Apr;7(2):145–53

69. Mildvan D. Implications of anemia in human immunodeficiency virus, cancer, and hepatitis C virus. Clin Infect Dis. 2003;37 Suppl 4:S293–6

70. Mildvan D, et al. Prevalence of anemia and correlation with biomarkers and specific antiretroviral regimens in 9690 human-immunodeficiency-virus-infected patients: findings of the Anemia Prevalence Study. Curr Med Res Opin. 2007 Feb;23(2):343–55

71. Volberding P, Levine AM, Dieterich D, et al. Anemia in HIV infection: clinical impact and evidence-based management strategies. Clin Infect Dis. 2004 May 15;38(10):1454–63. Epub 2004 Apr 27

72. Grinspoon S, Carr A. Cardiovascular risk and body-fat abnormalities in HIV-infected adults. N Engl J Med. 2005 Jan 6;352(1):48–62

73. Lichtenstein KA. Redefining lipodystrophy syndrome: risks and impact on clinical decision making. J Acquir Immune Defic Syndr. 2005 Aug 1;39(4):395–400

74. Saint-Marc T, Partisani M, Poizot-Martin I, et al. Fat distribution evaluated by computed tomography and metabolic abnormalities in patients undergoing antiretroviral therapy: preliminary results of the LIPOCO study. AIDS. 2000 Jan 7;14(1):37–49

75. Saves M, Raffi F, Capeau J, et al. Factors related to lipodystrophy and metabolic alterations in patients with human immunodeficiency virus infection receiving highly active antiretroviral therapy. Clin Infect Dis. 2002 May 15;34(10):1396–405. Epub 2002 Apr 22

76. Bacchetti P, Gripshover B, Grunfeld C, et al. Fat distribution in men with HIV infection. J Acquir Immune Defic Syndr. 2005;40:121–131

77. Fat Redistribution and Metabolic Change in HIV Infection (FRAM) Writing Team. Fat distribution in women with HIV infection. J Acquir Immune Defic Syndr. 2006 Aug 15;42(5):562–71

78. Hadigan C, Meigs JB, Wilson PW, et al. Prediction of coronary heart disease risk in HIV-infected patients with fat redistribution. Clin Infect Dis. 2003 Apr 1;36(7):909–16. Epub 2003 Mar 20

79. Miller J, Carr A, Emery S, et al. HIV lipodystrophy: prevalence, severity and correlates of risk in Australia. HIV Med. 2003 Jul;4(3):293–301

80. Lichtenstein KA, Ward DJ, Moorman AC, et al. Clinical assessment of HIV-associated lipodystrophy in an ambulatory population. AIDS. 2001 Jul 27;15(11):1389–98

81. Bogner JR, Vielhauer V, Beckmann RA, et al. Stavudine versus zidovudine and the development of lipodystrophy. J Acquir Immune Defic Syndr. 2001 Jul 1;27(3):237–44

82. van Vonderen MG, et al. 4th IAS Conference. Sydney, 2007. Abstract TuPeB077

83. Lazzaretti R, et al. 4th IAS Conference. Sydney, 2007. Abstract WeAB303

84. Carr A, Ory D. Does HIV cause cardiovascular disease? PLoS Med. 2006 Nov;3(11):e496

85. Mallon PW, Miller J, Kovacic JC, et al. Effect of pravastatin on body composition and markers of cardiovascular disease in HIV-infected men–a randomized, placebo-controlled study. AIDS. 2006 Apr 24;20(7):1003–10

86. Carr A, Workman C, Carey D, et al. Lancet. 2004 Feb 7;363(9407):429–38

87. Valantin MA, Aubron-Olivier C, Ghosn J, et al. Polylactic acid implants (New-Fill) to correct facial lipoatrophy in HIV-infected patients: results of the open-label study VEGA. AIDS. 2003 Nov 21;17(17):2471–7

88. Levan P, Nguyen TH, Lallemand F, et al. Correction of facial lipoatrophy in HIV-infected patients on highly active antiretroviral therapy by injection of autologous fatty tissue. AIDS. 2002;16:1985–1987

89. Guaraldi G, De Fazio D, Orlando G, et al. Facial lipohypertrophy in HIV-infected subjects who underwent autologous fat tissue transplantation. Clin Infect Dis. 2005 Jan 15;40(2):e13–5. Epub 2004 Dec 21

90. CDC. Prevalence of overweight and obesity among adults with diagnosed diabetes–United States, 1988–1994 and 1999–2002. MMWR Morb Mortal Wkly Rep. 2004 Nov 19;53(45):1066–8

91. Amorosa, et al. A Tale of 2 Epidemics: The Intersection between Obesity and HIV Infection in the Urban United States (CROI 2004). San Francisco, CA. Abstract 879

92. C Hadigan, Yawetz S, Thomas A, et al. Metabolic effects of rosiglitazone in HIV lipodystrophy: a randomized, controlled trial. Ann Intern Med. 2004 May 18;140(10):786–94

93. Gavrila A, Hsu W, Tsiodras S, et al. Improvement in highly active antiretroviral therapy-induced metabolic syndrome by treatment with pioglitazone but not with fenofibrate: a 2×2 factorial, randomized, double-blinded, placebo-controlled trial. Clin Infect Dis. 2005 Mar 1;40(5):745–9. Epub 2005 Feb 7

94. Schutt M, Meier M, Meyer M, et al. The HIV-1 protease inhibitor indinavir impairs insulin signalling in HepG2 hepatoma cells. Diabetologia. 2000 Sep;43(9):1145–8

95. Noor MA, Seneviratne T, Aweeka FT, et al. Indinavir acutely inhibits insulin-stimulated glucose disposal in humans: a randomized, placebo-controlled study. AIDS. 2002 Mar 29;16(5):F1–8

96. Blass SC, Ellinger S, Vogel M, et al. Overweight HIV Patients with Abdominal Fat Distribution Treated with Protease Inhibitors are at High Risk for Abnormalities in Glucose Metabolism – A Reason for Glycemic Control. Eur J Med Res. 2008 May 26;13(5):209–14

97. Manuthu EM, Joshi MD, Lule GN, Karari E. Prevalence of dyslipidemia and dysglycaemia in HIV infected patients. East Afr Med J. 2008 Jan;85(1):10–7

98. Schambelan M, Benson CA, Carr A, et al. Management of metabolic complications associated with antiretroviral therapy for HIV-1 infection: recommendations of an International AIDS Society-U.S. panel. J Acquir Immune Defic Syndr. 2002 Nov 1;31(3):257–75

99. Schwartz EJ, et al. Highly active antiretroviral therapy and the epidemic of HIV+ end-stage renal disease. J Am Soc Nephrol. 2005 Aug;16(8):2412–20. Epub 2005 Jun 29

100. Lucas GM, Mehta SH, Atta MG, et al. End-stage renal disease and chronic kidney disease in a cohort of African American HIV-infected and at-risk HIV-seronegative participants followed between 1988 and 2004. AIDS. 2007 Nov 30;21(18):2435–43

101. Szczech L, Hoover DR, Feldman JG, et al. Association between renal disease and outcomes among HIV-infected women receiving or not receiving antiretroviral therapy. Clin Infect Dis. 2004 Oct 15;39(8):1199–206. Epub 2004 Sep 27

102. Herman ES, Klotman PE. HIV-associated nephropathy: Epidemiology, pathogenesis, and treatment. Semin Nephrol. 2003 Mar;23(2):200–8

103. Martins D, Tareen N, Norris KC. The epidemiology of end-stage renal disease among African Americans. Am J Med Sci. 2002 Feb;323(2):65–71

104. Freedman, Soucie JM, Stone SM, Pegram S. Familial clustering of end-stage renal disease in blacks with HIV-associated nephropathy. Am J Kidney Dis. 1999 Aug;34(2):254–8

105. Abbott KC, Hypolite I, Welch PG, Agodoa LY. Human immunodeficiency virus/acquired immunodeficiency syndrome-associated nephropathy at end-stage renal disease in the United States: patient characteristics and survival in the pre highly active antiretroviral therapy era. J Nephrol. 2001 Sep–Oct;14(5):377–83

106. Hailemariam S, Walder M, Burger HR, et al. Renal pathology and premortem clinical presentation of Caucasian patients with AIDS: an autopsy study from the era prior to antiretroviral therapy. Swiss Med Wkly. 2001 Jul 14;131(27–28):412–7

107. Monahan M, Tanji N, Klotman PE, et al. HIV-associated nephropathy: an urban epidemic. Semin Nephrol. 2001 Jul;21(4):394–402

108. Gallant JE, DeJesus E, Arribas JR, et al. Tenofovir DF, emtricitabine, and efavirenz vs. zidovudine, lamivudine, and efavirenz for HIV. N Engl J Med. 2006 Jan 19;354(3):251–60

109. Rawlings MK, Klein, Klingler ET, Queen E, et al. Impact of Drug Therapy and co-morbidities on the Development of Renal Impairment in HIV-Infected Patients. Results of a Cardio Retrospective Database Study.

110. Marconi P, Lorenzini P, Corpolongo A, et al. Black race and degree of immunisuppression predict rate of proteinuria before and after combination antiretroviral treatment (cART) in Italian HIV-infected population. XVII International AIDS Conference. Mexico City; 2008 Poster THEP0197

111. Palella F, Li X, Kingsley L, et al. Proteinuria, glomerular filtration rate reductions, and associated factors among HIV-infected and -uninfected men in the Multicenter AIDS Cohort Study. 15th CROI; 2008; Boston. Abstract 973

112. Fine DM, Perazella MA, Lucas GM, Atta MG. Kidney biopsy in HIV: beyond HIV-associated nephropathy. Am J Kidney Dis. 2008 Mar;51(3):504–14. Epub 2008 Feb 7

Men Who Have Sex with Men of Color in the Age of AIDS: The Sociocultural Contexts of Stigma, Marginalization, and Structural Inequalities

Leo Wilton

Introduction

Current State of the AIDS Epidemic in MSM of Color Communities

Nearly three decades since the onset of AIDS epidemic in the United States (U.S.), men who have sex with men (MSM) have represented a significant disproportionate number of cases of HIV and AIDS.[1] Within this context, MSM refer to gay, bisexually, and heterosexually identified men who engage in sexual behavior with other men. With the advent of HIV antiretroviral therapies (e.g., HAART or highly active antiretroviral therapies), AIDS-related morbidity and mortality in MSM initially decreased during the 1990s.[2] Yet, recent epidemiological data have demonstrated that there has been an accelerated increase in rates of HIV and AIDS, as well as other sexually transmitted infections (STIs) in MSM.[1] For instance, in 2005, MSM represented 71% of the overall HIV infections among adult and adolescent males in the U.S.; MSM also accounted for the highest HIV transmission category, 67% of male infections, compared to 15% for heterosexual transmission and 13% for injection drug use.[3]

MSM of Color (identified as Asian/Pacific Islander, black, Latino, and Native American/Alaska Native men) have been significantly impacted by the AIDS epidemic in the United States.[4–9] Much of the HIV epidemiological data have demonstrated that black and Latino MSM – in particular – have experienced substantial disproportionate rates of HIV and AIDS in the U.S., with the rates among black MSM comparable to some of the highest rates observed in some resource-limited countries.[10] By race/ethnicity, of the 207,810 MSM cases of HIV/AIDS in 2005,

L. Wilton
State University of New York at Binghamton, College of Community and Public Affairs, Department of Human Development, P.O. Box 6000, Binghamton, NY 13902, U.S.
E-mail: lwilton@binghamton.edu

V. Stone et al. (eds.), *HIV/AIDS in U.S. Communities of Color*.
DOI: 10.1007/978-0-387-98152-9_10, © Springer Science + Business Media, LLC 2009

32% represented black MSM, compared to 50% for white MSM, 16% for Latino MSM, 1% for Asian/Pacific Islander MSM, and less than 1% for Native American/Alaska Native MSM.[3] However, incidence and prevalence rates of HIV/AIDS have been underestimated in specific racial/ethnic groups, including Asian/Pacific Islander and Native American communities, due to inadequate methodological approaches (e.g., research design, measurement, and sampling procedures) including but not limited to misclassification of racial/ethnic groups, surveillance systems not collecting data on specific groups, and failure to disaggregate within-group data to assess specific HIV-related health disparities.[8, 11, 12]

In a large-scale epidemiological investigation of MSM ($n = 1,767$) in five urban, U.S. cities (Baltimore, Los Angeles, Miami, New York City, and San Francisco), 46% of black men tested positive for HIV when compared to men from other racial/ethnic groups (white men = 21%; Latinos = 17%; Multiracial men = 19%; Asian/Pacific Islander, Native America/Alaska Native, and Other men = 13%).[13] Significantly, in this study, 67% of black men were unaware of their HIV positive status when compared to the overall sample (white men = 18%; Latinos = 48%; Multiracial men = 50%; Asian/Pacific Islander, Native American/Alaska Native and Other men = 50%).[13] Moreover, in terms of younger MSM (YMSM), in a large-scale cross-sectional, multisite, epidemiological study (e.g., Young Men's Survey) of 3,492 YMSM between the ages of 15 and 22 from seven urban cities in the U.S., HIV prevalence rates were higher among blacks (14.1%), Latinos (6.9%), and men of mixed race (especially those respondents of black racial backgrounds) (12.6%) than among whites (3.3%).[10] Based on the findings from Phase Two of the Young Men's Survey that enrolled 2,942 MSM (aged 23–29), HIV prevalence rates were as follows: black MSM (32%), Latino MSM (14%), and white MSM (7%).[14]

Significantly, according to the CDC,[15] current surveillance trends for 2001–2006 indicated that overall rate of HIV/AIDS diagnoses for MSM in the U.S. increased by 8.6%, although there was a decline in HIV/AIDS diagnoses in other HIV transmission categories (e.g., high-risk heterosexual contact, injection-drug use (IDU), and MSM/IDU). By race/ethnicity, the surveillance data showed that: (1) the overall rate of HIV/AIDS diagnoses increased by 12.4% for black MSM; (2) the rate of HIV/AIDS diagnoses for younger black MSM (aged 13–24) increased by 93.1%, which was equivalent to a twofold increase when compared to white MSM within the same age group; and (3) the rate of HIV/AIDS diagnoses for Asian/Pacific Islander MSM (aged 13–24) increased by 255.6%, which represented the largest proportionate increase by race/ethnicity for MSM. These current trends have been indicative of a consistent and substantial increase in the incidence and prevalence of HIV and AIDS among MSM of Color in the U.S.

Overall, the AIDS epidemic has had a significant impact on MSM of Color communities since its onset in the 1980s in the U.S.[16] Nonetheless, there has been a significant void in HIV prevention research on MSM of Color communities in relation to AIDS epidemic.[4, 6, 16–21] Within this context, the objective of this chapter is to better understand the factors that have led to the disproportionately high HIV incidence and prevalence rates in MSM of Color communities. Thus, this chapter will examine: (1) theoretical approaches to HIV prevention in MSM of Color communities with specific focus on the role of stigma, marginalization, and structural inequalities in MSM of Color communities; (2) factors associated with disproportionate HIV infection rates and HIV sexual behavior in MSM of Color; (3) assessment of current HIV prevention strategies; (4) revised HIV testing, prevention, and risk-reduction strategies; and (5) psychosocial support and mental health needs of MSM of Color. In particular, this chapter will be nested within culturally relevant conceptualizations for MSM of Color that articulates the significance of a paradigm shift in the field of public health that integrates core theoretical premises of interdisciplinarity, intersectionality, and structural inequalities. Parallel to these fundamental ideas, this work will provide praxis – theoretical applications and strategies for engaging the intersection of race/ethnicity, gender, sexuality, and social class – that transcend traditional ways of thinking, and provide focus to culture-specific contexts associated with AIDS epidemic in MSM of Color communities.

Theoretical Approaches to HIV Prevention in MSM of Color Communities

The Role of Stigma, Marginalization, and Structural Inequalities

A key element in addressing HIV-related health disparities for MSM of Color relates to the development of theoretical frameworks that are grounded within culturally relevant conceptualizations.[6, 12, 19, 21–25] Within this context, a critical analytic framework for HIV prevention research – including theory, methodologies, and praxis – incorporates a connection to the interface of racial, gender, sexual, and social class politics.[26] Thus, a major part of this work calls for a paradigm shift that links HIV prevention within intersectional and interdisciplinary discourses that correspond with sociocultural factors that are relevant to life experiences of MSM of Color.[21] In particular, the concepts of stigma, marginalization, and structural inequalities provide a theoretical framework to examine the complexities of the AIDS epidemic, as situated in the everyday, lived experiences of MSM of Color.

Building on the work of Cohen,[27] these fundamental ideas provide a conceptual framework for addressing asymmetrical power relationships (i.e., power inequalities) in communities of color, including those that incorporate sociohistorical and -political experiences of "exclusion and marginalization" based on race/ethnicity, gender, sexuality, and social class. Further, as articulated by Cohen,[27] a major component of these critical analyses relates to the duality of examining macro (e.g., external processes) and micro (e.g., internal processes) structures that have an impact on communities of color in relation to AIDS epidemic. For example, macrolevel processes involve marginalization associated with larger social structures (e.g., structural inequalities based on legal, political, economic, and educational social structures such as institutionalized racism) and microlevel processes relate to "secondary marginalization" within communities of color (e.g., based on gender and sexuality).[27] Therefore, the integration of transformative discourses in the area of AIDS that provide intersectional and interdisciplinary analyses serves as significant interventions in the field of public health. As such, this scholarly work must be at the center of the discourse through incorporating critical, innovative, and transformative analyses that interrogate and challenge hegemonic, Eurocentric, patriarchal, and heteronormative discourses that pathologize communities of color.[21]

Within this context, one critical question to pose is: How does scholarly research or the production of knowledge contribute to the current state of AIDS epidemic in MSM of Color communities, particularly in relation to their substantial disproportionate rates of HIV and AIDS in the U.S.? In the field of public health, the building of knowledge in HIV prevention research has been based, in part, on epistemological/theoretical frameworks in biomedical and social science research that have not incorporated interdisciplinary and intersectional approaches in the study of HIV-related health disparities in a systematic or substantive way for MSM of Color communities.[6, 18, 21, 28, 29] In particular, the work of Mullings and Schulz[29] is relevant here and provides an account of the significance of incorporating intersectional approaches as a mechanism to better understand and to develop theoretical formulations that address health disparities within the sociocultural contexts of communities: ".... Intersectional theory views race, gender, class [and sexuality] not as fixed and discrete categories or as properties of individuals but as social constructs that both reflect and reinforce unequal relationships between classes, racial groups, genders, [and sexualities]" (p. 373).[29]

Core theoretical paradigms in areas of public health and social science research that relate to HIV prevention have been primarily based on Western/Eurocentric theoretical or conceptual frameworks that focus on individual behavior (e.g., social cognitive theoretical frameworks).[30] As a result, the production of knowledge in HIV prevention research has often been shaped within an insular disciplinary context, thus maintaining a disconnection from transformative scholarly inquiries as well as sociocultural realities of lived experiences of MSM of Color communities. Thus, building on the work of Collins,[31] as situated through an intersectional theoretical conceptualization, one of the major problematic implications of this logic is that multiple identities of MSM of Color (e.g., racial, gender, and sexual identities) have been negatively constructed and pathologized through theoretical frameworks that have not adequately integrated the sociohistorical, -political, -economic, and -cultural contexts that have been integral to the cultural specificities of their lived experiences.[28]

The Problematic of SES as a Singular Discourse

Within this context, in public health, socioeconomic status (SES) has served as a primary predictor of health outcomes and has been incorporated as a key logic to account for disparate incidence and prevalence in the morbidity and mortality of health.[32] This logic has been, in part, used in the area of HIV prevention to account for the HIV-related health disparities in communities of color.[21] Based on the work of a number of scholars,[33,34] when controlling for social class in research on health outcomes (e.g., AIDS, cancer, diabetes), racial disparities often remain constant. Consequently, one of the key problematic limitations related to the utilization of social class as part of a core singular unit of analysis in health outcomes in communities of color links with the marginalization of the impact of the intersectional nature of race-, gender-, social class-, and sexuality-based structural inequalities.[35] For example, the logic of social class does not account for the racialization of social class as reflected in the incidence and prevalence of health disparities in communities of color.[34] Also, through incorporating the theoretical lens of Cohen's[27] work on marginalization, the intersectional nature of structural inequalities based on race/ethnicity, gender, social class, and sexuality relate to the disproportionate number of people of color that have been impacted by AIDS epidemic in the U.S.

Further, another major limitation of the SES discourse in public health involves the absence or peripheralization of the sociohistorical and -political impact of marginalization based on racial hierarchies in the U.S. (e.g., institutionalized racism).[36] Historically, several scholars have challenged the hegemonic, Eurocentric theoretical paradigms that have been utilized in research on communities of color.[33,37] For example, as articulated by Washington,[38] the historical legacy of cultural mistrust has been a central theme related to the health experiences (e.g., medical experimentation of black men and black women) of black communities in the U.S. Other researchers also have studied the historical trajectory and role of medical abuse in communities of color.[39] A recent significant illustration of medical abuse has been documented in black and Latino/ children living with HIV in foster care in the New York Metropolitan area; these youth of color were mandated by a child welfare agency to take highly toxic and experimental HIV drug medicines.[38] More specifically, over the years, several scholars[40] have documented the cumulative effects of the Tuskegee Syphilis study that was conducted on black men to study untreated tertiary syphilis in Macon County, Alabama from 1932 through 1972 by the U.S. Public Health Service. Researchers also have investigated cultural mistrust and cultural beliefs about AIDS-related genocide in communities of color.[41–43] In particular, as MSM of Color have experienced a significant impact of the AIDS epidemic, cultural mistrust and cultural beliefs about genocide have had an impact on HIV prevention as a result of the historical experiences with the medical establishment,[43,44] including the Tuskegee Syphilis Study.[45]

A Critique of Syndemic Theoretical Conceptualizations

Based on syndemic theory, the term "syndemic" has been conceptualized as the intersection of multiple areas of health or epidemics that have an impact on the health of communities.[46] In relation to MSM, Stall[47,48] posited that the interaction of several health factors, including substance abuse, depression, childhood sexual abuse, and intimate partner violence, related to increased HIV risk in urban MSM.

One of the major strengths of this scholarly work involves moving the field of public health beyond a unicentric level of analysis to a multifaceted structural level that engages the interrelationships of overlapping epidemics that have an impact on the current state of the AIDS epidemic in MSM. Nonetheless, a significant theoretical and empirical limitation of this area of scholarly inquiry relates to the void regarding the cultural specificities for MSM of Color at the core of this analysis, particularly in relation to the salient sociocultural health factors (e.g., racism and homophobia) that provide the basis for addressing HIV related disparities and developing culturally applicable HIV prevention interventions for this group of men. Within this context, based on the theoretical concept of marginalization, Cohen[27] articulated the salient role of intersectional influences on the AIDS epidemic in black communities: "AIDS touches on, or is related to, many other issues confronting, in particular, poor black communities: health care, poverty, drug use, homelessness" (p. 34). In this regard, the work of Cohen[27] serves as an intersectional and interdisciplinary theoretical framework to examine HIV prevention in MSM of Color communities. Further, the scholarly works of several researchers provide the basis for the incorporation of intersectional analyses related to overlapping epidemics in communities of color.[4, 25, 49–51]

Integrating Interdisciplinary and Intersectional Approaches in Health Disparities

Building on interdisciplinary and intersectional theoretical approaches, an integral component to the study of health disparities in MSM of Color communities is the incorporation and application of epistemological/theoretical frameworks and methodologies based on racial/ethnic/cultural studies (e.g., African Diaspora Studies, Latino/a Studies, Asian Diaspora Studies, Native American Studies), gender studies, queer/lesbian/gay/bisexual studies, and sexuality studies.[21] One of the objectives in utilizing the scholarly work of these areas in the study of health disparities relates to the development of epistemological/theoretical frameworks that provide the basis for incorporating the socio–historical, -political, -economic, and -cultural contexts that have been integral in communities of color. As such, theoretical and methodological approaches based on these scholarly areas work to juxtapose theory and practice that are grounded in culturally relevant conceptualizations, which are fundamental to the lived experiences of MSM of Color. According to Schulz et al.,[35] "Central to this intersectional theory is the tenet that racism and sexism, as well as other forms of oppression,... operate as mutually reinforcing systems of inequality" (p. 371). These areas provide a critical approach to the work on health disparities that engage a critique of service at macro and micro levels with respect to the sociopolitical processes that influence structural inequalities in MSM of Color communities. This paradigm shift has the promise of providing opportunities to engage intellectually rigorous dialogues regarding the centrality of social justice perspectives as well as the interrogation of knowledge to incorporate intersectional and interdisciplinary approaches within the domain of health disparities.

One current illustration of the innovative and groundbreaking scholarly research on MSM of Color communities that incorporates culturally grounded theoretical, methodological, and community-centered approaches has related to research on house-ball communities.[52] This work provides originality within the context of integrating intersectional and interdisciplinary perspectives that are integrated into the core of the analysis within the context of HIV prevention. According to researchers, house-ball communities have been conceptualized as a network or group of individuals that are connected through houses, which serve as familial, cultural, and supportive systems (e.g., fictive kin) for MSM of Color (with a particular focus on black, Latino, and transgender individuals). In this ethnographic investigation, the researchers examined the critical role that house-ball communities have served in building home and kinship networks, including a core value of articulating the importance of gender and sexuality expression as an integral part of an individual's racial, gender, and sexual identities. As such, this work is particularly relevant for groups that have experienced multiple forms of marginalization based on the intersection of racial, gender, social class, and heteronormative hierarchies as well as those that manifest in customary HIV prevention interventions developed for MSM of Color. According to Arnold and Bailey,[52] the findings of this study demonstrated that house-ball communities have assumed a salient leadership role in providing HIV prevention "intraventions" (e.g., prevention work that occurs organically within the context of communities) for groups that often have experienced stigma and discrimination.

In this regard, in a community study involving MSM of Color associated with the house ball community in the New York Metropolitan Area ($n = 504$), findings demonstrated that: (1) slightly more than half of the sample had not tested for HIV within the last year prior to assessment; (2) the majority of the respondents that tested HIV positive (17%) were unaware of their HIV positive status (73%); and (3) based on a subsample of respondents ($n = 371$) who reported having a male sexual partner within the last year prior to evaluation, an HIV positive status was associated with being black, 29 years of age or older, and a lack of HIV testing.[53] Further, house-ball communities have served as large scale, social networks in the U.S. for individuals often disenfranchised from accessing HIV prevention programs.[53] The implications of this work for providing culturally applicable HIV prevention "intraventions" for MSM of Color communities represent transformative approaches in the field of public health.

Sociocultural Factors as Innovative Theoretical Frameworks

Connected to stigma, marginalization, and structural inequalities, recent research has examined the effect of sociocultural factors on HIV sexual risk behavior in MSM of Color.[4,54] In one study, Diaz et al.[4] have incorporated the concept of social oppression as a core domain to account, in part, for the disproportionate health-related disparities in HIV, based on their work with a probability sample of 912 Latino gay men surveyed from three U.S. cities. Diaz et al.[4] provided an intersectional, tripartite model that found empirical support for the impact of socio-cultural factors (e.g., racism, homophobia, and poverty) on HIV sexual risk behavior in Latino gay men. Findings demonstrated that social oppression based on racism, poverty, and homophobia related to sexual experiences that provided the context for HIV sexual risk behavior. Specifically, higher levels of social oppression (e.g., racism, poverty, and homophobia) and psychological distress were predictive of Latino gay men engaging in risky sexual situations.

Further, based on this work, social oppression influenced HIV sexual risk behavior in that Latino gay men were more likely to engage in sexual experiences that were challenging to negotiate safer sexual practices. For example, according to Diaz et al.,[4] "Men who were more discriminated and psychologically distressed were more likely to participate in sexual situations under the influence of drugs or alcohol, to engage in sex as a way to alleviate anxiety and stress, and to be with partners who resisted condom use, among others" (p. 265). Taken together, the experience of challenging "sexual situations" mediated the influence of social oppression (e.g., racism, poverty, and homophobia) on HIV sexual risk behavior.[4] Further, in a community based sample of Asian/Pacific Islander gay men, findings showed that the lack of social support in modulating the effects of racism, homophobia, and anti-immigrant discrimination related to increased HIV sexual risk behavior (e.g., UAI) in the men.[9] These research investigations provide theoretical and empirical support in examining the impact of racism, homophobia, poverty, and immigration status as these intersectional domains manifest in the lives of MSM of Color.

Factors Related to HIV Sexual Risk Behavior in MSM of Color

Overview of HIV Related Risk Factors in MSM of Color

According to the CDC,[1] current surveillance data have demonstrated that approximately 60,000 new HIV infections occur each year in the U.S., and MSM account for a significant proportionate rate of new HIV infections. In this context, HIV behavioral research on MSM has shown that unprotected anal intercourse (UAI) with ejaculation with an HIV/STI-infected sexual partner has served as a key risk factor for HIV/STI transmission and/or coinfection.[16] For HIV-positive MSM, the practice of UAI with ejaculation has been associated with the risk of acquiring or transmitting another strain of HIV virus (e.g., HIV superinfection) as well as STI-infection.[55] Research has differentiated four levels of HIV sexual risk behavior in MSM: (1) unprotected receptive anal intercourse (URAI), (2) unprotected insertive anal intercourse (UIAI), (3) unprotected receptive oral intercourse (UROI), and (4) unprotected insertive oral intercourse (UIOI).[56]

Sexually transmitted infections (STIs), including Chlamydia, gonorrhea, syphilis, herpes, and Hepatitis B, have increased significantly among MSM of Color, particularly in urban cities in the U.S.[57] Importantly, the presence of an STI increases the biological vulnerability for the acquisition and transmission of HIV.[58] For HIV positive men, STIs (e.g., gonorrhea, nongonococcal urethritis, Herpes simplex virus type 2) may have deleterious effects on their current health status (e.g., immune system functioning) and contribute to an increase in viral load.[59] Biomedical research also has shown that acute HIV infection (e.g., significant levels of HIV virus in the blood or other bodily fluids) occurs during the initial phase of HIV infection.[60] Clearly, early diagnosis and treatment of HIV have predicted increased quality of life for persons living with HIV and AIDS.[2]

Building Formative Research on MSM of Color

Since the beginning of AIDS epidemic, there has been a substantial void in scientific research on MSM of Color, which has, to a considerable extent, contributed to inadequate theoretical/epistemological frameworks as well as formative research in most areas of their lives.[18] More specifically, as HIV epidemiological data have demonstrated that MSM of Color experience persistent HIV-related health disparities in the U.S., there has been a dearth of scholarly research that has systematically investigated factors associated with HIV sexual risk (and protective) behaviors in this group of men. However, recent trends in research on HIV-related health disparities have indicated that: (1) MSM of Color (e.g., Asian, black, and Latino MSM) are more likely to have unrecognized HIV infection and advanced disease (i.e., AIDS) at the time of their HIV diagnosis; (2) MSM of Color have been less likely to have HIV testing on a consistent basis; and (3) MSM of Color have had inadequate access to HIV care including HIV antiviral therapies.[2,7,61,62]

The development of a systematic base of scientific research in the area of HIV-related health disparities that focus on MSM of Color has been germane to addressing the considerable limitations in the field of public health. In this regard, the current state of HIV prevention research poses substantial challenges for conducting research on Asian/Pacific Islander (API) MSM as a result of the perception that the AIDS epidemic has not had a significant impact on API communities based on their reported prevalence rates of HIV and AIDS in the U.S.[12,19] However, researchers have challenged this premise and articulated the importance of providing a more sophisticated level of analysis to this issue through assessing HIV incidence rates, HIV testing patterns, and HIV sexual risk behaviors for API MSM.[64] For example, API MSM accounted for 67% of adolescent and adult male cases of HIV and AIDS among Asian Pacific Islanders, which represented the largest proportion in HIV transmission categories for this group (e.g., high-risk heterosexual contact, 16%; injection drug use, 11%; MSM/IDU, 4%).[3] Moreover, there have been significant increases in HIV incidence rates for API MSM, as evidenced by recent epidemiological data that reported a 255.6% increase for younger API MSM (aged 13–24) during the 2001–2006 period.[15] These data are indicative of the need to develop cross-sectional and longitudinal studies to have a better understanding of the structural pathways that relate to the incidence of HIV transmission risk among API MSM.

Community studies on API MSM have demonstrated increasing incidence and prevalence rates of HIV and AIDS, as well as other STIs (e.g., gonorrhea and syphilis), in the U.S. based on work related to HIV testing patterns, HIV sexual risk behavior, and access to culturally competent health care.[19] In a study of young, API MSM ($n = 908$) recruited from community venues in two cities (e.g., San Diego and Seattle) in the U.S., Do et al.[64] investigated recent HIV testing patterns in relation to prevalence, trends, and factors associated with HIV testing in the sample. Findings indicated that the role of ethnicity, familiarity and perceived connection to HIV testing locations, racial and sexual identities, having a primary partner, increased levels of social support, and the report of recent UAI were factors that were related to recent HIV testing. In another study, Do et al.[61] assessed HIV testing patterns and unrecognized HIV infection among 495 young API MSM in San Francisco. Results demonstrated that previous HIV testing was associated with being older, identifying with a gay sexual identity, having had an STI, higher frequency of lifetime sexual partners, and a higher level of acculturation. Also, approximately one quarter of the sample reported not having had prior HIV testing (e.g., based on perceived low risk and anxiety regarding HIV testing results); findings also indicated that of the 2.6% of the sample that tested HIV positive, the majority of the respondents were unaware of their HIV positive status. On the basis of available research in this area, considerable implications for the provision of culturally and linguistically competent HIV testing and prevention services are needed.[65] For example, for API MSM, cultural worldviews (e.g., cultural beliefs and values) regarding sexuality influence the contexts and processes associated with sexual behavior[19] and HIV testing practices.[64] As such, these factors are fundamental in transcending barriers to HIV prevention and care, particularly those that are representative of culturally appropriate strategies for API MSM.

In relation to black MSM, in a formative meta-analytic investigation, researchers examined 12 hypotheses as a method to identify factors related to their increased HIV infection rates.[66] The hypotheses that were examined were as follows: (1) sexual risk; (2) sexual identity/disclosure; (3) substance use; (4) STI history; (5) HIV testing patterns; (6) biological vulnerability to HIV; (7) penis circumcision; (8) HAART use; (9) sex with HIV-positive partners; (10) sexual networks; (11) incarceration history; and (12) anorectal douching. Notably, findings showed that black MSM engaged in comparable rates of HIV sexual risk behavior (e.g., UAI and number of sexual partners) and substance use as compared to men from other racial/ethnic backgrounds. Findings also demonstrated that black MSM had higher rates of STIs, lower frequencies of HIV testing patterns, and were less likely to be aware of their HIV positive serostatus.

Similarly, another current study[7] that examined HIV-related health disparities reported that black MSM, as compared to white MSM, showed lower substance use, fewer sexual partners, and were less likely to disclose same gender sexual behavior. Also, in this study, racial differences were not found in UAI, commercial sex work, HIV testing history, or sex with an HIV-positive sexual partner. Taken together, these formative research investigations pose considerable implications regarding the state of knowledge in HIV prevention research for black MSM in that the focus has shifted from an emphasis on individual behavior to include an examination of the social and structural factors that have an impact on HIV-related health disparities. In this regard, the next steps in the development of scholarly research on HIV-related health disparities among black MSM involves incorporating intersectional and interdisciplinary approaches that are culturally relevant for black MSM.

More specifically, as a strategy to develop scholarly research on black MSM that serves to curtail their substantial HIV prevalence rates, researchers from the Black Gay Men's Research Group[18] have posited that a vision for research on black MSM incorporates several guiding principles in the development and implementation of this work: (1) research must be conducted in an efficient manner; (2) research needs to be developed, implemented, and applied principally by black MSM researchers; (3) research needs to examine the cultural complexities and specificities of the intersectional identities of black MSM; (4) research should be funded through a multiplicity of resources that will have a meaningful impact on the state of the AIDS epidemic for black MSM; and (5) research must be conducted in combination with organizations and individuals reflective of black MSM.

From a theoretical perspective, much of the research on Latino MSM has focused on the significant role that cultural worldviews (e.g., cultural beliefs, values, and norms) have had on HIV risk and protective behaviors.[4] This scholarly research has served a critical role in providing intersectional and interdisciplinary theoretical and empirical contributions to the discourse on HIV-related health disparities for Latino MSM.[67] Building on the research in this area, the concepts of familismo (e.g., family-centeredness) and machismo (e.g., conceptions of masculinity) as well as the influence of religiosity and spirituality have been fundamental concepts that have had an impact on the social constructions of gender and sexuality (e.g., gender role socialization) for Latino MSM.[22] In this regard, cultural conceptualizations of gender (e.g., machismo) have had an impact on power differentials in relationships (e.g., the sexual role during anal intercourse), which may have an influence on HIV risk or protective behaviors.[68] Moreover, the intersectional role of marginalization (e.g., racism, poverty, homophobia, immigration status) has had an impact on the physical health and psychological well-being of Latino MSM.[69] As will be discussed later in the section on immigration status, the process of immigration and acculturation have provided complexities to the discourse on HIV-related health disparities for Latino MSM.[70]

Studies on Latino MSM have focused on several factors in relation to HIV sexual risk behavior including but not limited to HIV disclosure,[71,72] acculturation,[73] role of the Internet,[74,75] ethnic identity,[76] substance use,[77] and the impact of social inequalities.[4] In a community based sample of Latino HIV positive gay and bisexual men, findings demonstrated that: (1) UAI (e.g., UIAI and URAI) was related to alcohol and illicit drug use during sex; (2) older age, higher levels of acculturation, and depression were associated with a greater frequency of sexual partners during URAI; and (3) seroconcordance in a relationship was predictive of UAI with a "most recent" sexual partner.[73] In another study, Ramirez-Valles et al.[78] reported that younger age, higher education, and substance use (e.g., club drugs or other illicit drugs) were predictive of respondents engaging in UAI based on a sample of 643 Latino MSM from Chicago and San Francisco. Further, Jarama et al.[68] found that communication patterns regarding HIV, sexual attraction, machismo, and experiences of discrimination (e.g., homophobia) were predictive of Latino MSM ($n = 250$) engaging in HIV risk behaviors; additionally, 62% of respondents reported having had one or more sexual partners, while less than half of the sample engaged in UAI with a casual sex partner, within the last 3 months prior to assessment.

Contextualizing Sex in MSM of Color Communities: The Role of Sexual Contexts and Networks

Recent research has shown that a number of sexual contexts have contributed to HIV sexual behavior in MSM of Color over the last few years.[79,80] Some of these contexts are related to the characteristics of sexual partners,[81–83] emergence of bareback sex (e.g., the intention to engage in condomless anal intercourse),[84] the use of the Internet in interfacing with sexual partners (e.g., sexual partners in cyberspace),[85] the use of substances (e.g., alcohol and illicit drugs before or during sex),[26,86] and perceived safer sex strategies (e.g., serosorting, seropositioning, withdrawal before ejaculation).[87,88] One of the strengths in conducting formative research on emerging trends and contextual factors associated with HIV sexual risk behavior in MSM of Color is that findings can be used to contribute to current scientific knowledge and the development of efficacious HIV prevention strategies. However, one of the research challenges in this area relates to the need to incorporate culturally appropriate methodologies based on strong collaborations with practitioners affiliated with community based organizations. This represents a major component of culturally competent HIV prevention work as communities provide perspectives that are relevant to the experiences of MSM of Color.

HIV prevention research has posited that sexual networks have had a significant impact on the disproportionate rate of HIV prevalence in MSM of Color communities.[89] Sexual networks have been conceptualized as a network of individuals that have been "linked directly or through sexual contact."[90] One factor that has been shown to influence sexual networks relates to the influence of partner characteristics on the incidence and prevalence of HIV in MSM of Color communities.[83] For example, some studies[81] have shown that MSM of Color tend to have romantic/sexual partners reflective of their racial/ethnic backgrounds. The primary issue here is that HIV transmission risk for MSM of Color increases exponentially because research has demonstrated that MSM of Color (e.g., Asian, black, and Latino) have higher frequencies of STIs, lower frequencies of consistent HIV testing, disproportionate rates of HIV infection, and higher levels of unrecognized HIV infection.[5,7,64] In terms of black MSM, acute HIV infection has been shown to result in higher viral load and lower CD4 counts, which serve as critical factors for HIV seroconversion.[7]

Therefore, MSM of Color, especially black MSM, have experienced a substantially higher risk of acquiring and transmitting HIV due to the high HIV prevalence in their sexual networks.

Experiences of Violence in the Context of HIV Prevention for MSM of Color Communities

Studies have provided empirical support for examining the relationship between multiplicative forms of violence, including childhood sexual abuse (CSA), intimate partner violence (IPV), and other kinds of victimization in relation to HIV sexual risk behavior[91,92] including MSM of Color.[93–95] These areas of scholarly inquiry have been significantly understudied in MSM of Color, although some research has emerged in this area.[96] For example, in a qualitative study of childhood sexual abuse (CSA) in black MSM, findings indicated a 32% prevalence rate in CSA, based on a sample from three geographic regions in the U.S.[97] Also, according to Fields et al.,[97] the contexts of CSA involved: (1) the experience of CSA from a familial individual (e.g., older male relative); (2) the attribution of "same sex desire" as a result of the experience of CSA; and (3) psychological distress (e.g., depression, suicidality) and substance use due to CSA. In another study, black and Latino gay- and nongay identifying MSM who reported histories of CSA, which often were connected to a history of trauma, related to HIV sexual risk behavior.[95] Moreover, Toro-Alfonso and Rodriguez-Madera[94] showed that IPV within relationships was related to HIV sexual risk behavior in Latino MSM. These research investigations provide empirical data for the significance of developing research studies to further examine the social contexts of how experiences of violence relate to HIV sexual risk behavior. Moreover, the implications of these studies for both medical and mental health providers relate to the development and implementation of mechanisms to assess violence-related experiences, particularly within the context of how these foci relate to HIV prevention.

Substance Use in Relation to HIV Sexual Risk Behavior in MSM of Color

Much of the HIV prevention research has demonstrated that the influence of substance use (e.g., alcohol and illicit drugs) has had an impact on HIV sexual risk behavior in MSM.[77,98,99] However, a limited number of intra- or within-group studies have specifically examined the relationship between substance use and HIV sexual risk behavior (e.g., UAI) in community-based samples of MSM of Color.[26] For example, Choi et al.,[86] in a study of 496 Asian/Pacific Islander MSM in the San Francisco Bay area, reported that UAI was related to "being high and buzzed" on ecstasy and poppers with sex; no relationship was found between "being high or buzzed" on alcohol, marijuana, gamma hydroxybutyrate (GHB), and crystal methamphetamine with sex. On the basis of qualitative narratives in a sample of Latino gay men in the San Francisco Bay Area, Diaz[100] reported that crystal methamphetamine use was related to HIV sexual risk behavior. Further, Wilton,[26] in a community-based sample of 481 black gay and bisexual men in the New York Metropolitan Area, found that the use of alcohol before or during sex was related to relationship status (e.g., having a primary and casual sexual partner), higher income, STI testing history, and higher number of male sex partners, and that recreational drug use before or during sex was associated with being younger, having a casual sex partner, HIV positive status, and reporting UAI with a male sex partner.

The Influence of Immigration Status on MSM of Color and Its Connection to HIV Prevention

The role of immigration status on the sexual health of MSM of Color has been an understudied domain in HIV prevention research.[22, 23, 67, 101] Much of the scholarly work in this area has focused on the experiences of Latino MSM and Asian MSM[65, 102] with a void in studies on Caribbean (e.g., English-speaking) MSM and African MSM.[103] Significantly, the process of immigration has been a critical factor in understanding how cultural worldviews (e.g., cultural values and beliefs) influence sexual attitudes and behavior[65] as well as impact access to healthcare, including HIV prevention and care, for immigrant groups.[104, 105]

More specifically, in a large-scale epidemiological study of Asian/Pacific Islanders, findings showed that while the largest proportion of those with AIDS resided in California (42.9%), New York (15.7%), and Hawaii (11%), a significant proportion (two-thirds) of Asian/Pacific Islanders reported their place of birth as outside of the U.S.[106] Ramirez et al.[78] found that HIV prevalence rates were significantly higher in a sample of Latino gay and bisexual men and transgender individuals in San Francisco that were born within the U.S. as compared to those respondents who were born outside of the U.S.; however, findings also demonstrated that HIV prevalence rates were higher for those respondents in Chicago whose place of birth was outside the U.S. as compared to individuals whose place of birth was in the U.S. In a study of Latino MSM from Miami who were born outside of the U.S., findings showed that higher levels of psychological distress and substance use (e.g., club drugs), greater number of sexual partners, having an HIV positive status (e.g., at the onset of immigration), and a higher level of acculturation to U.S. culture related to HIV sexual risk behavior (e.g., UAI).[102]

This emerging area of research provides considerable implications for increasing the scholarly focus on the experiences and processes associated with immigration for MSM of Color that explore the complexities of the social contexts of sexuality and how these factors relate to sexual health.[54, 67, 107] In terms of immigration, contextual factors involving identity (e.g., racial, gender, and sexual identities) as well as stigma and discrimination (e.g., based on immigration status) need to be addressed in HIV prevention research and services for MSM of Color.[22] Indeed, a sustained emphasis on addressing how social structures have an impact on health care inequities for MSM of Color are critically significant, especially those that examine the role of discrimination based on legal status (e.g., undocumented individuals) in the U.S.[106] Also, the development, implementation, and assessment of culturally congruent HIV prevention and testing services (e.g., pre/post-test counseling), including the provision of linguistically competent services, needs to be integrated into HIV prevention and care.[108]

Transgender Women of Color and their HIV Prevention Needs

Much of the HIV prevention research that has been conducted on transgender (Male-to-Female) women, particularly transgender women of color, has demonstrated that this group experiences a considerable disproportionate incidence and prevalence rate of HIV and AIDS in the U.S.[109–112] In a recent systematic review of HIV prevalence and risk behaviors for transgender individuals in the U.S,[113] major findings showed that: (1) calculated rates of HIV infection for transgender women indicated a high prevalence (e.g., 27.7% of MTFs tested HIV positive and 11.8% of MTFs self-reported an HIV positive status); (2) transgender women reported significant rates of HIV sexual risk behavior (e.g., UAI, higher frequency of casual partners, and commercial sex work); (3) URAI, a primary risk for HIV transmission, was calculated at 44.1% for transgender women; and (4) black transgender women demonstrated increased HIV infection rates (e.g., 56.3% tested HIV positive and 30.8% self-reported an HIV positive status). Studies also have reported that transgender women have experienced health-related risks, including HIV risk behavior, through the administration of nonprescribed hormones (e.g., liquid subcutaneous silicon injections) by nonmedical providers as a method to feminize their physical appearance (e.g., face, breasts, thighs, buttocks).[114]

There has been an emergence of community based research that has focused on transgender women of color in relation to examining correlates of HIV sexual risk behavior.[115] Nemoto et al.[109] conducted a study of 312 transgender women of color (e.g., Asian, black, and Latina) in San Francisco and examined URAI by partner status. The results of the study showed that respondents who engaged in URAI with both primary partners and casual sex partners reported drug use before sex; however, respondents who had URAI with casual partners also were more likely to have an HIV positive status. Additionally, black transgender women from lower socioeconomic backgrounds were more likely to have engaged in URAI during commercial sex work.[109] In another study, Operario and Nemoto[116] found that Asian/Pacific Islander transgender women who engaged in URAI were more likely to report commercial sex work and have a history of attempted suicide; commercial sex work also was related to substance use before or during sex and a college level education, while illicit drug use related to commercial sex work. Further, in a qualitative study of transgender women of color that focused on contextual factors associated with HIV risk behavior (substance use and sexual behaviors), findings indicated that respondents engaged in HIV risk behavior with sexual partners as a way to affirm their gender identity and to provide "emotional connection" with their sexual partners. However, at the same time, respondents also discussed how the need for economic stability often had an impact on whether they would engage in HIV risk behavior during commercial sex work.[109]

On the basis of current HIV prevention research, large-scale epidemiological studies need to be conducted to assess HIV seroprevalence rates among transgender women of color in the U.S, particularly those that differentiate regional characteristics. As such, HIV behavioral research investigations are needed to describe patterns and characteristics of HIV risk and protective behaviors as well as to examine the interrelationships among a number of variables including but not limited to sexual and substance use behaviors, psychological factors (e.g., suicidality, depression, coping), and access to services. Further, qualitative investigations utilizing ethnographic fieldwork, focus groups, and individual interviews, need to be conducted to better understand how contextual factors work in the lives of transgender women of color. For example, qualitative studies need to explore how social constructions of gender and sexuality within culturally relevant frameworks relate to barriers in accessing culturally competent transgender health care (including HIV prevention and care). An integral part of this work calls for an examination of how stigma and discrimination (e.g., the intersection of racialized and genderized forms of stigma) relate to lived experiences of transgender women of color within inter- and intragroup domains. These multimethod methodological approaches will provide critical formative data as a basis for the development of culturally grounded HIV prevention interventions for transgender women of color that will address HIV-related health disparities.

Moving Beyond Current HIV Prevention Strategies

Assessment of Current HIV Prevention Strategies for MSM of Color

As the significant increase in HIV infection rates in MSM of Color communities in the U.S. has been well substantiated,[15] empirical research has demonstrated that HIV behavioral prevention interventions (e.g., individual-, group-, and community-level interventions) have had a positive impact on decreasing HIV sexual risk behavior (e.g., UAI and number of sexual partners) and increasing protective behaviors (e.g., condom use) in MSM.[117] Yet, the field of public health has been at crossroads in the development of culturally specific HIV prevention strategies for MSM of Color.[6, 118] In this context, there has been a void in culturally applicable, evidence-based, HIV prevention interventions that have been developed and implemented for MSM of Color.[24, 119, 120] According to the CDC,[121] development and implementation of DEBIs (Diffusion of Evidence-Based Effective Behavioral Interventions) have served to distribute high quality HIV prevention interventions (e.g., best evidence and promising evidence interventions) in the U.S., particularly for those individuals at a significant risk for the transmission of the HIV virus. However, there has been an absence of HIV behavioral interventions that have demonstrated effectiveness as a DEBI in the category of best-evidence or promising-evidence for MSM of Color with the exception of an HIV prevention intervention for API MSM.[122] It should be noted that, at the time of the publication of this chapter, the *Many Men, Many Voices* (*3MV*) HIV/STI behavioral intervention for black MSM was in the evaluation phase to determine the efficacy of the intervention. Nonetheless, *3MV* intervention represents one HIV behavioral intervention for black MSM, although the state of the AIDS epidemic calls for multiple prevention interventions for black MSM.

As an innovative, culturally grounded intervention, the *3MV* intervention has been conceptualized as an integrated HIV/STI group-level behavioral intervention for black MSM who identify as HIV negative and serostatus unknown. The primary objectives of *3MV* intervention are as follows: (1) to prevent the transmission of HIV/STIs through reducing HIV sexual risk behavior (e.g., UAI); (2) to increase protective sexual behaviors (e.g., condom use); (3) to promote influencing factors that relate to HIV sexual risk behavior (e.g., HIV/STI knowledge, perceived HIV/STI risk, identity, self-efficacy/behavioral intentions for condom use); (4) to increase health care seeking behaviors (e.g., HIV/STI testing); and (5) to increase mutual monogamy with a sexual partner who is not HIV positive. The core innovative elements of *3MV* intervention relate to the focus on dual-identity processes (e.g., racial and sexual identities), the integration of HIV/STIs as a mechanism for HIV seroconversion, and the influence of gender role socialization on HIV protective and risk behavior as manifested in power dynamics in relationships [e.g., sexual roles during anal intercourse including insertive ("top") and receptive ("bottom") anal intercourse]. Another critical dimension of the *3MV* intervention relates to the emphasis on safer sex strategies (e.g., outer course, mutual masturbation, etc). These contextual factors provide the basis for the cultural applicability of the intervention for Black MSM.

There have been other HIV prevention interventions for MSM of Color that have been published in HIV prevention research;[119, 120, 123–125] however, these interventions are not a part of the DEBI initiative. Two of these interventions (group- and community-level interventions) were developed for Black MSM,[119, 124] while other interventions (group-level) were designed for Latino MSM[123, 125] as well as Black and Latino MSM and MSMW (men who have sex with men and women) with histories of childhood sexual abuse.[120] On the basis of available HIV prevention research, there have been no published HIV prevention interventions for Native American MSM. It is beyond the scope of this chapter to provide a description of the aforementioned interventions. However, the issue of what constitutes an effective intervention needs to be raised for critical discussion, particularly since there may be effective interventions for MSM of Color that are not congruent with criteria established by the CDC as a DEBI.

As the field of public health has moved toward the development of evidence-based interventions as a method to strengthen prevention interventions,[126] one of the outcomes of this work that needs to be addressed relates to "structural imped-iments" that communities experience in the development, implementation, and assessment of their programs, including the emphasis on what constitutes scientific evidence (e.g., randomized controlled trials, quasi-experimental research designs, prospective cohort studies, etc.).[127] Also, there is a dire need to challenge the pos-itivist paradigm of quantitative methodological approaches as the primary source of what constitutes scientific evidence, including the incorporation of qualitative methodological approaches as a core element in the assessment of HIV prevention interventions.[18,28] As such, the issue of scientific evidence raises critical questions, as articulated by Buchanan and Allegrante,[127] that have been germane to commu-nities regarding the role of ethics and "... the rights of community members to be involved in the decisions about the goals and methods of community research, since such intervention research holds the potential to affect their lives in ways both intended and unintended" (p. 82). Therefore, a hierarchy of evidence-based standards[127] for HIV prevention interventions poses a critical tension experienced by communities, particularly those of MSM of Color, that have been disenfran-chised based on racial, gender, social class, and sexuality based hierarchies. As such, these hierarchies have been embedded as a part of core processes associated with evidence-based interventions, including posing critical implications for acquiring and maintaining funding of HIV prevention interventions for MSM of Color.[108]

Another persistent challenge in HIV prevention research has related to the devel-opment and implementation of HIV prevention strategies, including individual, group, community, and structural level interventions, for MSM of Color that incor-porate culturally grounded theoretical conceptualizations based on cultural beliefs, values, and norms of their respective MSM of Color communities.[6,21,22,24] A sig-nificant part of this work involves researchers that are representative of MSM of Color communities and maintain values that are congruent with those communi-ties.[18] Parallel to this process, the development of HIV prevention strategies need to be based on culturally congruent formative research in MSM of Color com-munities with respect to theoretical formulations, methodological approaches, and application of knowledge in the respective communities. This represents a major area of concern because formative studies on MSM of Color communities have been in the process of emerging in scholarly research. However, there have been several structural challenges that relate to the development of scholarly research on MSM of Color communities by MSM of Color researchers (e.g., racism and homophobia associated with acquiring adequate levels of funding for research inves-tigations).[18] Further, based on the work of social movements in the U.S. (e.g., Civil Rights, Gay Liberation, Feminist), there has been a developing network of MSM of Color researchers. In this regard, one significant strategy for moving HIV pre-vention research forward is to develop scholarly research experiences for MSM of Color researchers that incorporate theoretical frameworks and methodologies nested in culturally relevant approaches reflective of MSM of Color communities. This ini-tiative would provide research opportunities for MSM of Color in the development of theoretically conceptualized and methodologically rigorous studies, which would be grounded in their communities.

At the present time, there has been an emphasis on the adaptation of existing interventions for MSM of Color that have served as a strategy to address their current HIV-related health disparities.[128] However, the adaptation of existing interventions provides an interim strategy to address the issue of the inadequate number of HIV prevention interventions for MSM of Color. Within this context, the development of innovative, well conceptualized, and efficacious HIV prevention interventions nested within cultural conceptual frameworks will be paramount to addressing the increasing HIV rates among MSM of Color.[6] However, the issue of time serves as a key factor in the development and implementation of HIV prevention interventions for MSM of Color. For example, the process of high quality intervention research occurs within a longer-term period. As such, formative research (e.g., focus groups, individual interviews, ethnographic fieldwork, and quantitative surveys) needs to be conducted on MSM of Color, which will be followed by the development, assessment, and implementation of the HIV prevention interventions. Therefore, at the current moment, one of the dilemmas in the field relates to the need to address the increasing HIV incidence and prevalence rates in MSM of Color communities. Yet, the question remains regarding the reason(s) for the void in culturally relevant HIV prevention interventions for MSM of Color post 25 years into the AIDS epidemic – perhaps, a focus on structural barriers that relate to these processes may move the field in the right direction.

What Does the Future Hold for HIV Prevention Interventions for MSM of Color?

In relation to the concept of adaptation in HIV prevention interventions, there has been an adapted, peer-based, community-level HIV prevention intervention that was developed, implemented, and assessed for young black MSM between ages of 18 and 30 in three North Carolina metropolitan areas (Raleigh, Greensboro, and Charlotte) from 2004 to 2005.[119] On the basis of the Popular Opinion Leader (POL) model as a part of the Diffusion of Innovation Theory, approximately 15% of black MSM from these communities were recruited and trained in HIV prevention risk and served as popular opinion leaders with their peers as a strategy to promote safer sex norms in their respective communities. The results of this community level HIV prevention intervention demonstrated significant decreases in URAI. For example, while the baseline data showed that 32.4% ($n = 284$) of young black MSM engaged in URAI, this number decreased to 23.6% at the 4-month measurement point, 24.4% at the 8-month measurement point, 18.0% at the 12-month measurement point. This initiative provides the basis for the development of community level HIV prevention interventions for MSM of Color communities.

A Community Level HIV Prevention Intervention for Young black MSM was developed based on the adaptation of the Mpowerment project (e.g., Mpowerment for Black MSM).[129] The Mpowerment Intervention was developed based on formative qualitative research methodologies. Currently, the Mpowerment Intervention for black MSM has been in the field to determine the efficacy of the intervention; the anticipated completion date for this outcome evaluation is 2010. The aim of the project is to assess the effectiveness of a community level HIV prevention intervention through a reduction in HIV sexual risk behavior (e.g., UAI and number of sexual partners) and an increase in HIV healthcare seeking behaviors (e.g., HIV testing) in young black MSM in the southwest region of the U.S. (e.g., Dallas and Houston, Texas). Other areas that will be assessed for intervention effectiveness include knowledge of HIV status as well as psychosocial and mental health factors. Since the Mpowerment Intervention will be conducted in Dallas and the comparison group will be Houston, the objective is to compare cross-sectional data in both areas for the pre- and post-intervention of Mpowerment.

With respect to HIV prevention strategies, there has been a trend toward the development of "intraventions"[52] in MSM of Color communities as a strategy to address their health-related HIV disparities. Currently, several community based organizations across the country have developed "intraventions in their respective communities," which refer to HIV prevention strategies that have been organically designed and implemented within their communities. Therefore, a major emphasis has been placed on the development of innovative, culturally relevant "ground level" or "home grown" HIV prevention "intraventions" for MSM of Color communities. An illustration of three community level "intraventions" that have been developed by community based organizations in this area involve: (1) Pride in the City (PITC), (2) The Love Ball, and (3) CRIBB. The PITC and Love Ball were conceptualized by People of Color in Crisis (POCC) in Brooklyn, New York and CRIBB (Creating Responsible Intelligent Black Brothers) was developed by the National AIDS Education and Services for Minorities, Inc. (NAESM) in Atlanta, Georgia.

Pride in the City (PITC)

Pride in the City (PITC) has been conceptualized as a community level HIV prevention intravention for the black lesbian, gay, bisexual, and transgender (LGBT) community in the New York Metropolitan Area. A major component of this intravention involves a large-scale sexual health-focused program that occurs within the context of a weekend including park and beach events. The primary aim of PITC is to cultivate a community oriented collective space that is culturally grounded within the context of black LGBT communities. As such, one of the key strategies is to provide access to HIV/STI counseling, testing, and prevention in combination with a focus on community norms that relate to the importance of sexual health. Through this community level HIV prevention intravention, several community based organizations (e.g., AIDS Service Organizations) engage in a collaborative process to provide HIV counseling, testing, and prevention to community members. This intravention poses considerable implications for the significance of providing access to HIV prevention and services for individuals who may experience marginalization within conventional healthcare settings.

The Love Ball

The Love Ball involves the engagement of members of the House Ball community in an innovative, culturally specific, community-level HIV prevention intravention. Research has shown that house-ball community members have experienced multiple forms of marginalization based on their racial/ethnic, gender, and sexual identities (Arnold & Bailey, in press). For example, members of house-ball communities may be disenfranchised from conventional HIV prevention and care (Murrill et al., 2008).[53] To address HIV-related health disparities within House Ball communities, *The Love Ball* works to affirm the racial/ethnic, gender, and sexual identities of the members involved with the house-ball community based on the theme of love. A major component of the intravention is to sponsor a ball where members compete in a competition. Moreover, HIV counseling and testing along with prevention messages are integrated within the context of the Ball. This initiative provided a context to offer HIV prevention services that are not routinely provided at community events.

CRIBB

The CRIBB initiative was conceptualized in 2007 to focus on the development of leadership on the national level for young black MSM between the ages of 18 and 25. In this pursuit, the focus of this program has been on the development of a new generation of researchers and community practitioners that undertake the work of transformative leadership with respect to having an impact on the AIDS epidemic in black MSM communities. This year-long initiative introduces a group of approximately 10–12 young black MSM representative of different regions of the country to concepts of leadership and community as a strategy to address HIV-related health disparities for younger black MSM. During the course of a year, CRIBB members participate in culturally grounded institutes and seminars that focus on aspects of the current state of the AIDS epidemic for black MSM, leadership, and community work. One of the major objectives of CRIBB has been for each member to participate in the development and implementation of a selected community project that focuses on HIV prevention intraventions in black MSM communities.

Raising the Bar of Competence: An Assessment of HIV Testing Strategies

Need for Revised HIV Testing, Prevention, and Risk Reduction Agenda

The core principles of the recently revised recommendations for HIV testing and prevention have worked to incorporate HIV testing as a component of routine medical care with health care providers and to reduce barriers to HIV testing.[130] The objectives of these principles are as follows: (1) incorporate HIV testing as a component of routine medical care with health care providers; (2) develop models for the diagnosis of HIV beyond health care settings; (3) promote secondary HIV prevention with individuals living with HIV and AIDS as a strategy to prevent new HIV infections, and (4) decrease perinatal HIV transmission. Specifically, according to the CDC,[121] the aim for HIV prevention has been to "reduce the number of new HIV infections and to eliminate racial and ethnic disparities by promotion of HIV counseling, testing, and referral and by encouraging HIV prevention among both persons living with HIV and those at high risk for contracting the virus" (p. 585). Clearly, the increasing rates of unrecognized HIV infections among MSM of Color needs to be addressed – particularly since research has indicated that approximately 50–70% of HIV positive individuals have transmitted new sexually transmitted HIV infections.[130]

One primary strategy for addressing HIV-related health disparities in the U.S. has been the development of the Partner Counseling and Referral Services (PCRS) initiative. According to Hogben et al.,[131] the aim of PCRS strategy is to reduce HIV transmission in the U.S. by a focus on engaging sexual partners of HIV positive individuals through HIV counseling and testing. The underlying objective of the PCRS strategy is to identify HIV positive individuals and to promote protective behaviors (e.g., condom use) that have an impact on HIV transmission. On the basis of the work of Hogben et al.,[131] current studies have reported preliminary evidence that indicates the effectiveness of the PCRS strategy in serving as a strategy in achieving their objectives. However, there has been incongruity between these recent preliminary findings and the increasing disproportionate HIV infection rates among MSM of Color.

Further, one of the major limitations of the PCRS initiative relates to the complexities of the critical role that stigma, marginalization, and structural inequalities have on HIV testing and counseling for MSM of Color communities, thus significantly undermining the effectiveness of this strategy. For example, having access to high quality, culturally competent HIV prevention and care (including HIV counseling and testing) has been a significant barrier for MSM of Color.[132-134] For example, Malebranche et al.[135] found that healthcare experiences of black MSM involving racial and sexual discrimination served as barriers to the utilization of healthcare and HIV testing; additionally, these experiences involving healthcare had an impact on provider-patient communication patterns and protective behaviors. The implications of the findings, as posed by Malebranche et al.,[135] relate to the importance of developing a cadre of healthcare providers reflective of communities of color based on race, gender, and sexuality, thus establishing core domains for cultural competencies in working with MSM of Color.

On the basis of the substantial recent HIV incidence rates among MSM of Color in the U.S., there is a dire need for the development and implementation of innovative, culturally relevant HIV testing and prevention strategies for MSM of Color. To address this problem, significant funding resources on the local, state, and federal levels need to be allocated to community based organizations in the development, implementation, and assessment of culturally relevant HIV testing procedures. In particular, there has been promising evidence[3] that indicates that gay pride of color programs and events sponsored by community based organizations have become an effective strategy for providing contexts for the development and implementation of culturally applicable models of HIV testing and prevention. Also, based on the work of Mayer et al.,[136] through community based organizations, a major part of this work can focus on accessing marginalized groups of individuals within MSM of Color communities (e.g., House Ball communities, commercial sex workers, incarcerated youth, homeless youth, etc.) who may be at significant risk for HIV transmission. In this pursuit, researchers that are reflective of MSM of Color communities need to provide the leadership in the development and implementation of HIV testing and prevention programmatic efforts.[135]

Psychosocial Support and Mental Health Needs for MSM of Color

As the AIDS epidemic enters a third decade, the current state of scholarly research regarding psychosocial and mental health issues for MSM of Color remains understudied.[95] According to the U.S. Surgeon General's Report, people of color have experienced barriers in accessing quality mental health services and care and have not been adequately represented in research in the area of mental health.[137] Similarly, MSM of Color have reported dissatisfaction with mental health services as a result of structural barriers including but not limited to heterosexism and homophobia.[138] Further, much of the extant research on the influence of racial/ethnic discrimination on mental health for people of color utilizing population based studies has found that the experience of racial/ethnic discrimination relates to increased psychological distress for people of color, including diagnosis of major depression, generalized anxiety disorder, and onset of substance use.[139] Similarly, population based studies of LGBT communities have shown that perceived discrimination (e.g., lifetime and daily discrimination) had a negative impact on their quality of life in addition to increases in current psychological distress and mental health disorders.[140] Other population based studies have reported a higher prevalence of mental health disorders, suicidal ideation, and substance use among lesbian, gay, and bisexual individuals as compared to heterosexual individuals.[141, 142] In this regard, population based studies of LGBT communities of color are needed to ascertain characteristics of mental health utilization as well as the prevalence of mental health and substance use morbidity.[143] Yet, there has been a significant void in population based studies that have focused on MSM of Color.

Sociocultural Factors in Relation to Mental Health for MSM of Color

Building on the work of several scholars,[144] stigma has been a core critical issue for MSM of Color. Specifically, the negotiation of racial, gender, and sexual identities juxtaposed with experiences of individual and institutionalized racism and homophobia have served as relevant culturally specific psychosocial issues for MSM of Color.[138] For example, according to Wheeler,[24] Black MSM have to work through the stressors associated with being a black male (e.g., racism, unemployment, incarceration, health issues) and that of being emotionally and/or sexually attracted to men (e.g., gender role expectations). A significant part of this work relates to the negotiation of relationships with significant others including family, friends, and sexual partners. Similarly, with respect to gender expression and socialization, Sandfort et al.[145] found that Latino gay and bisexual men who identified as effeminate reported greater psychological distress in addition to instances of homophobia as compared to those who did not identify as effeminate. Further, in a qualitative study of Black and Latino HIV-positive MSM who reported a history of childhood sexual abuse, findings showed that the sociocultural context of the men's lives was central to their lived experiences. For example, predominant themes related to sexual identity, role of family and cultural expectations regarding children, gender role socialization, influence of substance use, religiosity and spirituality, and HIV-related stigma, marginalization, and barriers to HIV care.[95]

On the basis of the work of Meyer,[146] the sociocultural model of minority stress in lesbian, gay, and bisexual (LGB) communities has provided a theoretical framework to examine the relationship between chronic stress and stigmatization, particularly as related to psychosocial distress. In particular, through the use of a distal-proximal domain, Meyer posited that the experiences of "minority" stressors for LGB individuals (e.g., expectations of stigma, internalized homophobia, and experiences of prejudice and discrimination) relate to mental health outcomes. As a part of minority stress processes, distal refers to experiences of prejudice, discrimination and violence based on sexual identity and proximal relates to experiences associated with "expectations of rejection, concealment, and internalized homophobia" (p. 248).[146] Additionally, with a specific focus on MSM of Color (e.g., Latino gay and bisexual men), researchers have developed theoretical models to examine the effects of social discrimination (e.g., racism, homophobia, poverty) in relation to psychological distress and resiliency.[144]

Further, the experiences of HIV-related stigma and discrimination both within and external to MSM of Color communities have served as relevant psychosocial issues for MSM of Color. For example, in a study of 301 Latino gay and bisexual men, Zea et al.[147] found that HIV disclosure was predictive of respondents reporting higher levels of social support which had an impact on their lower depression and self-esteem. Similarly, Peterson et al.[148] reported that greater psychosocial resources mediated the relationship between stress and depressed mood in a community sample of Black gay, bisexual, and heterosexual men. Within this context, MSM of Color living with HIV and AIDS have to negotiate their HIV positive status involving issues of disclosure to romantic and sexual partners, families, friends, health care providers, as well as other significant others.[132] HIV positive MSM of Color also have to manage the stressors of stigma within MSM Communities of Color (e.g., issues of rejection and discrimination). Therefore, HIV prevention interventions need to address the stigmatization of HIV positive MSM of Color by HIV negative MSM of Color. For example, Diaz[149] found high levels of HIV-related stigma among Latino HIV negative MSM and high levels of psychological distress associated with the experiences of HIV related stigma for Latino HIV positive MSM.

Summary

Since the onset of AIDS epidemic, MSM of Color communities have experienced considerable HIV-related health disparities in the U.S. There has been a substantial void in scholarly research on MSM of Color within the context of the AIDS epidemic. There have been significant limitations in the conceptual frameworks utilized in research on HIV-related health disparities for MSM of Color. Traditional models used in research on HIV-related health disparities have not integrated to a substantial degree culturally relevant conceptualizations at the core of the work. Thus, the objective of this chapter was to examine the factors that contribute to the significant incidence and prevalence rates of HIV and AIDS in MSM of Color communities. In particular, the concepts of stigma, marginalization, and structural inequalities were posed as a theoretical framework to examine HIV-related health disparities in MSM of Color communities. A basic premise of this work involves a paradigm shift that integrates intersectional and interdisciplinary theoretical and methodological approaches in the study of HIV related health disparities in MSM of Color communities. One of the core ideas put forth in the development of this work relates to a focus on the intersection of race, gender, social class, and sexual politics within the context of HIV prevention in MSM of Color communities.

References

1. Centers for Disease Control and Prevention. *HIV/AIDS Surveillance Report, 2006, 18,* 1–46. U.S. Department of Health and Human Services: Atlanta, GA; 2008
2. Hall HI, Byers RH, Ling Q, Espinoza L. Racial/ethnic and age disparities in HIV prevalence and disease progression among men who have sex with men in the United States. *American Journal of Public Health.* 2007; 97: 1060–1066

3. Centers for Disease Control and Prevention. *HIV/AIDS Surveillance Report, 2005, 17*, 1–55. U.S. Department of Health and Human Services: Atlanta, GA; 2007

4. Diaz RM, Ayala G, Bein E. Sexual risk as an outcome of social oppression: data from a probability sample of Latino gay men in three U.S. cities. *Cultural Diversity and Ethnic Minority Psychology.* 2004; 10: 255–267

5. Koblin BA, Torian LV, Guilin V, Ren L, MacKellar DA, Valleroy LA. High prevalence of HIV infection among young men who have sex with men in New York City. *AIDS.* 2000; 14: 1793–1780

6. Mays VM, Cochran SD, Zamudio A. HIV prevention research: are we meeting the needs of African American men who have sex with men? *Journal of Black Psychology.* 2004; 30: 8–105

7. Millet GA, Flores SA, Peterson JL, Bakeman R. Explaining disparities in HIV infection among Black and White men who have sex with men: a meta-analysis of HIV risk behaviors. *AIDS.* 2007; 21: 2083–2091

8. Vernon I. *Prevention of HIV Infection in Native American Communities.* Paper presented at the National Institutes of Health, Office of AIDS Research Advisory Council: Bethesda, MA; 2007

9. Yoshikawa H, Wilson PAD, Chae DH, Cheng J. Do family and friendship networks protect against the influence of discrimination on mental health and HIV risk among Asian and Pacific Islander gay men? *AIDS Education and Prevention.* 2004; 16: 68–83

10. Valleroy LA, MacKellar DA, Karon JM, Rosen DH, McFarland W, Shehan DA, et al. HIV prevalence and associated risks in young men who have sex with men. *Journal of the American Medical Association.* 2000; 284: 198–204

11. Fieland KC, Walters KL, Simoni JM. Determinants of health among two-spirit American Indians and Alaska Natives. In: Meyer IH, Northridge ME, eds. *The Health of Sexual Minorities: Public Health Perspectives on Lesbian, Gay, Bisexual, and Transgender Populations.* New York: Springer, 2007, pp. 268–300

12. Nemoto T, Wong FY, Ching A, Chung CL, Bouey P, Herncikson M, et al. HIV seroprevalence, risk behaviors, and cognitive factors among Asian and Pacific Islander American men who have sex with men: a summary and critique of empirical studies and methodological issues. *AIDS Education and Prevention.* 1998; 10: 31–47

13. Centers for Disease Control and Prevention. HIV prevalence, unrecognized infection, and HIV testing among men who have sex with men – five U.S. cities, June 2004–April 2005. *Morbidity and Mortality Weekly Report.* 2005; 54: 597–601

14. Centers for Disease Control and Prevention. HIV incidence among young men who have sex with men – seven U.S. cities, 1994–2000. *Morbidity and Mortality Weekly Report.* 2001; 50: 440–444

15. Centers for Disease Control and Prevention. Trends in HIV/AIDS diagnoses among men who have sex with men – 33 states, 2001–2006. *Morbidity and Mortality Weekly Report.* 2008; 57: 681–686

16. Wilton L. Perceived health risks and psychological factors as predictors of sexual risk-taking within HIV positive gay male seroconcordant couples. *Dissertation Abstracts International.* 2001; 61(7-B): 3867

17. Bing EG, Bingham T, Millett GA. Research needed to more effectively combat HIV among African American men who have sex with men. *Journal of the National Medical Association.* 2008; 100: 52–56

18. Black Gay Research Group. *Black Gay Research Agenda.* Black Gay Men's Research Group and National Black Gay Men's Advocacy Coalition: New York; 2007

19. Choi KH, Yep GA, Kumekawa E. HIV prevention among Asian and Pacific Islander American men who have sex with men: a critical review of theoretical models and directions for future research. *AIDS Education and Prevention.* 1998; 10: 19–30

20. Peterson JL, Coates TJ, Catania JA, Middleton L, Hilliard B, Hearst N. High-risk sexual behavior and condom use among gay and bisexual African American men. *American Journal of Public Health.* 1992; 82: 1490–1494

21. Wilton L. *The Absence of Color in Black Gay Men's Experiences – It's a Paradox: Thinking About HIV and AIDS*. Paper presented to the New York State Department of Health, AIDS Institute: Albany, NY; 2006

22. Diaz RM. *Latino Gay Men and HIV: Culture, Sexuality, and Risk Behavior*. Routledge Press: New York; 1997

23. Padilla M, Castellanos D, Guilamo-Ramos V, Reyes AM, Sanchez ML, Soriano MA. Stigma, social inequality, and HIV risk disclosure among Dominican male sex workers. *Social Science & Medicine*. 2008; 67: 380–388

24. Wheeler DP. Exploring HIV prevention needs for nongay-identified Black and African American men who have sex with men: a qualitative exploration. *Sexually Transmitted Diseases*. 2006; 33: S11–S16

25. Zea MC, Reisen CA, Diaz RM. Methodological issues in research on sexual behavior with Latino gay and bisexual men. *American Journal of Community Psychology*. 2003; 31: 281–291

26. Wilton L. Correlates of substance use in relation to sexual behavior in Black gay and bisexual men: implications for HIV prevention. *Journal of Black Psychology*. 2008; 34: 70–93

27. Cohen C. *The Boundaries of Blackness: AIDS and the Breakdown of Black politics*. University of Chicago Press: Chicago; 1999

28. Wyatt GE, Williams JK, Myers HF. African American sexuality and HIV/AIDS: recommendations for future research. *Journal of the National Medical Association*. 2008; 100: 44–51

29. Mullings L, Schulz AJ. Intersectionality and health: an introduction. In: Schulz AJ, Mullings L, eds. *Gender, Race, Class, and Health: Intersectional Approaches*. New York: John Wiley & Sons, Inc, 2005, pp. 3–20

30. Airhihenbuwa CO, Okonor TA. Toward evidence-based and culturally appropriate models for reducing global health disparities: an Africanist perspective. In: Wallace BC, ed. *Toward Equity in Health: A New Global Approach to Health Disparities*. New York: Springer, LLC, 2008, pp. 47–60

31. Collins PH. *Black Sexual Politics: African Americans, Gender, and the New Racism*. Routledge Press: New York; 2005

32. Smedley BD, Stith AY, Nelson AR. *Unequal Treatment: Confronting Racial and Ethnic Disparities in Health Care*. National Academies Press: Washington, D.C.; 2002

33. Williams RA. Historical perspectives on health care disparities: is the past prologue? In: Williams RA, ed. *Eliminating Healthcare Disparities in America: Beyond the IOM Report*. Totowa, NJ: Humana Press, 2007, pp. 3–19

34. LaVeist T. *Minority Populations and Health: An Introduction to Health Disparities in the U.S.*. Jossey-Bass: San Francisco; 2005

35. Schulz AJ, Freudenberg N, Daniels J. Intersections of race, class, and gender in public health interventions. In: Schulz AJ, Mullings L, eds. *Gender, Race, Class, and Health: Intersectional Approaches*. New York: John Wiley & Sons, Inc, 2005, pp. 371–393

36. Smedley A. *Race in North America: The Origin and Evolution of a Worldview*, 3rd edition. Westview Press: Boulder, CO; 2007

37. Krieger N. Studies of difference: theoretical underpinnings of the medical controversy of black-white differences in the United States, 1830–1870. In: LaVest TA, ed. *Race, Ethnicity, and Health: A Public Health Reader*. San Francisco, CA: John Wiley & Sons, 2002, pp. 11–33

38. Washington HA. *Medical Apartheid: The Dark History of Medical Experimentation on Black Americans from Colonial Times to the Present*. New York: Harlem Moon Press; 2008

39. Briggs L. *Reproducing Empire: Race, Sex, and U.S. Imperialism in Puerto Rico*. University of California Press: Berkeley; 2002

40. Brandt AM. Racism and research: the case of the Tuskegee Syphilis experiment. In: Reverby SM, ed. *Tuskegee's Truths: Rethinking the Tuskegee Syphilis Study*. Chapel Hill, NC: University of North Carolina Press, 2000, pp. 15–33

41. Bird ST, Bogart L. Conspiracy beliefs about HIV/AIDS and birth control among African Americans: Implications for the prevention of HIV, other STIs, and unintended pregnancy. *Journal of Social Issues.* 2005; 61: 109–126

42. Klonoff EA, Landrine H. Do blacks believe HIV/AIDS is a governmental conspiracy against them? *Preventive Medicine.* 1999; 28: 451–457

43. Ross MW, Essien EJ, Torres I. Conspiracy beliefs about the origin of HIV/AIDS in four racial/ethnic groups. *Journal of Acquired Immune Deficiency Syndromes.* 2006; 41: 342–344

44. Silvestre AJ, Hylton JB, Johnson LM, Houston C, Witt M, Jacobson L, et al. Recruiting minority men who have sex with men for HIV research: results from a 4-city campaign. *American Journal of Public Health.* 2006; 96: 1020–1027

45. Thomas SB, Quinn SC. The Tuskegee Syphilis Study, 1932–1972: implications for HIV education and AIDS risk education programs in the Black community. *American Journal of Public Health.* 1991; 81: 1498–1505

46. Singer M. AIDS and the health crisis of the U.S. urban poor: the perspective of critical medical anthropology. *Social Science and Medicine.* 1994; 39: 931–948

47. Stall R, Mills TC, Williamson J, Hart T, Greenwood G, Paul J, et al. Association of co-occurring psychosocial health problems and increased vulnerability to HIV/AIDS among urban men who have sex with men. *American Journal of Public Health.* 2003; 93: 939–942

48. Stall R. *An Update on Syndemic Theory Among Urban Gay Men.* Paper presented at the American Public Health Association: Washington, DC; 2007

49. Fullilove R. *African Americans, Health Disparities and HIV/AIDS: Recommendations for Confronting the Epidemic in Black America.* National Minority AIDS Council: Washington, DC; 2006

50. Harawa N, Adimora A. Incarceration, African Americans and HIV: advancing a research agenda. *Journal of the National Medical Association.* 2008; 100: 57–62

51. Jones KT, Johnson WD, Wheeler DP, Gray P, Foust E, Gaiter J. The North Carolina Men's Health Initiative Study Team. Nonsupportive peer norms and incarceration as HIV risk correlates for young Black men who have sex with men. *AIDS & Behavior.* 2008; 12: 41–50

52. Arnold EA, Bailey MM. Constructing home and family: how the ballroom community supports African American GLBTQ youth in the face of HIV/AIDS. *Journal of Gay and Lesbian Social Services.* 2009, in press

53. Murrill CS, Liu K, Guilin V, Colon ER, Dean L, Buckley LA, et al. HIV prevalence and associated risk behaviors in New York's house ball community. *American Journal of Public Health.* 2008; 98: 1074–1080

54. Choi KH, Hudes ES, Steward WT. Social discrimination, concurrent sexual partnerships, and HIV risk among men who have sex with men in Shanghai, China. *AIDS & Behavior.* 2008; 12(1): 71–77

55. Ghosn J, Thibault V, Delaugerre C, Fontaine H, Lortholary O, Rouzioux C. Sexually transmitted hepatitis c virus superinfection in HIV/hepatitis c virus co-infected men who have sex with men. *AIDS.* 2008; 22: 658–661

56. Vittinghoff E, Douglas J, Judon F, McKirnan D, MacQueen K, Buchbinder SP. Per-contact risk for human immunodeficiency virus transmission between male sexual partners. *American Journal of Epidemiology.* 1999; 150: 306–311

57. Buchacz K, Klausner JD, Kerndt PR, Shouse RL, Onorato I, McElroy PD, et al. HIV incidence among men diagnosed with early syphilis in Atlanta, San Francisco, and Los Angeles, 2005 to 2005. *Journal of Acquired Immune Deficiency Syndromes.* 2008; 47: 234–240

58. Corey L, Wald A, Celum CL, Quinn TC. The effects of herpes simples virus-2 on HIV-1 acquisition and transmission: a review of two overlapping epidemics. *Journal of Acquired Immune Deficiency Syndromes.* 2004; 35: 435–445

59. Kaul R, Pettengell C, Seth PM, Sunderji S, Biringer A, MacDonald K, et al. The genital tract immune milieu: an important determinant of HIV susceptibility and secondary transmission. *Journal of Reproductive Immunology,* 2008; 77: 32–40

60. Keele BF, Giorgi EE, Salazar-Gonzalez JF, Decker JM, Pham KT, Salazar MG, et al. Identification and characterization of transmitted and early founder virus envelopes in primary

HIV-1 infection. *Proceedings of the National Academy of Sciences of the United States of America*. 2008; 105: 7552–7557

61. Do TD, Chen S, McFarland W, Secura GM, Behel SK, MacKellar DA, et al. HIV testing patterns and unrecognized HIV infection among young Asian and Pacific Islander men who have sex with men in San Francisco. *AIDS Education and Prevention*. 2005; 17: 540–544

62. Manning SE, Thorpe LE, Ramaswamy C, Hajat A, Marx MA, Karpati AM, et al. Estimation of HIV prevalence, risk factors, and testing frequency among sexually active men who have sex with men, aged 18–64 years – New York City, 2002. *Journal of Urban Health*. 2007; 84: 212–225

63. Raymond HF, Chen S, Truong HM, Knapper KB, Klausner JD, Choi KH, et al. Trends in sexually transmitted diseases, sexual risk behavior, and HIV infection among Asian/Pacific Islander men who have sex with men, San Francisco, 1999–2005. *Sexually Transmitted Diseases*. 2007; 34: 262–264

64. Do TD, Hudes ES, Proctor K, Han CS, Choi KH. HIV testing trends and correlates among young Asian and Pacific Islander men who have sex with men in two U.S. cities. *Sexually Transmitted Diseases*. 2006; 45: 77–84

65. Chng CL, Wong FY, Park RJ, Edberg MC, Lai DS. A model for understanding sexual health among Asian American/Pacific Islander men who have sex with men (MSM) in the United States. *AIDS Education and Prevention*. 2003; 15: 21–38

66. Millett GA, Peterson JL, Wolitski R, Stall R. Greater risk for HIV infection of Black men who have sex with men: a critical literature review. *American Journal of Public Health*. 2006; 96: 1007–1019

67. Carrillo H. *The Night is Young: Sexuality in Mexico in the Time of AIDS*. University of Chicago Press: Chicago; 2001

68. Jarama SL, Kennamer JD, Poppen PJ, Hendricks M, Bradford J. Psychosocial, behavioral, and cultural predictors of sexual risk for HIV infection among Latino men who have sex with men. *AIDS & Behavior*. 2005; 9: 513–523

69. Marin BV. HIV prevention in the Hispanic community: sex, culture, and empowerment. *Journal of Transcultural Nursing*. 2003; 14: 186–192

70. Bianchi FT, Reisen CA, Zea MC, Poppen RJ, Shedlin MG, Penha NM. The sexual experiences of Latino men who have sex with men who migrated to a gay epicenter in the U.S. *Culture, Health, & Sexuality*. 2007; 9: 505–518

71. Poppen PJ, Reisen CA, Zea MC, Bianchi FT, Echeverry JJ. Serostatus disclosure, seroconcordance, partner relationship, and unprotected anal intercourse among HIV-positive Latino men who have sex with men. *AIDS Education and Prevention*. 2005; 17: 227–237

72. Zea MC, Reisen CA, Poppen RJ, Bianchi FT, Echeverry RJ. Predictors of disclosure of human immunovirus-positive serostatus among Latino gay men. *Cultural Diversity and Ethnic Minority Psychology*. 2007; 13: 304–312

73. Poppen PJ, Reisen CA, Zea MC, Bianchi FT, Echeverry JJ. Predictors of unprotected anal intercourse among HIV-positive Latino gay and bisexual men. *AIDS & Behavior*, 2004; 8: 379–389

74. Carballo-Dieguez A, Miner M, Dolezal C, Rosser BR, Jacoby S. Sexual negotiation, HIV-status disclosure, and sexual risk behavior among Latino men who use the internet to seek sex with other men. *Archives of Sexual Behavior*. 2006; 35: 463–481

75. Fernandez MI, Warren JC, Varga LM, Pardo G, Hernandez N, Bowen GS. Cruising in cyber space: Comparing internet chatroom versus community venues for recruiting Hispanic men who have sex with men to participate in prevention studies. *J Ethn Subst Abuse*. 2007; 6: 143–162

76. Warren JC, Fernandez MI, Harper GW, Hidalgo MA, Jamil OB, Torres RS. Predictors of unprotected sex among young sexually active African American, Hispanic, and White MSM: the importance of ethnicity and culture. *AIDS & Behavior*. 2008; 12: 459–468

77. Dolezal C, Carballo-Dieguez A, Nieves-Rosa L, Diaz F. Substance use and sexual risk behavior: Understanding their association among four ethnic groups of Latino men who have sex with men. *Journal of Substance Abuse*. 2000; 11: 323–336

78. Ramirez-Valles J, Garcia D, Campbell RT, Diaz RM, Heckathorn DD. HIV infection, sexual risk behavior, and substance use among Latino gay and bisexual men and transgender persons. *American Journal of Public Health*. 2000; 98: 1036–1042

79. Eaton LA, Kalichman SC, Cain DN, Cherry C, Stearns HL, Amaral CM, et al. Serosorting sexual partners and risk for HIV among men who have sex with men. *American Journal of Preventive Medicine*. 2007; 33: 479–485

80. Horvath KJ, Rosser BR, Remafedi G. Sexual risk taking among young Internet-using men who have sex with men. *American Journal of Public Health*. 2008; 98: 1059–1067

81. Berry M, Raymond HF, McFarland W. Same race and older partner selection may explain higher HIV prevalence among Black men who have sex with men. *AIDS*. 2007; 21: 249–350

82. Bingham TA, Harawa NT, Johnson DF, Secura GM, Valleroy LA. The effect of partner characteristics of HIV infection among African American men who have sex with men in the Young Men's Survey, Los Angles, 1999–2000. *AIDS Education and Prevention*. 2003; 15: 39–52

83. Choi KH, Operaio D, Gregorich SE, McFarland W, MacKellar D, Valleroy L. Age and race mixing patterns of sexual partnerships among Asian men who have sex with men: implications for HIV transmission and prevention. *AIDS Education and Prevention*. 2003; 15: 53–65

84. Mansergh G, Marks G, Colfax GN, Guzman R, Rader M, Buchbinder S. "Barebacking" in a diverse sample of men who have sex with men. *AIDS*. 2002; 16: 653–659

85. Rosser BR, Miner MH, Bockting WO, Ross MW, Konstan J, Gurak L, et al. HIV risk and the internet: results of Men's Internet sex (MINTS) study. *AIDS & Behavior*. 2008

86. Choi KH, Operaio D, Gregorich SE, McFarland W, MacKellar D, Valleroy L. Substance use, substance choice, and unprotected anal intercourse among young Asian American and Pacific Islander men who have sex with men. *AIDS Education and Prevention*. 2002; 17: 418–429

87. Berry M, Raymond HF, Kellogg T, McFarland W. The internet, HIV serosorting and transmission risk among men who have sex with men, San Francisco. *AIDS*. 2008; 30: 787–789

88. Parsons JT, Schrinshaw EW, Wolitski RJ, Halkitis PN, Purcell DW, Hoff CC, et al. Sexual harm reduction practices of HIV-seropositive gay and bisexual men: serosorting, strategic positioning, and withdrawal before ejaculation. *AIDS*. 2005; 19: S13–S25

89. Centers for Disease Control and Prevention. Use of social networks to identify persons with undiagnosed HIV infection – seven U.S. cities, October 2003–September 2004. *Morbidity and Mortality Weekly Report*. 2004; 54: 601–605

90. Adimora AA, Schoenbach VJ. Social context, sexual networks, and racial disparities in rates of sexually transmitted infections. *Journal of Infectious Diseases*. 2005; 191: 1007–1019

91. Wyatt GE, Myers HF, Williams JK, Kitchen CR, Loeb T, Carmona JV, et al. Does a history of trauma contribute to HIV risk for women of color? implications for prevention and policy. *American Journal of Public Health*. 2005; 92: 660–665

92. Wyatt GE, Myers HF, Loeb TB. Women, trauma, and HIV: an overview. *AIDS & Behavior*. 2004; 8: 401–403

93. Simoni JM, Walters KL, Balsam KF, Meyers SB. Victimization, substance use, and HIV risk behaviors among gay/bisexual/two-spirit and heterosexual American Indian men in New York City. *American Journal of Public Health*. 2006; 96: 2240–2245

94. Toro-Alfonso J, Rodriguez-Madera S. Domestic violence in Puerto Rican gay male couples: perceived prevalence, intergenerational violence, addictive behaviors, and conflict resolution skills. *Journal of Interpersonal Violence*. 2004; 19: 639–654

95. Williams JK, Wyatt E, Resell J, Peterson J, Asuan-O'Brien A. Psychosocial issues among gay- and non-gay-identifying HIV-seropositive African American and Latino MSM. *Cultural Diversity and Ethnic Minority Psychology*. 2004; 10: 268–286

96. Arreola S, Neilands TB, Pollack LM, Paul JP, Catania JA. Higher prevalence of childhood sexual abuse among Latino men who have sex with men than non-Latino men who have sex with men: data from the Urban Men's Health Study. *Child Abuse & Neglect*. 2005; 29: 285–290

97. Fields S, Malebranche D, Feist-Price S. Childhood sexual abuse in Black men who have sex with men: results from three qualitative studies. *Cultural Diversity and Ethnic Minority Psychology.* 2008; 14: 385–390

98. Fernandez MI, Bowen GS, Varga LM, Collazo JB, Hernandez N, Perrino T, et al. High rates of club drug use and risky sexual practices among Hispanic men who have sex with men in Miami, Florida. *Substance Use & Misuse.* 2005; 40: 1347–1362

99. Operario D, Choi KH, Chu PL, McFarland W, Secura GM, Behel S, et al. Prevalence and correlates of substance use among young Asian Pacific Islander men who have sex with men. *Prevention Science.* 2006; 7: 19–29

100. Diaz RM. Methamphetamine use and its relation to HIV risk: data from Latino gay men in San Francisco. In: Meyer IH, ed. *The Health of Sexual Minorities: Public Health Perspectives on Lesbian, Gay, Bisexual, and Transgender Populations.* New York: Springer, 2007, pp. 584–603

101. Huang ZJ, Wong FY, De Leon JM, Park RJ. Self-reported HIV testing behaviors among a sample of Southeast Asians in an urban setting in the United States. *AIDS Education and Prevention*, 20, 65–77

102. Akin M, Fernandez MI, Bowen GS, Warren JC. HIV risk behaviors of Latin American and Caribbean men who have sex with men in Miami, Florida, U.S. *Pan American Journal of Public Health.* 2008; 23: 341–348

103. Hutchinson C. *Comparing Stigma Management Among Men who have Sex with Men in Barbados, West Indies and the San Francisco Bay Area.* University of California at Berkeley: Berkeley, CA; 2005

104. Morin SF, Carrillo H, Steward WT, Maiorana A, Trautwein M, Gomez CA. Policy perspectives on public health for Mexican migrants in California. *Journal of Acquired Immune Deficiency Syndromes.* 2004; 37: S252–S259

105. Organista KC, Carrillo H, Ayala G. HIV prevention with Mexican migrants: review, critique, and recommendations. *Journal of Acquired Immune Deficiency Syndromes.* 2004; 37: S227–S239

106. Zaidi IF, Crepaz N, Song R, Wan CK, Lin LS, Hu DJ, et al. Epidemiology of HIV/AIDS among Asians and Pacific Islanders in the United States. *AIDS Education and Prevention.* 2005; 17: 405–417

107. Choi KH, Ning Z, Gregorich SE, Pan QC. The influence of social and sexual networks in the spread of HIV and syphilis among men who have sex with men in Shanghai, China. *Journal of Acquired Immune Deficiency Syndromes.* 2007; 45: 77–84

108. Ayala G, Chion M, Diaz RM, Heckert AL, Nuno M, del Pino HE, et al. Accion mutua (shared action): a multipronged approach to delivering capacity-building assistance to agencies serving Latino communities in the United States. *Journal of Public Health Management Practice.* 2007; 13: S33–S39

109. Nemoto T, Operario D, Keatley J, Han L, Soma T. HIV risk behaviors among male-to-female transgender persons of color in San Francisco. *American Journal of Public Health.* 2004; 94: 1193–1199

110. Operario D, Soma T, Underhill K. Sex work and HIV status among transgender women: Systematic review and meta-analysis. *Journal of Acquired Immune Deficiency Syndromes.* 2008; 48: 97–103

111. Sausa LA, Keatley J, Operario D. Perceived risks and benefits of sex work among transgender women of color in San Francisco. *Archives of Sexual Behavior.* 2008; 36: 768–777

112. Sugano E, Nemoto T, Operario D. The impact of exposure to transphobia on HIV risk behavior in a sample of transgendered women of color in San Francisco. *AIDS & Behavior.* 2006; 10: 217–225

113. Herbst JH, Jacobs ED, Finlayson TJ, McKleroy VS, Neumann MS, Crepaz N, et al. Estimating HIV prevalence and risk behaviors of transgender persons in the United States: a systematic review. *AIDS & Behavior.* 2008; 12: 1–17

114. Lawrence AA. Transgender health concerns. In: Meyer IH, Northridge ME, eds. *The Health of Sexual Minorities: Public Health Perspectives on Lesbian, Gay, Bisexual, and Transgender Populations.* New York: Springer, 2008, pp. 473–585

115. Garofalo R, Deleon J, Osmer E, Doll M, Harper GW. Overlooked, misunderstood and at-risk: exploring the lives and HIV risk of ethnic minority male-to-female transgender youth. *Journal of Adolescent Health.* 2006; 38: 230–236

116. Operario D, Nemoto T. Sexual risk behavior and substance use among a sample of Asian Pacific Islander transgendered women. *AIDS Education and Prevention.* 2005; 17: 430–433

117. Herbst JH, Beeker C, Matthew A, McNally T, Passin WF, Kay LS, et al. The effectiveness of individual-, group-, and community-level HIV behavioral risk-reduction interventions for adult men who have sex with men: a systematic review. *American Journal of Preventive Medicine.* 2007; 32: S38–S67

118. Wheeler DP, Lauby JL, Liu K, Van Sluytman LG, Murrill C. A comparative analysis of sexual risk characteristics of Black men who have sex with men or with men and women. *Archives of Sexual Behavior.* 2008; 37(5): 697–707

119. Jones KT, Gray P, Whiteside O, Wang T, Bost D, Dunbar E, Foust E, et al. Evaluation of an HIV prevention intervention adapted for Black men who have sex with men. *American Journal of Public Health.* 2008; 98: 1043–1050

120. Williams JK, Wyatt GE, Rivkin I, Ramamurthi HC, Li X, Liu H. Risk reduction for HIV-positive African American and Latino men with histories of childhood sexual abuse. *Archives of Sexual Behavior.* 2008; 37(5): 763–772

121. Centers for Disease Control and Prevention. Twenty-five years of HIV/AIDS – United States, 1981–2006. *Morbidity and Mortality Weekly Report.* 2006; 55: 585–589

122. Choi KH, Lew S, Vittinghoff E, Catania JA, Barrett DC, Coates TJ. The efficacy of brief group counseling in HIV risk reduction among homosexual Asian and Pacific Islander men. *AIDS.* 1996; 10: 81–87

123. Carballo-Dieguez A, Dolezal C, Leu CS, Nieves L, Diaz F, Decena C, et al. A random-ized controlled trial to test an HIV-prevention intervention for Latino gay and bisexual men: Lessons learned. *AIDS Care.* 2005; 17: 314–328

124. Peterson JL, Coates TJ, Catania J, Hauck WW, Acree M, Daigle D, et al. Evaluation of an HIV risk reduction intervention among African American homosexual and bisexual men. *AIDS.* 1996; 3: 319–325

125. Toro-Alfonso J, Varas-Diaz N, Andujar-Bello I. Evaluation of an HIV/AIDS prevention inter-vention targeting Latino gay men and men who have sex with men in Puerto Rico. *AIDS Education and Prevention.* 2002; 14: 445–456

126. Wallace BC. The forces driving and embodied within a new field of equity in health. In: Wallace BC, ed. *Toward Equity in Health: A New Global Approach to Health Disparities.* New York: Springer, LLC, 2008, pp. 1–40

127. Buchanan DR, Allegranate JP. What types of public health proposals should agencies be funding and what types of evidence should matter? Scientific and ethical considerations. In: Wallace BC, ed. *Toward Equity in Health: A New Global Approach to Health Disparities.* New York: Springer, LLC, 2008, pp. 81–96

128. Jones KT, Wilton L, Millett G, Johnson WD. Theoretical considerations for culturally relevant HIV prevention interventions for Black men who have sex with men (MSM): formu-lating the Black MSM stress severity and resiliency model. In: McCree D, Jones KT, O'Leary A, eds. *AIDS Among African Americans: A Community in Crisis.* New York: Springer, in press

129. Kegeles S. *A Community Level HIV Prevention Intervention for Young Black MSM.* Center for AIDS Prevention Studies: San Francisco; 2007

130. Branson BM, Handsfield HH, Lampe MA, Janssen RS, Taylor AW, Lyss SB, et al. Revised recommendations for HIV testing of adults, adolescents, and pregnant women in health care settings. *Morbidity and Mortality Weekly Report.* 2006; 55: 1–17

131. Hogben M, McNally T, McPheeters M, Hutchinson AB, & Task Force on Community Preventive Services. The effectiveness of HIV partner counseling and referral services in increasing identification of HIV-positive individuals: a systematic review. *American Journal of Preventive Medicine.* 2007; 33: S89–S100

132. Wheeler DP. Working with positive men: HIV prevention with black men who have sex with men. *AIDS Education and Prevention.* 2005; 17: 102–115

133. Wilson PA, Yoshikawa H. Improving access to health care among African American, Asian and Pacific Islander, and Latino lesbian, gay, and bisexual populations. In: Meyer IH, Northridge ME, eds. *The Health of Sexual Minorities: Public Health Perspectives on Lesbian, Gay, Bisexual, and Transgender Populations*. New York: Springer, 2007, pp. 607–637

134. Wilton L. *Experiences of Racism, Homophobia, and Discrimination in a Community Based Sample of Black Gay and Bisexual Men: Implications for HIV Prevention*. Paper presented at The Second Annual Health Disparities Conference, Teachers College, Columbia University: New York, NY; 2007, March

135. Malebranche DJ, Peterson JL, Fullilove RE, Stackhouse RW. Race and sexual identity: perceptions about medical culture and healthcare among Black men who have sex with men. *Journal of the National Medical Association*. 2004; 96: 97–107

136. Mayer KH, Mimiaga MJ, VanDerwarker R, Goldhammer H, Bradford JB. Fenway community health's model of integrated, community-based LGBT care, education, and research. In: Meyer IH, Northridge ME, eds. *The Health of Sexual Minorities: Public Health Perspectives on Lesbian, Gay, Bisexual, and Transgender Populations*. New York: Springer, 2008, pp. 693–715

137. United States Department of Health and Human Services. *Mental Health: Culture, Race, and Ethnicity – A Supplement to Mental Health: A Report of the Surgeon General*. U.S. Department of Health and Human Services: Rockville, MD; 2001

138. Greene B. Ethnic-minority lesbians and gay men: Mental health and treatment issues. *Journal of Consulting and Clinical Psychology*. 1994; 62: 243–251

139. Williams DR, Neighbors HW, Jackson JS. Racial/ethnic discrimination and health: findings from community studies. *American Journal of Public Health*. 2003; 93: 200–208

140. Mays VM, Cochran SD. Mental health correlates of perceived discrimination among lesbian, gay, and bisexual adults in the United States. *American Journal of Public Health*. 2001; 91: 1869–1876

141. Gilman SE, Cochran SD, Mays VM, Hughes M, Ostrow D, Kessler RC. Risk of psychiatric disorders among individuals reporting same-sex sexual partners in the national comorbidity survey. *American Journal of Public Health*. 2001; 91: 933–939

142. Cochran SD, Ackerman D, Mays VM, Ross MW. Prevalence of non-medical drug use and dependence among homosexually active men and women in the U.S. population. *Addiction*. 2004; 99: 989–998

143. Cochran SD, Mays VM, Alegria M, Ortega A, Takeuchi D. Mental health and substance use disorders among Latino and Asian American lesbian, gay, and bisexual adults. *Journal of Consulting and Clinical Psychology*. 2007; 75: 785–794

144. Diaz RM, Ayala G, Bein E, Henne J. The impact of homophobia, poverty, and racism on the mental health of gay and bisexual Latino men: findings from 3 U.S. cities. *American Journal of Public Health*. 2001; 91: 927–931

145. Sandfort TG, Melendez RM, Diaz RM. Gender nonconformity, homophobia, and mental distress in Latino gay and bisexual men. *Journal of Sex Research*. 2007; 44: 181–189

146. Meyer I. Prejudice and discrimination as social stressors. In: Meyer IH, Northridge ME, eds. *The Health of Sexual Minorities: Public Health Perspectives on Lesbian, Gay, Bisexual, and Transgender Populations*. New York: Springer, 2007, pp. 242–267

147. Zea MC, Reisen CA, Poppen RJ, Bianchi FT, Echeverry RJ. Disclosure of HIV status and psychological well-being among Latino gay and bisexual men. *AIDS & Behavior*. 2005; 9: 15–26

148. Peterson JL, Folkman S, Bakeman R. Stress, coping, HIV status, psychosocial resources, and depressive mood in African American gay, bisexual, and heterosexual men. *American Journal of Community Psychology*. 1996; 24: 461–487

149. Diaz R. In our own backyard: HIV/AIDS stigmatization in the Latino gay community. In: Teunis N, Herdt G, eds. *Sexual Inequalities and Social Justice*. Berkeley, CA: University of California Press, 2007, pp. 50–65

HIV Prevention and Heterosexual African American Women

Gina M. Wingood, Christina Camp, Kristin Dunkle, Hannah Cooper, and Ralph J. DiClemente

Epidemiology of HIV/AIDS Among African American Women

Early in the epidemic, HIV infection and AIDS were diagnosed among relatively few women and female adolescents. Currently, women account for more than 25% of all new HIV/AIDS diagnoses in the U.S. Heterosexually acquired HIV/AIDS is the predominant route of transmission for African American women. Among African American women diagnosed with HIV/AIDS during 2001–2004, 78% contracted the infection via heterosexual contact.[1,2] Unfortunately, African American women are being devastated by the HIV/AIDS epidemic. Thus, designing effective HIV prevention programs for this population is crucial. Theoretical frameworks are critical components of HIV prevention programs because they serve as guides for developing the core elements, vignettes, and activities of HIV prevention interventions.

Theoretical Frameworks Assessing Women's Risk of HIV

Many theories have been used to design HIV prevention interventions including Social Cognitive Theory, AIDS Risk Reduction Model, and the Information Motivation Behavior Model. One theoretical framework underlying several proven evidence-based HIV prevention efforts for African American women is the theory of Gender and Power.[3] Later we discuss the Theory of Gender and Power, and describe a research study, known as *SHAWL (the Social Health of African American Women)*, to investigate the theory's application to understanding African American women's HIV risk.

G.M. Wingood (✉)
Emory University, Rollins School of Public Health,
Department of Behavioral Sciences and Health Education, Atlanta, GA, U.S.
E-mail: gwingoo@sph.emory.edu

V. Stone et al. (eds.), *HIV/AIDS in U.S. Communities of Color*.
DOI: 10.1007/978-0-387-98152-9_11, © Springer Science + Business Media, LLC 2009

The Social Health of African American Women

To facilitate our understanding of how risk factors and exposures influence African American women's risk of HIV, the chapter authors conducted a nationally representative random-digit dial telephone household survey of 1,509 women between October 2006 and May 2007. Potential participants who self-reported being female, African American, or white, of age 20–45, and unmarried or not currently in any relationship equivalent to marriage were eligible for inclusion.

Sampling employed a dual-frame design, incorporating two selection stages without stratification in each frame. The larger frame was designed to provide coverage of the eligible population (both white and African American) on a national basis, defined as all counties with an eligible household incidence of 10% or greater; this frame included 1,096 of 3,140 counties. The second frame targeted areas containing a high density of African American women and was restricted to counties with a household incidence of African American women of 7% or greater. Within each residential household contacted, a female adult in the target age range was selected via simple random sampling, and screened for remaining eligibility criteria. Those agreeing to participate were compensated $50 for completing the assessment. A total of 1,068 interviews were completed with African American women. Analysis is currently in its initial stages. Since the aim of the study was to assess variables known to increase exposure to HIV risk among African American women, the primary study outcomes were unprotected sexual intercourse, defined as the number of times they had vaginal sex with a steady partner in the past 3 months and the number of times they used condoms during vaginal sex with a steady partner in the past 3 months. A second study outcome, having multiple sexual partners, was defined as the number of different male sexual partners (men other than the women's steady partner) a woman has had in the past 6 months. In addition to these outcome variables, a range of critical risk factor and exposure variables related to the Theory of Gender and Power were assessed.

The Theory of Gender and Power: An Overview

The theory of Gender and Power is a social structural model that attempts to understand women's risk as a function of three different interlinked structures (none of which can be independent of the others) that characterize the gendered relationships between men and women. These three structures are (1) the sexual division of labor, which examines economic inequities that favor men, (2) the sexual division of power, which examines inequities and abuses of authority and control in relationships and institutions that favor men, and (3) the structure of cathexis, which examines social norms and affective attachments.

The three structures exist at two levels, the societal and the institutional level. The societal level is the highest level in which the three social structures are embedded. The three structures are rooted in society through numerous abstract, historical, and sociopolitical forces that consistently segregate power and ascribe norms on the basis of gender-determined roles. The three structures are also evident at a lower level, the institutional level. Social institutions include, but are not limited to, families, relationships, religious institutions, the medical system, and the media. The social structures are maintained within institutions through social mechanisms such as unequal pay for comparable work, the imbalance of control within relationships, and the degrading images of women as portrayed in the media. The presence of these and other social mechanisms constrain women's daily life by producing gender-based inequities in women's economic potential, in their control of resources, and in gender-based expectations.

Each Structure Comprises Exposures and Risk Factors

The gender-based inequities and disparities in expectations that arise from each of the three structures (sexual division of labor, sexual division of power, structure of cathexis) generate different "risk factors" and "exposures" that influence women's risk for HIV. While the term *risk factor* is traditionally used to denote *any influence* that enhances risk for HIV, the theory of Gender and Power reserves this term specifically to denote intrapersonal variables that emanate from within women and influence their risk for HIV. We define *exposures* as variables that are external to women, which may influence their sexual risk behavior. Exposures include, but are not limited to, having an abusive male partner, and having limited pool of available partners. Later, we define each structure in the theory and variables assessed as part of the *SHAWL* study. We also further refine the theory of Gender and Power by bringing macrosocial factors into focus (Fig. 1). We define macrosocial factors as dimensions of "the social, economic, and political environments that shape and constrain individual, community, and societal health outcomes."[4] These factors have also been referred to as "structural determinants of health" and "contextual factors." In the theory of Gender and Power, macrosocial factors are conceptualized as a domain of exposures. Consonant with exposures within this theory, macrosocial exposures arise from the sexual division of labor, the sexual division of power, and cathexis. We bring this domain of exposures into focus here because macrosocial factors are widely posited to be potent determinants of racial/ethnic disparities in sexually transmitted HIV. To date, however, empirical investigations lag behind these propositions.

HIV-Related Factors Associated with the Sexual Division of Labor

The inequities resulting from the sexual division of labor are manifested as economic exposures and risk factors. According to the sexual division of labor, as the economic inequity between men and women increases and favors men (making

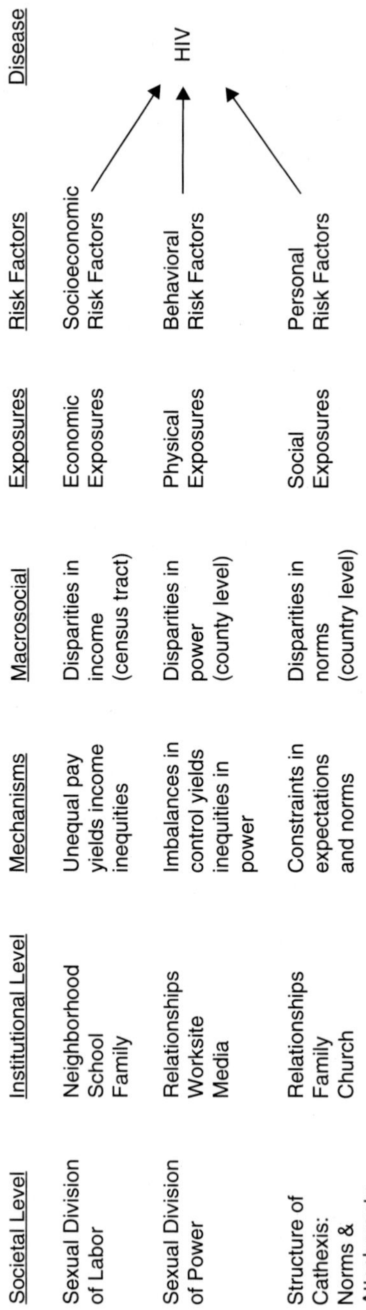

Societal Level	Institutional Level	Mechanisms	Macrosocial	Exposures	Risk Factors	Disease
Sexual Division of Labor	Neighborhood School Family	Unequal pay yields income inequities	Disparities in income (census tract)	Economic Exposures	Socioeconomic Risk Factors	HIV
Sexual Division of Power	Relationships Worksite Media	Imbalances in control yields inequities in power	Disparities in power (county level)	Physical Exposures	Behavioral Risk Factors	
Structure of Cathexis: Norms & Attachments	Relationships Family Church	Constraints in expectations and norms	Disparities in norms (country level)	Social Exposures	Personal Risk Factors	

Fig. 1 Influence of theory of Gender and Power on women's HIV risk

women more dependent on men), women will be at greater risk for HIV. Nearly 1 in 4 African Americans live in poverty.[5] Socioeconomic problems associated with poverty including having a limited education,[6] having a lower income,[7] being underemployed,[8–10] having limited access to high-quality health care,[11] consuming alcohol,[8–10, 12] and using noninjection drugs[13, 14] have all been associated with increased HIV risk behaviors among African American women. Other individual-level factors associated with African American women's risk of HIV include having personal attitudes and beliefs unsupportive of safer sex[15, 16] and having a low perceived risk of HIV infection.[17]

Thus, several of the exposures and risk factors examined as part of the *SHAWL* study included residing in a poor neighborhood, income disparities between women and their partners, being younger, unemployed, and having a limited education. Plans to elaborate exposures within the Theory of Gender and Power include intensifying efforts to explore the role of select macrosocial processes, arising from the sexual division of labor in shaping African American girls' and women's risk of HIV. These processes include local rates of poverty, wealth, high school graduation, and income inequality.

HIV-Related Factors Associated with the Sexual Division of Power

The inequities resulting from the sexual division of power are manifested as physical exposures and behavioral risk factors. According to the sexual division of power, as the power inequity between men and women increases and favors men, women's sexual choices and behavior may be constrained enhancing their risk for HIV. Numerous studies have demonstrated that having poor communication skills,[8–10, 16] having a male partner who abuses drugs or alcohol,[18, 19] having a sexually[20] and/or physically abusive male partner,[21, 22] having a male partner who disapproves of practicing safer sex,[8–10] and having an older male partner[23] all significantly increase African American women's HIV risk.

Thus, several of the exposures and risk factors examined as part of the *SHAWL* study included, but not be limited to, partner-related and institutional factors, such as having a sexually, emotionally, or physically abusive partner, having an older partner, having a partner who has concurrent partners, having a partner who has had male sexual partners, and having a partner who has had a history of incarceration. In addition to the partner-related exposures, experiences of racial and gender discrimination were assessed as well as HIV-associated behavioral risk factors such as binge drinking, drug use practices, and assertive communication self-efficacy. Plans to refine the Theory of Gender and Power include incorporating macrosocial processes that arise from and capture the sexual division of power, such as, local male to female sex ratios among African Americans, rates of violence against women (both sexual and domestic), and rates of racially motivated hate crimes.

HIV-Related Exposures and Risk Factors Associated with the Structure of Cathexis

The inequities resulting from the structure of cathexis (i.e., social norms and affective attachments) are manifested as social exposures and as personal risk factors. According to the structure of cathexis, women who are more accepting of conventional social norms and beliefs will be at greater risk of HIV. Exposures examined as part of the *SHAWL* study included, but were not limited to, having an older partner, having a partner who desires a pregnancy, having a limited partner pool, being in a long-term relationship, and risk factors such as possessing conservative or traditional gender norms, and perceived stigma associated with various sexual experiences (e.g., asking partner for a condom, asking doctor to conduct an STD exam) was assessed. Plans to refine the Theory of Gender and Power include incorporating macrosocial processes that arise from and capture social norms and affective attachments, including local marriage rates and rates of religious congregation membership among African American adults.

The Theory of Gender and Power is the underlying theoretical framework to several evidence-based HIV interventions. We will now describe several of these evidence-based interventions, and illustrate the application of the theory when it was applied.

HIV Prevention Interventions for Heterosexual African American Women

To reduce African American women's vulnerability to HIV, the examination of risk factors and exposures associated with women's HIV risk must be accompanied by effective behavioral prevention efforts. Since 2000, the Centers for Disease Control and Prevention (CDC) has identified a number of HIV interventions with proven evidence of effectiveness that have been designed, implemented, and evaluated with predominantly African American women.[24] This chapter will focus on five HIV prevention intervention studies that have been conducted since 2000. All of these trials included at least 70% African American women in the sample and used a randomized controlled trial with at least a 6-month follow-up to evaluate the efficacy of the intervention. HIV prevention studies that apply the Theory of Gender and Power articulate the manner in which the intervention applied this theoretical framework.

In 2002, Ehrhardt[25] et al. published a study that assessed the short- and long-term effects of a gender-specific group intervention for women on unsafe sexual encounters and strategies for protection against HIV/STD infection. Family planning clients ($N = 360$) from a high HIV seroprevalence area in New York City were randomized to an eight-session intervention, a four-session intervention, or a control condition and followed at 1, 6, and 12 months postintervention. This gender-specific intervention was designed to decrease unsafe sexual practices among women. It was based on the AIDS Risk Reduction Model, which was modified to enhance its gender-specificity. The eight- and four-session interventions shared the same format, consisting of 2 hour, small group sessions. The four-session version of the intervention was developed with the objective of making it as similar to the longer version as possible except for the time spent on the group exercises. The following sequence of topics was covered in each intervention, with one topic per session in the longer intervention and two topics per session in the shorter version:[1] Why should I care about getting STDs and HIV?;[2] How do I avoid partners who do not care?;[3] What is the best way to protect myself?;[4] How can I find out if we are infected?;[5] How do I ask my partner to use protection?;[6] How do I influence my partner to use protection?;[7] How do I refuse sex or unprotected sex?; and[8] How do I continue protecting myself and others?

Using an intention-to-treat analysis, women who were assigned to the eight-session group had about twice the odds of reporting decreased or no unprotected vaginal and anal intercourse compared with controls at 1 month (OR = 1.93, 95% confidence interval [CI] = 1.07, 3.48, $P = 0.03$) and at 12-month follow-up (OR = 1.65, 95% CI = 0.94, 2.90, $P = 0.08$). Relative to controls, women assigned to the eight-session condition reported during the previous month approximately three-and-a-half ($P = 0.09$) and five ($P < 0.01$) fewer unprotected sex occasions at 1- and 12-month follow-up, respectively. Women in the eight-session group also reduced the number of sex occasions at both follow-ups and had a greater odds of first-time use of an alternative protective strategy (refusal, mutual testing) at 1-month follow-up. Results for the four-session group were in the expected direction but overall were inconclusive. Thus, gender-specific interventions of sufficient intensity can promote short- and long-term sexual risk reduction among women in a family planning setting.

In 2003, Sterk et al. published a study to evaluate the effectiveness of an HIV intervention for African American women who use crack cocaine.[26] Two-hundred sixty-five women (aged 18–59 years) were randomly assigned to a four-session enhanced motivation condition, a four-session enhanced negotiation intervention, or to the National Institute on Drug Abuse standard condition (which emphasizes epidemiology of the local HIV epidemic, HIV knowledge, and HIV risk and preventive behaviors). The enhanced intervention conditions were conducted in individual sessions; the theory of Gender and Power was one of the theoretical frameworks used in this study; however, it was unclear how the theory was applied.

Session 1 of the motivation condition emphasized the local HIV epidemic, sex and drug-related risk behaviors, HIV risk reduction strategies, and the impact of race and gender on HIV risk and protective factors. The session ended with the request to the participant to consider why she would be motivated to change her life. *Session 2* commenced by reviewing the participant's change list, and short- as well as long-term goals were discussed. Following this discussion, short-term goals for behavior change were set. *Session 3* addressed the participant's experiences with the intended short-term behavioral change, including her sense of control and feelings of ambivalence. *Session 4* reviewed the prior session and introduced the delivery of risk reduction messages tailored to the participant's level of readiness for change.

Session 1 of the enhanced negotiation condition was similar to that described for the motivation condition. However, the session ended with a specific skills-training component of condom use and safe injection, and intended behavioral changes were discussed. In *Session 2*, the list of possible behavioral changes and the level of control were reviewed and general communication skills and strategies to develop assertiveness were discussed. Following this discussion, short-term goals for communication, gaining control, and developing assertiveness were set. *Session 3* introduced the negotiation and conflict strategies. *Session 4* was built on the previous sessions, including the development of tailored negotiation and conflict resolution styles.

A substantial proportion of women reported no past 30-day crack use at 6-month follow-up (100%–61%, $P < 0.001$). Significant ($P < .05$) decreases in the frequency of crack use; the number of paying partners; the number of times vaginal, oral, or anal sex was had with a paying partner; and sexual risks, such as trading sex for drugs were reported over time. Significant ($P < 0.05$) increases in male condom use with sex partners were observed, as well as decreases in casual partners' refusal of condoms. Findings suggest that combined components of the culturally appropriate, gender-tailored intervention may be most effective at enhancing preventive behavior among similar populations.

In 2004, Wechsberg et al. published the results of a randomized, three-arm trial for out-of-drug treatment African American women who used crack ($N = 620$), and women were assessed at 3- and 6-months follow-up.[27] Participants were randomized to one of the three arms: a woman-focused HIV intervention for crack abusers, a revised National Institute on Drug Abuse standard intervention, and a control group. The woman-focused intervention addressed drug dependence as a form of "bondage" and was designed to facilitate greater independence and increase personal power and control over behavior choices as well as life circumstances. The intervention contained psychoeducational information and skills training on reducing HIV risk and drug use, presented within the context of African American women's lives in the inner city, where pervasive poverty and violence limit women's options and increase the likelihood of poor (i.e., high-risk) behavior choices.

All the three groups reported significant reductions in the proportion of women having any unprotected sex in the past 30 days between baseline and 3- and 6-month follow-up. Although the woman-focused group demonstrated greater reductions in unprotected sex than the standard-NIDA intervention and control groups at 3 months, these results were not statistically significant at the 0.05 level. However, at 6 months, this trend was statistically significant relative to controls, with fewer woman-focused group participants reporting any unprotected sex in the past 30 days (odds ratio [OR] = 0.62, $P = 0.03$). All study conditions demonstrated significant reductions in the proportion of women reporting trading sex for money or drugs in the past 30 days between baseline and 3- and 6-month follow-up. Both intervention groups showed significant reductions in the percentage of women who traded sex compared with control subjects, with the standard-R group (OR = 0.48, $P = 0.007$) having slightly stronger effects than the woman-focused group (OR = 0.58, $P = 0.046$) at 3-month follow-up. At 6 months, these trends in reduction continued, although they were not statistically significant. At 3 months, the odds of being homeless were the lowest in the woman-focused group (OR $= 0.35$, $P = 0.0002$). In multiple logistic regression analysis controlling for full-time employment at baseline, the odds of being employed full time at 3 months were significantly higher in the woman-focused group relative to both controls (OR $= 2.53$; $P = 0.0027$) and the standard-R group (OR $= 2.02$, $P = 0.0175$). The study concluded that a woman-focused intervention can successfully reduce risk and facilitate employment and housing and may effectively reduce the frequency of unprotected sex in the longer term.

In 2004, Drs. Wingood and DiClemente published a randomized controlled trial of the *WILLOW* (Women Involved In Life Learning from Other Women) intervention, which included 366 women living with HIV in Alabama and Georgia.[32] Participants were randomized to either a four-session intervention condition or a four-session comparison condition that focused on adherence and nutrition for women living with HIV. The Theory of Gender and Power was applied in *WILLOW* and application of the theory highlighted social conditions prevalent in the lives of women living with HIV such as having limited practical support (i.e., money for food, childcare), having violent domestic partners, being stigmatized as an HIV transmitter, receiving limited social support from kin and nonkin, and communicating nonassertively about safer sex. *Session 1* of the four-session intervention emphasized gender pride by discussing the joys and challenges of being a woman and by acknowledging the accomplishments of women in society. This session also sought to assist women in identifying people in their social network who have provided social support and in recognizing the essential qualities of supportive network members. *Session 2* discussed ways of maintaining supportive network members, encouraged women to seek new network members, and informed participants about how to disengage from network members who were not supportive of healthy behaviors. Peer educators emphasized that social support could be requested without having to disclose their serostatus. *Session 3* enhanced awareness of HIV transmission risk behaviors and debunked common myths regarding HIV prevention for people living with HIV ("If both partners are HIV positive it is OK to have unprotected sex"). This session also taught participants communication skills for negotiating safer sex, reinforced the benefits of using condoms consistently, and peer educators modeled proper condom use skills. *Session 4* taught women to distinguish between healthy and unhealthy relationships, discussed the impact of abusive partners on safer sex, and informed women of local shelters for women in abusive relationships.

Over the 12-month follow-up, women in the *WILLOW* intervention, relative to the comparison group, reported fewer episodes of unprotected vaginal intercourse (1.8 vs. 2.5; $P = 0.022$), were less likely to report never using condoms (OR $= 0.27$; $P = 0.008$), had a lower incidence of bacterial infections (chlamydia and gonorrhea) (OR $= 0.19$; $P = 0.006$), and reported higher HIV knowledge and condom use self-efficacy. In addition, the intervention reported more network members (biologically related kin or nonkin who provide social support), fewer beliefs that condoms interfere with sex, fewer partner-related barriers to condom use, and demonstrated greater skill in using condoms. This is the first trial to demonstrate reductions in risky sexual behavior, incident bacterial STDs, and enhanced HIV-preventive psychosocial and structural factors among women living with HIV.

In 2004, Drs. DiClemente and Wingood published the results of a randomized, two-arm, single blind, controlled trial of sexually experienced African American females ($N = 522$), 14–18 years of age, conducted at a family medicine clinic.[28] Participants in this study, known as *SIHLE* (*Sistas, Informing Healing, Living and Empowering*), completed a self-administered survey and a personal interview, demonstrated condom application skills, and provided vaginal swab specimens for STD testing at baseline and at 6- and 12-months postintervention. The Theory of Gender and Power[3] is one of the theoretical frameworks guiding the design and implementation of the SIHLE intervention. *Session 1* activities were created to highlight HIV-related social processes prevalent in the lives of African American female adolescents. Through the examination of poetry written by African American women, discussion of challenges and joys of being an African American female, exposure to artwork from African American women, identifying African American role models, and prioritizing personal values participants were empowered to raise their expectations of what it is to be a woman cognizant of her sexuality regardless of how society may view them. Also this session stressed the importance of completing educational requirements, developing career goals, and writing effective professional resumes, and it was designed to be economically empowering. *Session 2* focused on providing information about STDs and HIV, including a discussion of behaviors that put them at risk for the diseases, and how the diseases can affect their goals and dreams. Correct condom skills were introduced as a means of lowering STD risk. Finally, participants discussed how "triggers" (e.g., having an older partner, gang involvement, sexually degrading media) could increase adolescents' HIV risk. *Session 3* provided the young women with the skills to properly use condoms and refuse risky sex. Through role-plays, women also learned how to eroticize condom use to develop their positive attitudes toward using condoms and enhance their male partner's acceptance of condom use. *Session 4* commenced by distinguishing healthy from unhealthy relationships and defining the words "abuse" and "respect." Subsequently, adolescents were taught coping skills to more effectively handle a verbally abusive or physically abusive partner. Participants were also taught coping skills to more effectively handle abuse that may occur as a consequence of introducing HIV/STD prevention practices (i.e., condom use) into the relationship.

Using population-averaged generalized estimating equations (GEE) analyses for the entire 12-month follow-up period, adolescents in the intervention, in contrast to the comparison group, were nearly twice as likely to report using condoms consistently in the 30 days preceding assessments (OR = 1.97; 95% CI = 1.25, 3.10; $P = 0.004$) and were more than twice as likely to report using condoms consistently in the 6 months preceding assessments (OR = 2.28; 95% CI = 1.50, 3.47; $P = 0.0001$). Adolescents in the HIV intervention also had a lower incidence of laboratory-confirmed chlamydia (OR = 0.17; 95% CI = 0.03, 0.93;

$P = 0.04$). Additionally, adolescents in the HIV intervention also had higher scores on measures of psychosocial mediators of HIV-preventive behaviors.

Disseminating HIV Prevention Interventions for African American Women

While the design, implementation, and evaluation of HIV prevention interventions for African American women is important, perhaps even more critical is the dissemination of these studies. In 2001, the Institute of Medicine published a report recommending that public health agencies use evidence-based HIV prevention interventions.[29] In accordance with the report, the CDC requires CDC-funded agencies, health-departments, and community-based agencies interested in implementing HIV prevention efforts to use evidence-based HIV behavioral interventions. Through CDC's Diffusion of Evidence-Based Intervention (DEBI) program, nationally, more than 650 agencies have received training in *SISTA*,[30] an evidence-based HIV prevention program for African American women.[31] In 1999, *SISTA* was cited as an evidence-based HIV intervention and published in the CDC's Compendium of HIV Prevention Interventions with Evidence of Effectiveness.[32] *SISTA* was a randomized controlled trial in which participants were randomized to a five-session intervention, a delayed control, or no HIV education condition. The theory of Gender and Power was the underlying theoretical framework for *SISTA*. The five-session intervention condition emphasized ethnic and gender pride, HIV risk-reduction information, sexual assertiveness and communication skills, proper condom use skills, and developing norms supportive of safer sex. Despite the delayed HIV education and control conditions, women in the intervention demonstrated increased consistent condom use, greater sexual communication, greater sexual assertiveness, and increased partner norms supportive of consistent condom use.

Agencies seeking certification in implementing *SISTA* can send two staff members to participate in a weeklong training. The 1-week *SISTA* training program is known as the *SISTA* Institute. Trainees in the *SISTA* Institute are provided training on the theoretical frameworks, core elements, intervention activities, and evaluation methods that comprise *SISTA*. Trainees graduating from the *SISTA* Institute are certified to implement this intervention. A technical assistance program has been created to provide additional training and address questions and concerns that may arise during the implementation of *SISTA* in the trainees' local communities. Individuals, who have been certified to implement *SISTA* through the *SISTA* Institute, are eligible to receive a 1-week training and certification to implement a newly published evidence-based HIV prevention program for African American female adolescents described earlier in this manuscript, known as *SIHLE*[28] and an evidence-based HIV intervention for women living with HIV, also described earlier in this manuscript, known as *WILLOW*.[33] All the three programs, *SISTA*, *SIHLE*, and *WILLOW*, target African American females and are designed to reduce HIV sexual risk behaviors and share similar theoretical, core, and methodological elements. Given their similarities, these programs are being promoted as a suite of HIV interventions for African American women. In an effort to accommodate and expand the intervention suite to new and emerging subpopulations of African American women, the designers of the suite (Drs. Gina Wingood and Ralph DiClemente) have tailored and are evaluating the efficacy of several of the interventions within this suite for use with other subgroups of African American women (i.e., female adolescents attending STD clinics, and young adult women receiving care at health maintenance organizations). Moreover, in an attempt to reach women across the African Diaspora the original researchers are currently adapting and evaluating the efficacy of interventions within the suite for use with women in sub-Saharan Africa and the Caribbean. In an era when fiscal and human resources are severely constrained by competing public health priorities, it would be cost- and time-prohibitive for many public and private sector agencies to develop and evaluate a new program for each subgroup for which they desire to administer an HIV prevention program. Perhaps, promoting clusters of technological innovations, such as an HIV intervention suite, may serve to facilitate adoption and diffusion of evidence-based HIV prevention programs.

Future Directions

While notable research, programs, and services designed to reduce HIV risk among African American women have been developed, public health researchers must expand their agenda. Among the new and emerging issues there is a need to:

1. Explore effective ways to design and implement social structural interventions, such as conducting interventions within faith-based communities to reduce African American women's risk of HIV.
2. Explore how combining behavioral interventions and biomedical interventions can be designed to reduce African American women's HIV risk.
3. Explore how effective primary and secondary HIV prevention interventions for women can be more widely disseminated to African American women at greatest risk.
4. Explore ways to design cost-effective HIV prevention interventions for African American women that can reduce risky sexual practices, as well as biological outcomes such as sexually transmitted infections.
5. Explore alternative formats for conducting and disseminating HIV interventions, such as the use of interactive multimedia.
6. Explore the role of macrosocial factors in shaping African American women's risk of HIV, identify effective interventions to reduce related vulnerabilities, and amplify resilience. Creating a new and expanded agenda to reduce and even halt the feminization of the HIV epidemic needs to be a public health priority. However, prior to creating a new agenda an assessment of the lessons learned from our current prevention efforts conducted among women is required. Several meta-analyses and reviews of HIV prevention programs conducted among

women have demonstrated that HIV prevention programs with African American women are effective. However, without a new vision and forward foresight the HIV epidemic will continue its devastating toll on the health of African American women nationally.

References

1. Centers for Disease Control & Prevention. Trends in HIV/AIDS diagnoses – 33 states, 2001–2004. *Morbidity & Mortality Weekly Report*, 2005; 54, 1149–1153
2. Centers for Disease Control & Prevention. HIV/AIDS Surveillance Report, 2004. Atlanta, GA: *U.S. Department of Health & Human Services*, 2005; vol. 16, pp. 1–46
3. Wingood GM, DiClemente RJ. Application of the theory of gender and power to examine HIV-related exposures, risk factors, and effective interventions for women. *Health Education & Behavior*, 2001; 27, 539–565
4. Blankenship KM, Bray SJ, Merson MH. Structural interventions in public health. *AIDS*, 2000; 4: S11–S21
5. U.S. Census Bureau. *Poverty: 1999. Census 2000 Brief*. Issued May 2003
6. Anderson JE, Brackbill R, Mosher WD. Condom use for disease prevention among unmarried U.S. women. *Family Planning Perspectives*, 1996; 28, 25–28
7. Peterson JL, Grinstead OA, Golden E, Catania JA, Kegeles S, Coates TJ. Correlates of HIV risk behaviors in black and white San Francisco heterosexuals: the population-based AIDS in multiethnic neighborhoods (AMEN) study. *Ethnicity & Disease*, 1992; 2, 361–370
8. Wingood GM, DiClemente RJ. Relationship characteristics associated with noncondom use among young adult African American women. *American Journal of Community Psychology*, 1998; 26, 29–53
9. Wingood GM, DiClemente RJ. The influence of psychosocial factors, alcohol, drug use on African American women's high-risk sexual behavior. *American Journal of Preventive Medicine*, 1998; 15, 54–59
10. Wingood GM, DiClemente RJ. Partner influences and gender-related factors associated with noncondom use among young adult African American women. *American Journal of Community Psychology*, 1998; 26, 29–51
11. Diaz T, Chu SY, Buehler JW, et al. Socioeconomic differences among people with AIDS: results from a multistate surveillance project. *American Journal of Preventive Medicine*, 1994; 10, 217–222
12. Graves KL, Hines AM. Ethnic differences in the association between alcohol and risky sexual behavior with a new partner: an event-based analysis. *AIDS Education and Prevention*, 1997; 9, 219–237
13. Fullilove R, Fullilove M, Bowser B, et al. Risk of sexually transmitted disease among black adolescent crack users in Oakland and San Francisco, Calif. *Journal of the American Medical Association*, 1990; 263, 851–855
14. Edlin BR, Erwin KL, Faruque S, et al. Intersecting epidemics: crack cocaine use and HIV infection among inner city young adults. Multicenter Crack Cocaine and HIV Infection Study Team. *New England Journal of Medicine*, 1994; 24, 1422–1427
15. Jemmott JB, Jemmott LS, Spears H, Hewitt N, Cruz-Collins M. Self-efficacy, hedonistic expectancies, and condom-use intentions among inner-city black adolescent women: a social cognitive approach to AIDS risk behavior. *Journal of Adolescent Health*, 1992; 13, 512–519
16. Catania JA, Coates TJ, Kegeles S, et al. Condom use in multi-ethnic neighborhoods of San Francisco: the population-based AMEN (AIDS in multi-ethnic neighborhoods) study. *American Journal of Public Health*, 1992; 82, 284–287
17. Nyamathi A, Bennett C, Leake B, Lewis C, Flaskerud J. AIDS-Related knowledge, perceptions, and behaviors among impoverished minority women. *American Journal of Public Health*, 1993; 83, 65–71

18. Sterk C. *Fast Lives: Women Who Use Crack Cocaine*. Philadelphia, PA: Temple University Press; 1999

19. Sterk CE. *Tricking and Tripping: Prostitution in the Era of AIDS*. Putnam Valley, NY: Social Change Press; 2000

20. Wyatt GE. The sociocultural context of African American and White American women's rape. *Journal of Social Issue*, 1992; 48, 77–91

21. Wingood GM, DiClemente RJ. The effects of an abusive primary partner on the condom use and sexual negotiation practices of African American women. *American Journal of Public Health*, 1997; 87, 1016–1018

22. Wingood GM, DiClemente RJ, Hubbard McCree D, Harrington K, Davies S. Dating Violence and African American Adolescent Females' Sexual Health. *Pediatrics*, 2001; 107, E72

23. Miller K, Clark L, Moore JS. Heterosexual risk for HIV among female adolescents: sexual initiation with older male partners. *Family Planning Perspectives*, 1997; 29, 212–214

24. Lyles CM, Kay LS, Crepaz N, et al. Best-Evidence Interventions: Findings from a systematic review of HIV behavioral interventions for U.S. populations at high risk, 2000–2004. *American Journal of Public Health*, 2007; 97, 133–143

25. Ehrhardt AA, Exner TM, Hoffman S, et al. A gender-specific HIV/STD risk reduction intervention for women in a health care setting: short- and long-term results of a randomized clinical trial. *AIDS Care*, 2002; 14, 147–161

26. Sterk CE, Theall KP, Elifson KW. Effectiveness of a risk reduction intervention among African American women who use crack cocaine. *AIDS Education & Prevention*, 2003; 15, 15–32

27. Wechsberg WM, Lam WK, Zule WA, Bobashev G. Efficacy of a woman-focused intervention to reduce HIV risk and increase self-sufficiency among African American crack abusers. *American Journal of Public Health*, 2004; 94, 1165–1173

28. DiClemente RJ, Wingood GM, Harrington KF, et al. Efficacy of an HIV prevention intervention for African American adolescent girls: a randomized controlled trial. *Journal of the American Medical Association*, 2004; 292, 171–179

29. Institute of Medicine. *Report Brief. No Time to Lose: Getting the Most From HIV Prevention*. Washington, DC: National Academies Press; 2001. Available at http://www.iom.edu

30. Prather C. Personal communications regarding progress of CDC disseminating SiSTA, 2005

31. DiClemente RJ, Wingood GM. A randomized controlled social skills trial: An HIV sexual risk-reduction intervention among young adult African American women. *Journal of the American Medical Association*, 1995; 274, 1271–1276

32. Centers for Disease Control & Prevention. HIV/AIDS Prevention Research Synthesis Project. Compendium of HIV Prevention Interventions with Evidence of Effectiveness. 1999

33. Wingood GM, DiClemente RJ, Mikhail I, et al. A randomized controlled trial to reduce HIV transmission risk behaviors and STDs among women living with HIV: The WILLOW Program. *Journal of Acquired Immune Deficiency Syndromes*, 1992; 37, S58–S67

Substance Abuse, HIV, and Mental Health Issues: Prevention and Treatment Challenges

Dionne J. Jones and George W. Roberts

Introduction

Two decades of research has established a link between substance abuse and HIV/AIDS, often referred to as the twin epidemics.[1,2] Additionally, substance abuse and mental disorders are often co-occurring conditions;[3] persons with substance use disorders are at elevated risk for mental health disorders and vice versa. People infected with HIV/AIDS and having co-occurring mental health and substance abuse disorders face enormous difficulty in accessing treatment and they often fail to receive adequate treatment for one or more of their illnesses.[4] People with triple diagnoses (substance abuse, mental health disorders, and HIV) represent a growing challenge to health care service providers. This is even more tenuous for racial/ethnic minorities who are disproportionately represented and impacted by these diseases.

This chapter presents data on the prevalence of drug use, mental illness, and HIV/AIDS among racial/ethnic minorities; addresses the link between substance abuse and HIV/AIDS; the link between mental disorder and HIV; and examines the effectiveness of HIV risk reduction strategies for drug-using populations. Further, the chapter discusses mental health issues and the needs of HIV-positive substance abusers and sets forth optimal management strategies for engaging the dually and triply diagnosed in treatment. Focus will be placed on racial/ethnic minorities, particularly African Americans, where appropriate.

D.J. Jones (✉)
Services Research Branch, Division of Epidemiology, Services & Prevention Research, National Institute on Drug Abuse, Bethesda, MD, U.S.
E-mail: djones1@nida.nih.gov

V. Stone et al. (eds.), *HIV/AIDS in U.S. Communities of Color*.
DOI: 10.1007/978-0-387-98152-9_12, © Springer Science + Business Media, LLC 2009

Prevalence of Drug Use, Mental Illness, and HIV/AIDS

There is diversity of drug use across racial and ethnic minority groups; the groups are not homogeneous. For instance, African Americans have lower prevalence rates of both licit and illicit substances during their early years compared with other racial/ethnic groups.[5] However, use by African Americans increases in late adolescence and escalates in adulthood.[5] An explanation of this complex dynamic is that family support, peer nonuse, and social skills in childhood may serve as protective factors for African American youth.[5] Hispanic youth start to use drugs earlier than others, but drop off in later adolescence at a rate similar to that of whites. The consequences of drug abuse and addiction disproportionately affect minority populations. For example, African Americans represent 13% of the U.S. population, but about one-half of new HIV/AIDS diagnoses in 33 states with long-term confidential name-based HIV reporting in 2005.[6] Similarly, with regard to the criminal justice system, African Americans represented 30% of local jail inmates, 42% of federal inmates incarcerated for a drug offense, 30% of persons on probation (drug offenses accounted for one-quarter of probation offenses), and 41% of parolees.[7]

Injection drug use has been a significant factor in HIV transmission since the beginning of the U.S. epidemic, accounting for slightly more than one-third (36%) of AIDS cases.[8] Although there have been sharp declines in the proportion of injection drug users (IDUs) with HIV/AIDS,[9] there is still a strong association between injection drug use and HIV transmission and acquisition among African Americans and men. In 2006, an estimated 36,817 new HIV/AIDS cases were diagnosed in 33 states with HIV reporting and 4,728 (12.8%) cases were attributed to injection drug use: 3,016 cases for males and 1,712 cases for females. African Americans accounted for 47.1% of all HIV/AIDS cases diagnosed in 2006, while Hispanics accounted for 29.2%.[10]

As of 2006, a total of 491,727 persons were living with HIV/AIDS in the 33 states based on confidential name-based HIV infection reporting. Injection drug use was a reported exposure mode for 92,547 (18.8%) of these persons with HIV/AIDS. African Americans and Hispanics accounted for 76.2% of all IDUs living with HIV/AIDS (54.5% and 21.6%, respectively) at the end of 2006. Injection drug use was a reported mode of exposure for 31,339 African American males and 19,136 African American females, and for 14,472 Hispanic males and 5,528 Hispanic females.[10]

High-risk heterosexual contact was the most frequently reported mode of transmission of HIV/AIDS among African American and Hispanic women in 2006 (44% and 52%, respectively). This category includes sex with an IDU or a bisexual male. Risk factors not reported or identified for HIV/AIDS cases reported in 2006 were equally high, representing 43% for African American women and 33% for Hispanic women.[10]

Given the significant numbers of IDUs who are living with HIV/AIDS, and the large numbers of African Americans and Hispanics who are exposed to HIV through injection drug use, comprehensive prevention services are needed for this population. As shown earlier, African American and Hispanic women are infected most often through high-risk heterosexual contact. Most preventive interventions have shown greater effects for reducing injection use rather than sexual risks, even though IDUs can transmit HIV through both behaviors.[11] Therefore, intensive research efforts should focus on developing risk reduction strategies that are effective for African American and Hispanic men and women who are at risk of acquiring and transmitting HIV through both sexual and injecting behaviors.

Mental illness is often associated with the acquisition, progression, and treatment of HIV/AIDS.[12–15] While there are no national estimates of the prevalence of mental disorders among people living with HIV, researchers have documented high rates of mental illness in HIV patients receiving medical care. For example, Bing et al. reported that 48% of adults in the HIV Cost and Services Utilization Study (HCSUS) were screened positively for a mental disorder.[16] Researchers at the University of Washington in Seattle also found that nearly 63% of the HIV-infected patients enrolled in their clinic were diagnosed with a mental disorder.[17] Using the Structured Clinical Interview for DSM-IV Disorders (SCID), Whetten et al. found that the most prevalent mental disorders among a largely African American sample of patients in North Carolina included major depression (58%), borderline personality disorder (38%), antisocial personality disorders (35%), and posttraumatic stress disorder (30%).[18]

A recent national estimate found that major depression is the most prevalent lifetime mental disorder.[19] Depression is also the most common mental disorder associated with HIV/AIDS. Studies have shown higher rates of lifetime and current depression among people living with HIV than among the general population.[20,21] Using national HCUS data, two studies reported rates of depression in 36% and 37%, respectively, of patients receiving medical care.[16,20] Depression is associated with factors such as trauma, childhood sexual abuse, and substance use, all of which can contribute to HIV risk.[14,22,23] Depression also has been found to be prevalent in certain groups such as African Americans, women, gay men, and substance users, who may be at greater risk for HIV transmission.[17,18,24–26]

Link Between Substance Abuse and HIV

Defining Terms

Drug use refers to casual or recreational use of drugs for pleasure and to feel good, or out of curiosity and through peer pressure. Drugs may also be used to enhance or improve athletic or cognitive performance.[3] Although drug users believe that they are in control of their use, many find this not to be the case as the drugs take over their lives. *Drug abuse* occurs when users continue to take the drug although they are aware that its use results in negative consequences for themselves and others. *Drug tolerance* is the most common response to repetitive use of the same drug and can be defined as the reduction in response to the drug after repeated administrations.[27]

Drug addiction is a chronic, relapsing brain disease. It is characterized by compulsive drug seeking and use, in spite of harmful consequences.[3] Drugs change the structure of the brain and the way it works – this is why addiction is considered a brain disease. Changes in the brain can be long-lasting and lead to harmful behaviors.[3]

Effects of Drugs on the Brain

Drugs target the brain's reward system by releasing dopamine, a neurotransmitter present in regions of the brain responsible for regulating movement, emotion, cognition, motivation, and feelings of pleasure.[3] When this system, which rewards our natural behavior, is overstimulated, it results in euphoria that drug abusers continually seek. Over time, drug abuse can lead to changes in neurons and brain circuits resulting in a reduction in the experience of pleasure; this leads the abuser to seek the drugs in larger quantities to experience the dopamine high.[28] Long-term exposure to drugs of abuse also impairs cognitive functioning and reduces control over behavior, which could lead to risky sexual behaviors. Risky sexual behaviors such as having multiple sex partners or not using condoms expose users to sexually transmitted infections including HIV/AIDS.

Drug Abuse Trajectories Among Minorities and High-Risk Behaviors

Drug abuse is a complex issue; it is the result of an interaction of multiple factors. Some factors related to substance abuse are personal (sensation seeking, impulsivity, depressive symptoms, low self-esteem),[29] familial (social support, monitoring),[30] relational (risk-taking partner, abusive, dating violence),[31] and environmental (drug availability, poverty, crime).[32]

Studies have shown an association between drug and alcohol use, partner violence, and sexually risky behaviors.[31,33] Women with multiple partners in the past 12 months and women who reported injecting drugs were significantly more likely to indicate having experienced a severe form of sexual intimate partner violence in the past 6 months.[31] Among a racially diverse sample of 152 adults (58% white, 27% black, 11% Hispanic, and 4% mixed/other) with serious mental illness receiving community mental health services, 70% reported childhood physical and/or sexual abuse and 32% reported both types of abuse.[33] An association was found between childhood abuse and HIV risk through drug abuse and adult victimization.[33] HIV interventions for persons with childhood abuse histories should include a component to address the trauma as well as the sexual risk behaviors.

Singer et al. used syndemic theory to understand the social and cultural contexts of African American and Hispanic heterosexual young adults in Hartford, CT in order to explain their high rates of sexually transmitted diseases.[34] Syndemic theory helps explain how multiple epidemics interact and develop under conditions of health and social disparity. That is, diseases and other health problems (e.g., malnutrition) often develop as a result of adverse social conditions (e.g., poverty, stigmatization, oppressive social relationships) that contribute to high-risk behavior. Their study led these researchers to conclude that the young adults in their sample used a "cultural logic" of risk assessment that is based on their experiences growing up in the inner city, which put them at high risk for STDs.[34] For example, the youth cited key features of their psychosocial life experiences that shaped their views, attitudes, and behaviors, such as coming of age, living in a broken home, experiencing domestic violence, having limited expectations about one's future, and having lack of expectation about living a long life, among others.[34] Interventions designed to deter early engagement in risky sexual behaviors and/or drug use, or to stop such behaviors or prevent relapse must, therefore, consider sociocultural and other related factors in their design and development.

Link Between Mental Disorders and HIV

Depression, anxiety, and severe mental illness (SMI) are most frequently diagnosed among HIV-infected persons.[17, 18, 35] Because depression may mimic or exacerbate somatic symptoms in chronic medical conditions, including HIV, patients are sometimes treated for a medical condition rather than for the depression.[35] Yet, depression, one of the most prevalent diagnoses among HIV-positive persons, particularly women,[35] has been treated efficaciously and safely with antidepressants when it is diagnosed.[36]

Persons with mental disorders are at heightened risk of contracting HIV infection as a result of their engagement in high-risk behaviors. Consequently, they have increased rates of sexually transmitted diseases and are at risk for hepatitis B and hepatitis C infection.[37] They are also at high risk for chronic medical disorders and are less likely to receive needed interventions that can be lifesaving. Recent studies have found the prevalence of HIV greater in people with SMI than in the general population.[35]

Effects of Mental Illness on HIV Treatment

A number of studies have documented the relationship between mental illness and initiating and adhering to HIV treatment. Research has shown that patients with mental illness begin highly active antiretroviral therapy (HAART) later than patients without a diagnosis of mental illness. For example, patients with a diagnosis of depression or anxiety experienced longer delays in initiating HAART than those who did not have a psychiatric diagnosis.[17] Patients with untreated mental illness were less than half as likely to begin treatment for HIV. However, the patients who were diagnosed and treated for mental illness were as likely to start HAART as those without mental illness.[17] Because there is evidence that some patients may avoid treatment for both their mental illness and HIV disease,[14] these findings suggest that treating mental illness may increase patient receptivity to HIV treatment. Thus, for patients with comorbid mental disorders and HIV, treatment of the mental disorder should be a primary goal in HIV care settings.

Even though a good deal of attention has focused on the role of depression in HIV treatment, there is further indication that mental illness, and particularly depression, is often underdiagnosed. Asch et al. examined medical records and found that providers did not diagnose 54% of patients who reported depression during the Composite International Diagnostic Interview (CIDI) survey.[20] Patients with providers who saw fewer numbers of HIV-infected patients were less likely to have an overlooked diagnosis of depression. Undiagnosed mentally ill patients are less likely to adhere to HIV treatment, and there is evidence that the consequences may be worse for HIV-infected women who are depressed.[25]

The stigma associated with the dual diagnosis of mental illness and HIV infection is a barrier to treatment and care. Fear of stigma causes many infected persons to disengage and retreat from seeking needed services and treatment. In addition to stigma, traumatic events and distrust have also been associated with poorer adherence to medication regimens and HIV risk behavior.[38] Moreover, dually and multiply diagnosed persons often experience increased disability and distress, poor coping skills, heightened psychosocial stress from poverty, homelessness, and incarceration, and continued risky behavior. Ultimately, these consequences increase the burden on clinical care and the service delivery system.[39]

Effectiveness of HIV Risk Reduction Strategies for Drug-Using Populations

The most effective HIV risk reduction strategies are seen in programs that incorporate multiple factors in the prevention intervention. Specifically, effective prevention programs take into consideration factors such as the race/ethnicity, gender, age, social and environmental context of the group targeted, and the subgroup of drugs used (e.g., crack smoking, injection drug use, etc.). Results from two large-scale multisite research projects funded by the National Institute on Drug Abuse (NIDA) to examine the effectiveness of risk reduction interventions suggested that multiple interventions are needed at multiple levels.[40] The research showed that a combination of community-based outreach, drug treatment, and network-based interventions were effective HIV risk reduction approaches.[40]

Interventions Using Community-Based Outreach

Community-based outreach takes an interventionist approach. Its focus is on service delivery with a public health interface. A number of interventions have focused on risk behavior change; they often incorporated aspects of models or theories of behavior change, and the primary focus of the intervention has been on beliefs and attitudes that influence behavior. Hierarchical risk-reduction messages, distribution of condoms and bleach kits, HIV testing, and treatment referrals were included in behavior change activities of outreach workers. As a result of these street-based interventions, IDUs stopped injecting drugs, reduced injection frequency, stopped reusing syringes and other equipment, and stopped crack use. Sex-related risks were also reduced and condom use increased.[40]

Other researchers developed gender-specific and culturally specific interventions that were effective.[41–43] To illustrate, after their participation in an enhanced woman-focused intervention, African American sex workers who were crack users reduced their crack use, the number of paying partners, and the number of sexual encounters with paying partners. They also increased their condom use.[41] In addition to culture and gender, interventions should also consider incorporating other contextual issues such as risk reduction related to violence, substance use, and comorbid conditions and simultaneously link the participants to housing, education, and skills for independence.[42]

Community-based outreach interventions lead to entry into drug treatment, which is associated with decreases in HIV transmission.[40] Pretreatment interventions may be effective in helping drug users to initiate treatment. A study involving African American crack-using women in a pretreatment intervention showed that these women reduced their crack use and were more likely to initiate treatment than women in the control group 3 months after the study ended.[44] Although these African American women were motivated to change their behavior, actual admission to treatment was low as a result of structural barriers.[43] This points to a clear need for sensitivity on the part of providers of treatment and care and for easy accessibility for persons needing and seeking care.

Similar risk reduction results were obtained in a study with men and women receiving outpatient psychiatric care for a mental illness.[45] Benefits included less unprotected sex, fewer casual sex partners, fewer new sexually transmitted infections, improved safer sex communications, improved HIV knowledge, more positive condom attitudes, stronger condom use intentions, and improved behavior skills.[45]

Drug Treatment Is Effective HIV Prevention

Drug abuse treatment is a protective factor for drug users and as such, it is deemed to be effective in preventing HIV/AIDS.[46] Drug users who enter and remain in treatment reduce their drug use, reduce HIV drug risk behaviors, and reduce HIV, hepatitis B virus, and hepatitis C infection rates. HIV risk reduction interventions in drug treatment programs were more effective in reducing HIV risk behaviors than standard drug treatment alone.[11] Some characteristics associated with such treatment effectiveness include interventions delivered later in the course of treatment, separate sessions for men and women, didactic lectures, training in self-control and coping skills, as well as the conduct of peer group counseling and discussion.[11]

Syringe exchange programs (SEPs) can facilitate entry into drug abuse treatment, and as such strong linkages should be established between SEPs and other effective drug abuse treatment programs.[47] Interventions should, therefore, be developed to encourage SEP participants (many of whom have high rates of substance use disorder but are hesitant about seeking treatment) to enroll in treatment.[48] HIV risk reduction interventions for IDUs in treatment can be optimized by targeting participants' risk reduction motivation and behavioral skills.[49]

Network-Based Interventions

Network-based interventions utilize peers or others in a social group to facilitate the intervention. Networks can be effective as HIV prevention interventions because they have been shown to be a source of HIV transmission.[50–52] Network members with a high level of perceived sexual risk were likely to engage in sexual risk behaviors.[50] Those who exchanged encouragement with multiple network leaders about using condoms were less likely to report engaging in unprotected sex, and those network members who talked about HIV risks with a greater number of network leaders were less likely to engage in unprotected sex in the past 6 months than those who did not have such conversations.[50]

Peers as role models to promote HIV risk reduction is an effective strategy in working with out-of-treatment drug users. This was confirmed in a study that compared a peer-delivered, enhanced intervention with the NIDA standard intervention for reducing HIV risk behaviors in out-of-treatment IDUs and crack cocaine users. While participants in both groups reduced their drug use, participants in the peer-enhanced intervention had greater reductions in crack use than participants in the NIDA standard intervention (83% vs. 76%; $p < 0.05$).[53] However, it was more difficult to change sexual risk behaviors than drug-using behaviors.[52]

Reflecting on an HIV intervention that utilized counseling of couples, focus groups, and meetings facilitated by drug users or staff, Neaigus concluded that network-based interventions had the potential for sustainable, large-scale risk reduction among IDUs.[51] Moreover, it was a cost-effective approach because of the multiplier effect of reaching drug users through their social networks.[51] Benefits also accrued to the peer leaders who were themselves former IDUs. Having received training as HIV peer educators to promote HIV prevention among their risk network members and others at risk of acquiring and transmitting HIV, a group of African American peer leaders developed HIV prevention skills themselves.[52] They reported a significant increase in condom use and in cleaning used needles with bleach.[52]

The foregoing data make it clear that multiple strategies are needed to access hard-to-reach out-of-treatment drug users and to facilitate their behavior change and entry into treatment. It is important to target participants' risk reduction motivation and behavioral skills rather than to employ passive informational approaches.[49] Further, optimal benefit can be achieved from interventions that focus on participants' risk reduction motivation within the sexual-related content, while placing equal emphasis on participants' risk reduction knowledge, motivation, and behavioral skills within the drug-related content. Multiple interventions are needed at multiple levels (individual, community, systems, legal, institutional). Settings for the interventions also have to be varied, e.g., in the streets, storefronts, clinics, and drug treatment centers. Finally, multiple risk behaviors have to be targeted, e.g., drug use, injection risk, and sexual behaviors.[39]

Mental Health Issues and Needs of HIV-Positive Substance Abusers

Persons diagnosed with HIV infection often have a variety of mental health issues and needs. Comorbid substance abuse is common among HIV-positive individuals with mental illness,[39,54] and persons dually diagnosed are at high risk for HIV infection.[55] Individuals with triple diagnoses tend to be poor and indecisive, cognitively impaired, and engage in risky behaviors.[4] Persons living with HIV, mental illness, and substance abuse are at elevated risk for other diseases (such as diabetes) due, in part, to the higher likelihood of engaging in health-compromising behaviors such as poor diet, eating too much, or having a sedentary life style. These multiple diagnoses disproportionately affect women, racial/ethnic minorities, and the economically disadvantaged.[39]

Accessing and Utilizing Services

There are inequalities in access to care and they vary across general medical, specialty mental health, and substance abuse treatment sectors.[56] Persons with mental health problems are often underdiagnosed for physical illnesses although they have high morbidity and mortality, and they tend not to seek or utilize health care services.[57]

A naturalistic longitudinal study of individuals with personality disorders concluded that minority participants, particularly Hispanic participants, were significantly less likely than white participants to receive a range of outpatient and inpatient psychosocial treatments and psychotropic medications. This indicates an urgent need to evaluate treatment assessment and delivery, cultural biases within the current diagnostic system, and possible variations in personality disorders across racial/ethnic groups.[58]

A longitudinal study addressing issues of service needs, service utilization, and access to care for 116 HIV-positive drug-abusing women in five cities found significant gaps between drug abuse treatment services for which the women expressed a need and the services they actually received.[59] HIV secondary prevention was also a critical need for the women, many of whom were engaging in risky behaviors that made them susceptible to reinfection, infection with other diseases, and transmission to others. Unfortunately, lack of funding was cited as a major barrier to the provision of more adequate services for the women.[59]

Treatment and services must be accessible and conveniently located in order to address the mental health issues and needs of HIV-positive patients. Treatment services have to be conducive and health care providers need to be culturally sensitive and empathetic – creating a caring environment free from bias and discrimination. Integrated treatment programs are more effective for persons with co-occurring substance abuse and mental health disorders than separate services.[54]

Benefits of Social Support

Social support refers to perceptions of, or experience with other people providing emotional support, material or tangible support and health-related support.[60] HIV-positive persons who perceived that they have social support are more willing to disclose their HIV status than those who do not perceive that they have such support. Stigma is associated with both fewer disclosures and less social support.[60]

Abstinence-oriented social support is associated with positive substance abuse treatment outcomes. For example, 59 opioid-dependent outpatients receiving methadone participated in a behavioral intervention that encouraged them to include drug-free family members or friends in their drug abuse treatment process.[61] These individuals facilitated the development of a supportive, nondrug-using social network. Approximately 78% of patients participating in the social support intervention achieved at least four consecutive weeks of abstinence; women responded better than men.[61]

Spirituality and involvement in religious organizations can provide social support for persons with dual or triple diagnosis. Among mentally ill African Americans, spirituality can be an effective tool for recovery. Spirituality offers emotional consolation, inspiration, guidance, and security.[62] A large proportion of severely mentally ill Puerto Rican women in a study reported that their religious or spiritual beliefs were critical to their coping, had influenced them to reduce risk, and/or provided them with needed social support.[63]

Similarly, spirituality and spiritually based coping with HIV among a group of 230 predominantly African American and Puerto Rican low-income HIV-positive women correlated positively with the frequency of HIV-related social support received, and correlated negatively with recent drug use.[64] Marcus et al. collaborated with a local church to develop a faith-based substance abuse and HIV/AIDS prevention program for African American adolescents. Participants in the intervention reported significantly less marijuana and other drug use and more fear of AIDS than a comparison group.[1] Religious institutions have tradition- ally been a source of social support for African American and other minority communities.

An example of material support is seen in a housing program, which provided permanent housing and support, along with assertive community treatment, and intensive case management for homeless people with mental illness. The result was a significant reduction in homelessness and hospitalization as well as improvements in other outcomes, such as well-being.[65]

Benefit can also be derived from social support for psychosocial factors such as depression, avoidant coping, and life stress, which may be related to disease pro- gression in HIV.[66, 67] Availability of social support was one of six factors related to depressive symptoms among HIV-positive women.[67] The other factors were the frequency of HIV symptoms, recent experiences of sadness/hopelessness, and the use of three coping strategies: living positively with HIV, isolation/withdrawal, and denial/avoidance.[67] Another study found an association between positive affect and physical health.[65] Conversely, greater negative mood and lower social sup- port were related to greater use of avoidance-oriented coping strategies. Patients on HAART who used such negative coping strategies tended to have poorer medication adherence and subsequently higher viral load.[68]

Optimal Management Strategies for the Dually and Triply Diagnosed

Intervention and treatment programs and services are not always readily avail- able for persons who are dually and triply diagnosed. These clients are sometimes excluded from services in one system because of the comorbid disorder(s) and told to return when the other problem is under control.[69] The appropriate psychiatric treatment with HIV-infected persons who have a comorbid psychiatric disorder can reduce their risk behaviors, improve treatment adherence and quality of life, and help decrease mortality.[70] A critical factor to the provision of appropriate treatment is accurate diagnosis.[70] For example, signs and symptoms of major depression tend to be masked by symptoms of other comorbidities found in HIV-positive patients.[70] However, for HIV treatment to be effective, persons infected with the virus must also have available and accessible mental health and substance abuse services.[16]

People living with HIV/AIDS, mental illness, and substance abuse disorders bear an added burden when they are forced to seek treatment and services from multiple service delivery systems, and this is, unfortunately, often the case. The development of strategies for treatment engagement is urgently needed. Services should be inte- grated utilizing an interdisciplinary approach and housed under one roof to address the needs of the whole person.[71] The burden should not be placed on clients to navigate multiple systems; such a fragmented approach is ineffective. An analysis of behavioral health services in medical settings in the U.S. indicated that behavioral health services such as mental health and substance abuse services, particularly when delivered as part of primary medical care, can be critical to improving the health of the population.[72]

Treatments for dual diagnosis would combine or integrate for interventions at the clinician level for mental illness and HIV or mental illness and substance use disorder. This means that the same clinician or team of clinicians would work in one setting to provide coordinated and comprehensive care for mental health and substance abuse to the client.[69] In this way, the services are seamless for the client who learns to manage both illnesses. Evidence suggests that provision of both mental health and substance abuse services promoted receipt of HIV care.[73] Treatment must, therefore, address the comorbidities of substance abuse and mental illness that influence the patient's behavior in order for antiretroviral therapies to be effective.

The effectiveness of integrated dual diagnosis treatments for clients with SMI and substance use disorders is supported by research studies using experimental and quasiexperimental designs.[69] A multisite research study, the HIV/AIDS Treatment Adherence, Health Outcomes and Cost Study (The Cost Study), was funded by six federal agencies to test models of integrated interventions for HIV primary care, mental health, and substance abuse. Findings from the multisite study are reported in eight papers that comprise a supplemental issue of *AIDS Care*.[39]

Critical components of integrated programs, several of which can be considered to be evidence-based practices, are staged interventions, assertive outreach, motivational interventions, counseling, social support interventions, long-term perspective, comprehensiveness, and cultural sensitivity and competence.[69] Consistent with this, findings from the Cost Study showed that comprehensive integrated treatment delivered for 18 months or more resulted in significant reduction in substance abuse, increased remission rates, reduction in hospital use, and other improvements in health outcomes.[74]

Integrated mental health and substance abuse treatment was provided for 1 year to 141 HIV-positive participants recruited through routine mental health and substance abuse screening at tertiary infectious disease clinics in North Carolina.[18] Participants were interviewed at 3-month intervals. Statistically significant decreases were found in participants' psychometric symptomology, illicit substance abuse, alcohol use, and inpatient hospital days at follow-up. Patients also reported fewer emergency room visits; they were more likely to receive antiretroviral medications and adequate psychotropic medication regimens. However, treatment participation did not result in changes in sexual risk, physical health, or medical adherence.[18]

A model of integrated services for HIV/AIDS, substance abuse, and mental health has been organized and implemented by the Holistic Native Network.[49] The Network is a collaboration of the Native American Health Center and Friendship House Association of American Indians, two community-based organizations located in San Francisco and Oakland, and services are provided to clients within the context of culture and community. Positive changes in quality of life have been reported by clients surveyed after 3 months in treatment. The program's success is credited to the fact that the spiritual, medical, and psychosocial needs of the Native American HIV-positive clients are being met.[75]

Barriers to integrated services exist at a number of levels (e.g., policy, program, clinical, consumer, and family) and impede implementation of integrated dual and triple diagnosis services. A major barrier is stigma associated with the three illnesses. Separate funding streams create another barrier, as does the lack of coordination among HIV-related medical, mental health, and substance abuse treatment facilities.[4] Indeed, substance abuse, mental health, and HIV-related organizations have different licensing and regulatory bodies and develop different professional cultures.[15] Some strategies to overcome the barriers suggested by Drake et al. are organizational and financing changes at the policy level, clarity of program mission with structural changes to support dual diagnosis services, training and supervision for clinicians, and dissemination of accurate information to consumers and families to support understanding, demand, and advocacy.[69] Others have suggested that optimal care can be provided to racial/ethnic minority patients if clinicians use a cultural competence framework, enhance patient–provider communication, diversify their clinical staff, proactively enhance receipt of HAART, and are attentive to issues related to adherence to HAART.[76]

In addition, ancillary services such as transportation assistance and case management can improve patients' involvement in their own medical care.[13,21] This view is widely shared. For example, a review of literature on integrated care for the Cost Study showed that there was support for a wide range of primary and ancillary services delivered by a multidisciplinary team employing a biopsychosocial approach.[13] Researchers at the Miriam Hospital in Providence, RI developed a model of integrated substance abuse counseling and referral for treatment within a primary care HIV-care setting.[77] Using a multidisciplinary approach, they provided linkages to treatment services for substance abuse and mental illness. In addition, participants received help with social service needs, including housing and medical coverage. Participants have also been referred to a variety of treatment modalities, including intensive outpatient services, methadone, buprenorphine, outpatient services, and residential as well as individual and group counseling.[77] This assistance facilitates continuity of care and optimal HIV treatment adherence.

Similarly, Bouis et al. created an integrated, multidimensional treatment model for persons triply diagnosed with substance abuse, mental disorder, and HIV. This treatment model is based on the transtheoretical model of behavior change as well as evidence-based practices used in treating persons dually diagnosed with substance abuse and mental disorders.[78] The interdisciplinary focus of the treatment model facilitated collaboration between the medical and behavioral health care professionals and offered comprehensive care that addressed a continuum of client needs that might have influenced the positive treatment outcomes.[78]

Conclusion

Dual and triple diagnoses are complex clinical problems affecting a diverse patient population, a disproportionate number of whom are racial/ethnic minorities. Patients with comorbid substance use disorders and mental illness are at elevated risk of contracting HIV/AIDS, and they are more likely to have negative treatment outcomes such as poor adherence and frequent hospitalizations.[71] Each condition must be addressed to influence the patients' behavior. To address the needs of multiply diagnosed patients, an integrated and multidisciplinary team must address patients' substance abuse and mental health issues and provide comprehensive HIV treatment and care.[71,79] The multidisciplinary team or network must be creative in their assessment and packaging of prevention interventions. Further, the team must be empathetic to the treatment needs of the patients based on the patients' level of tolerance, motivation, and abilities.[79]

Undoubtedly, persons with a dual diagnosis of mental disorder and substance abuse should receive more intense HIV prevention intervention than persons with a single diagnosis of substance abuse disorder.[55] Persons who are dually diagnosed tend to engage in more high-risk behaviors, which place them at elevated risk of contracting HIV.[55] Indeed, these risky behaviors may be a reflection of the poverty, high-risk environments, and overall poor health and medical care often seen in SMI persons.[37] Successful treatment approaches must address the comorbidities of substance abuse and mental illness that influence the patient's behavior so as to maximize the effectiveness of antiretroviral therapies.[55] Further research is needed to understand the independent and joint effects of substance abuse and mental illness on HIV outcomes, and to better inform adherence interventions for HIV-infected persons.[35]

References

1. Marcus MT, Walker T, Swint JM, Smith BP, Brown C, Busen N, Edwards T, Liehr P, Taylor WC, Williams D, von Sternberg K. Community-based participatory research to prevent substance abuse and HIV/AIDS in African American adolescents. J Interprof Care. 2004; 18(4): 347–359

2. Gabel LL, Pearsol JA. The twin epidemics of substance use and HIV: a state-level response using a train-the-trainer model. Fam Pract. 1993; 10(4): 400–405

3. National Institute on Drug Abuse (NIDA). Drugs, Brains, and Behavior: The Science of Addiction. Bethesda, MD: U.S. Department of Health and Human Services, National Institutes of Health, February 2007

4. Caslyn RJ, Klinkenbert WD, Morse GA, Miller J, Cruthis R. Recruitment, engagement, and retention of people living with HIV and co-occurring mental health and substance use disorders. AIDS Care. 2004; 16(Suppl. 1): S56–S70

5. National Institute on Drug Abuse (NIDA). Drug Use Among Racial/Ethnic Minorities. Revised Ed. Bethesda, MD: U.S. Department of Health and Human Services, National Institutes of Health, 2003

6. Centers for Disease Control and Prevention. HIV/AIDS Fact Sheet, HIV/AIDS Among African Americans, 2006. Atlanta, GA: U.S. Department of Health and Human Services, Centers for Disease Control and Prevention, 2008

7. Blankenship KM, Smoyer AB, Bray SJ, Mattocks K. Black–White disparities in HIV/AIDS: the role of drug policy and the corrections system. J Health Care Poor Underserved. 2005; 16(4 Suppl. B): 140–156

8. Centers for Disease Control and Prevention. Drug-Associated HIV Transmission Continues in the United States. Atlanta, GA: U.S. Department of Health and Human Services, Centers for Disease Control and Prevention, May 2002

9. Centers for Disease Control and Prevention. Trends in HIV/AIDS diagnoses – 33 States, 2001–2004. MMWR Morb Mort Wkly Rep. 2005; 54(45): 1149–1153

10. Centers for Disease Control and Prevention. HIV/AIDS Surveillance Report 2006, Vol. 18. Atlanta, GA: U.S. Department of Health and Human Services, Centers for Disease Control and Prevention, 2008

11. Pendergast ML, Urada D, Podus DJ. Meta-analysis of HIV risk-reduction interventions within drug abuse treatment programs. J Consult Clin Psychol. 2001; 69: 389–405

12. Angelino AF, Treisman GJ. Management of psychiatric disorders in patients infected with human immunodeficiency virus. Clin Infect Dis. 2001; 33: 847–856

13. Soto TA, Bell J, Pillen MB. Literature on integrated HIV care: a review. AIDS Care. 2004; 16(Suppl. 1): S43–S55

14. Treisman GJ, Angelino AF, Hutton HE. Psychiatric issues in the management of patients with HIV infection. JAMA. 2001; 286(22): 2857–2864

15. Walkup J, Blank MB, Gonzalez JS, Safren S, Schwartz R, Brown L, Wilson I, Knowlton A, Lombard F, Grossman C, et al. The impact of mental health and substance abuse factors on HIV prevention and treatment. J Acquir Immune Defic Syndr. 2008; 47(Suppl. 1): S15–S19

16. Bing EG, Burnam MA, Longshore D, Fleishman JA, Sherbourne CD, London AS, Turner BJ, Eggan F, Beckman R, Vitiello B, Morton SC, Orlando M, Bozzette SA, Ortiz-Barron L, Shapiro M. Psychiatric disorders and drug use among human immunodeficiency virus-infected adults in the United States. Arch Gen Psychiatry. 2001; 58: 721–728

17. Tegger MK, Crane HM, Tapia KA, Uldall KK, Holte SE, Kitahata MM. The effect of mental illness, substance use, and treatment for depression on the initiation of highly active antiretroviral therapy among HIV-infected individuals. AIDS Patient Care STDS. 2008; 22(3): 233–243

18. Whetten K, Reif S, Ostermann J, Pence BW, Swartz M, Whetten R, Conover C, Bouis S, Thielman N, Eron J. Improving health outcomes among individuals with HIV, mental illness, and substance use disorders in the Southeast. AIDS Care. 2006; 18(Suppl. 1): S18–S26

19. Kessler RC, Berglund P, Demler O, Jin R, Merikangas KR, Walters EE. Lifetime prevalence and age-of-onset distributions of DSM-IV disorders in the National Comorbidity Survey Replication. Arch Gen Psychiatry. 2005; 62(6): 593–602

20. Asch SM, Kilbourne AM, Gifford AL, Burnam MA, Turner B, Shapiro MF, Bozzette SA. Underdiagnosis of depression in HIV: who are we missing? J Gen Intern Med. 2003; 18(6): 450–460

21. Klinkenberg WD, Sacks S. HIV/AIDS Treatment Adherence, Heath Outcomes and Cost Study Group. Mental disorders and drug abuse in persons living with HIV/AIDS. AIDS Care. 2004; 16(Suppl. 1): S22–S42

22. Brief DJ, Bollinger AR, Vielhauer MJ, Berger-Greenstein JA, Morgan EE, Brady SM, Buondonno LM, Keane TM. Understanding the interface of HIV, trauma, post-traumatic stress disorder, and substance use and its implications for health outcomes. AIDS Care. 2004; 16(Suppl. 1): S97–S120

23. Kalichman SC, Benotsch EG, Rompa D, Gore-Felton C, Austin J, Juke W, DiFonzo K, Buckles J, Kyomugisha F, Simpson D. Unwanted sexual experiences ad sexual risks in gay and bisexual men: associations among revictimization, substance use, and psychiatric symptoms. J Sex Res. 2001; 38(1): 1–9

24. Atkinson JH, Grant I. Natural history of neuropsychiatric manifestations of HIV disease. Psychiatr Clin North Am. 1994; 17(1): 17–33

25. Cook JA, Grey D, Burke J, Cohen MH, Gurtman AC, Richardson JL, Wilson TE, Young MA, Hessol NA. Depressive symptoms and AIDS-related mortality among a multisite cohort of HIV-positive women. Am J Public Health. 2004; 94(7): 1133–1140

26. Perdue T, Hagan H, Thiede H, Valleroy L. Depression and HIV risk behavior among Seattle-area injection drug users and young men who have sex with men. AIDS Educ Prev. 2003; 15(1): 81–92

27. Hardman JG, Limbird LE, Gilman AG. Goodman and Gilman's The Pharmacological Basis of Therapeutics, 100 edition. 2001, p. 624

28. Volkow ND, Fowler JS, Wang GJ. The addicted human brain viewed in the light of imaging studies: brain circuits and treatment strategies. Neuropharmacology. 2004; 47(Suppl. 1): 3–13

29. Hendershot CS, Stoner SA, George WH, Norris J. Alcohol use, expectancies, and sexual sensation seeking as correlates of HIV risk behavior in heterosexual young adults. Psychol Addict Behav. 2007; 21(3): 365–372

30. National Institute on Drug Abuse (NIDA). Preventing Drug Use among Children and Adolescents: A Research-Based Guide for Parents, Educators, and Community Leaders. Second Ed. Bethesda, MD: U.S. Department of Health and Human Services, National Institutes of Health, 2003

31. El-Bassel N, Gilbert L, Wu E, Chang M, Gomes C, Vinocur D, Spevack T. Intimate partner violence prevalence and HIV risks among women receiving care in emergency departments: implications for IPV and HIV screening. Emerg Med J. 2007; 24(4): 255–259

32. Freisthler B, Gruenewald PJ, Johnson FW, Treno AJ, Lascala EA. An exploratory study examining the spatial dynamics of illicit drug availability and rates of drug use. J Drug Educ. 2005; 35(1): 15–27

33. Meade CS, Kershaw TS, Hansen NB, Sikkema KJ. Long-term correlates of childhood abuse among adults with severe mental illness: adult victimization, substance abuse, and HIV sexual risk behavior. AIDS Behav. 2007; (e-pub ahead of print), DOI 10.1007/s10461-007-9326-4

34. Singer MC, Erickson PI, Badiane L, Diaz R, Ortiz D, Abraham T, Nicolaysen AM. Syndemics, sex and the city: understanding sexually transmitted diseases in social and cultural context. Soc Sci Med. 2006; 63(8): 2010–2021

35. Chander G, Himelhoch S, Moore RD. Substance abuse and psychiatric disorders in HIV-positive patients. Drugs. 2006; 66(6): 769–789

36. Repetto MJ, Petitto JM. Psychopharmacology in HIV-infected patients. Psychosom Med. 2008; 70(5): 585–592

37. Rosenberg SD, Goodman LA, Osher FC, Swartz MS, Essock SM, Butterfield MI, Constantine NT, Wolford GL, Salyers MP. Prevalence of HIV, Hepatitis B, and Hepatitis C in people with severe mental illness. Am J Public Health. 2001; 91: 31–37

38. Whetten K, Reif S, Whetten R, Murphy-McMillan LK. Trauma, mental health, distrust, and stigma among HIV-positive persons: implications for effective care. Psychosom Med. 2008; 70(5): 531–538

39. Stoff DM, Mitnick L, Kalichman S. Research issues in the multiple diagnoses of HIV/AIDS, mental illness and substance abuse. AIDS Care. 2004; 16(Suppl. 1): S1–S5

40. Coyle SL, Needle RH, Normand J. Outreach-based HIV prevention for injecting drug users: a review of published outcome data. Public Health Rep. 1998; 113(Suppl. 1): 19–30

41. Sterk CE, Theall KP, Elifson KW. Effectiveness of a risk reduction intervention among African American Women who use Crack Cocaine. AIDS Educ Prev. 2003; 15(1): 15–32

42. Wechsberg WM, Lam WK, Zule W, Hall G, Middlesteadt R, Edwards J. Violence, homelessness, and HIV risk among crack-using African American women. Subst Use Misuse. 2003; 38(3–6): 669–700

43. Wingood GM, DiClemente RJ. Enhancing adoption of evidence-based HIV interventions: promotion of a suite of HIV prevention interventions for African American women. AIDS Educ Prev. 2006; 18(4 Suppl. A): 161–170

44. Wechsberg WM, Zule WA, Riehman KS, Luseno WK, Lam WK. African American crack abusers and drug treatment initiation: barriers and effects of a pretreatment intervention. Subst Abuse Treat Prev Policy. 2007; 2: 10

45. Carey MP, Carey KB, Maisto SA, Gordon CM, Schroder KEE, Vanable PA. Reducing HIV-risk behavior among adults receiving outpatient psychiatric treatment: results from a randomized controlled trial. J Consult Clin Psychol. 2004; 72(2): 252–268

46. Metzger DS, Navaline H, Woody GE. Drug abuse treatment as AIDS prevention. Public Health Rep. 1998; 113(Suppl. 1): 97–106

47. Brooner R, Kidorf M, King V, Beilenson P, Svikis D, Vlahov D. Drug abuse treatment success among needle exchange participants. Public Health Rep. 1998; 113(Suppl. 1): 129–139

48. Kidorf M, Disney E, King V, Kolodner K, Beilenson P, Brooner RK. Challenges in motivating treatment enrollment in community syringe exchange participants. J Urban Health. 2005; 82(3): 456–467

49. Copenhaver MM, Lee IC. Optimizing a community-friendly HIV risk reduction intervention for injection drug users in treatment: a structural equation modeling approach. J Urban Health. 2006; 83(6): 1132–1142

50. El-Bassel N, Gilbert L, Wu E. A social network profile and HIV risk among men on methadone: do social networks matter? J Urban Health. 2006; 83(4): 602–613

51. Neaigus A. The network approach and interventions to prevent HIV among injection drug users. Public Health Rep. 1998; 113(Suppl. 1): 140–150

52. Latkin CA. Outreach in natural settings: the use of peer leaders for HIV prevention among injecting drug users' networks. Public Health Rep. 1998; 113(Suppl. 1): 151–159

53. Cottler LB, Compton WM, Abdallah AB, Cunningham-Williams R, Abram F, Fichtenbaum C, Dotson W. Peer-delivered interventions reduce HIV risk behaviors among out-of-treatment drub abusers. Public Health Rep. 1998; 113(Suppl. 1): 31–41

54. Parry CD, Blank MB, Pithey AL. Responding to the threat of HIV among persons with mental illness and substance abuse. Curr Opin Psychiatry. 2007; 20(3): 235–241

55. Dausey DJ, Desai RA. Psychiatric comorbidity and the prevalence of HIV infection in a sample of patients in treatment for substance abuse. J Nerv Ment Dis. 2003; 191(1): 10–17

56. Burnam MA, Bing EG, Morton SC, Sherbourne C, Fleishman JA, London AS, Vitiello B, Stein M, Bozzette SA, Shapiro MF. Use of mental health and substance abuse treatment services among adults with HIV in the United States. Arch Gen Psychiatry. 2001; 58: 729–736

57. McCabe MP, Leas L. A qualitative study of primary health care access, barriers and satisfaction among people with mental illness. Psychol Health Med. 2008; 13(3): 303–312

58. Bender DS, Skodol AE, Dyck JR, Markowitz JC, Shea MT, Yen S, Sanislow CA, Pinto A, Zanarini MC, McGlashan TH, Gunderson JG, Daversa MT, Grilo CM. Ethnicity and mental health treatment utilization by patients with personality disorders. J Consult Psychol. 2007; 75(6): 992–999

59. Weissman G, Melchior L, Huba G, Smereck G, Needle R, McCarthy S, Jones A, Genser S, Cottler L, Booth R, et al. Women living with drug abuse and HIV disease: drug abuse treatment access and secondary prevention issues. J Psychoactive Drugs. 1995; 27(4): 401–411

60. Smith R, Rossetto K, Peterson BL. A meta-analysis of disclosure of one's HIV-positive status, stigma and social support. AIDS Care. 2008; 20(10): 1266–1275 (e-pub. June 27, 2008)

61. Kidorf M, King VL, Neufeld K, Stoller KB, Peirce J, Brooner RK. Involving significant others in the care of opioid-dependent patients receiving methadone. J Subst Abuse Treat. 2005; 29(1): 19–27

62. Perdue B, Johnson D, Singley D, Jackson C. Assessing spirituality in mentally ill African Americans. ABNF J. 2006 Spring; 17(2): 78–81

63. Loue S, Sajotovic M. Spirituality, coping, and HIV risk and prevention in a sample of severely mentally ill Puerto Rican women. J Urban Health. 2006; 83(6): 1168–1182

64. Simoni JM, Martone MG, Kerwin JF. Spirituality and psychological adaptation among women with HIV/AIDS: implications for counseling. J Couns Psychol. 2002; 49(2): 139–147

65. Nelson G, Aubry T, Lafrance A. A review of the literature on the effectiveness of housing and support, assertive community treatment, and intensive case management interventions for persons with mental illness who have been homeless. Am J Orthopsychiatry. 2007; 77(3): 350–361

66. Pressman SD, Cohen S. Does positive affect influence health? Psychol Bull. 2005; 131(6): 925–971

67. Moneyham L, Murdaugh C, Phillips K, Jackson K, Tavakoli A, Boyd M, Jackson N, Vyavaharkar M. Patterns of risk of depressive symptoms among HIV-positive women in the southeastern United States. J Assoc Nurses AIDS Care. 2005; 16(4): 25–38

68. Weaver KE, Llabre MM, Durán RE, Antoni MH, Ironson G, Penedo FJ, Schneiderman N. A stress and coping model of medication adherence and viral load in HIV-positive men and women on highly active antiretroviral therapy (HAART). Health Psychol. 2005; 24(4): 385–392

69. Drake RE, Essock SM, Shaner A, Carey KB, Minkoff K, Kola L, Lynde D, Osher FC, Clark RE, Rickards L. Implementing dual diagnosis services for clients with severe mental illness. Psychiat Serv. 2001; 52(4): 469–476

70. Treisman G, Angelino A. Interrelation between psychiatric disorder and the prevention and treatment of HIV infection. Clin Infect Dis. 2007; 45: S313–S317

71. Douaihy AB, Jou RJ, Gorske T, Salloum IM. Triple diagnosis: dual diagnosis and HIV disease, Part 1. AIDS Read. 2003; 13(7): 331, 332, 339–341

72. Blount A, Schoenbaum M, Kathol R, Rollman BL, Thomas M, O'Donohue W, Peek CJ. The economics of behavioral health services in medical settings: a summary of the evidence. Prof Psychol Res Pr. 2007; 38(3): 290–297

73. Weaver MR, Conover CJ, Proescholdbell RJ, Arno PS, Ang A, Ettner SL. Utilization of mental health and substance abuse care for people living with HIV/AIDS, chronic mental illness, and substance abuse disorders. J Acquir Immune Defic Syndr. 2008; 47(4): 449–458

74. The HIV/AIDS Treatment Adherence, Health Outcomes and Cost Study Group. The HIV/AIDS treatment adherence, health outcomes and cost study: conceptual foundations and overview. AIDS Care. 2004; 16(Suppl. 1): S6–S21

75. Nebelkopf E, Penagos M. Holistic Native network: integrated HIV/AIDS, substance abuse, and mental health services for Native Americans in San Francisco. J Psychoactive Drugs. 2005; 37(3): 257–264

76. Stone VE. Optimizing the care of minority patients with HIV/AIDS. Clin Infect Dis. 2004; 38: 400–404

77. Zaller N, Gillani FS, Rich JD. A model of integrated primary care for HIV-positive patients with underlying substance use and mental illness. AIDS Care. 2007; 19(9): 1128–1133

78. Bouis S, Reif S, Whetten K, Scovil J, Murray A, Swartz M. An integrated, multidimensional treatment model for individuals living with HIV, mental illness, and substance abuse. Health Soc Work. 2007; 32(4): 268–278

79. Goldsmith RJ, Garlapati V. Behavioral interventions for dual-diagnosis patients. Psychiatr Clin North Am. 2004; 27(4): 709–725

African Americans and HIV Clinical Research

Kimberly Smith and William D. King

African Americans are significantly overrepresented among individuals with HIV/AIDS in the U.S. This fact has been well documented and publicized.[1] It is much less well known that African Americans are underrepresented in research on HIV/AIDS in the U.S. A recent search of publications listed on Medline revealed over 94,000 articles published between 1996 and July 2008 in the area of HIV-1 and AIDS. Of these, only 1.7% refer to African Americans and/or Blacks.[2] This is a slight increase over that of a similar review published in 2000, which revealed that less that 1% of the AIDS-related literature in Medline through 1999 related explicitly to African Americans.[3] This is despite the fact that of the 1,014,797 cases of AIDS reported to the CDC through 2001, African Americans accounted for 40.4% of the total, and nearly 60% of women, heterosexuals, and children suffering with this disease.[1] Furthermore, of the 36,817 newly diagnosed cases of HIV reported to the CDC in 2006, African Americans accounted for 49%.[1]

One of the primary reasons for the underrepresentation of African Americans in medical literature on HIV/AIDS is that African Americans are less likely to participate in clinical trials. A study published in the New England Journal of Medicine revealed that 14% of adults receiving HIV care participated in clinical trials and 24% received experimental medications. Blacks were 50% less likely to be clinical trial participants or receive experimental medications compared with whites. Among those who sought experimental medications, Caucasians received them more often than Blacks (77 vs. 69%; $p = 0.03$).[4] According to the Adult AIDS Clinical Trials Group (AACTG) Annual Report 2002, African Americans comprised 47.6% of national AIDS cases in July 2000–2001, while 27.7% accrued in AACTG clinical trial sites.[5] More recently, the Supplement to HIV and AIDS Surveillance (SHAS) Project reported that 17% of the 6,892 HIV-infected subjects in the study had been in a clinical trial; however, in the adjusted model, African Americans were 20% less

K. Smith (✉)
Section of Infectious Diseases, Rush University Medical Center, Chicago Il
E-mail: ksmith2@rush.edu

V. Stone et al. (eds.), *HIV/AIDS in U.S. Communities of Color*.
DOI: 10.1007/978-0-387-98152-9_13, © Springer Science + Business Media, LLC 2009

likely to report clinical trial participation (OR 0.80, 95% CI 0.6–0.9) than White non-Hispanics.[6] This lack of participation in clinical trials likely results from many factors including a lack of trust in the medical establishment on the part of African American patients, lack of access to research institutions where clinical research takes place, and stereotypes regarding African American's willingness and appropriateness for participation in clinical trials. The effect of this underrepresentation is that African Americans have less access to state-of-the art drugs and treatment strategies. And importantly, data from research in which African Americans are not adequately represented may not be directly applicable to African Americans, may underrecognize differences between African Americans and other groups, and may not address issues that disproportionately impact African Americans. This chapter will (1) review the recent literature on participation of African Americans in HIV clinical trials and compare it to other research areas, (2) discuss the barriers to clinical trial participation, and (3) discuss strategies to improve clinical trial participation among African American and other underrepresented groups.

African Americans and HIV Clinical Trials

In the early years of the HIV epidemic clinical trials of treatment for HIV and HIV/AIDS related diseases enrolled white males primarily. For example, one of the key early studies of the AACTG comparing immediate versus delayed therapy with zidovudine in HIV-infected persons with CD4 cell counts of 500 or more included 1,637 patients of whom 90% were white males.[7] This study enrolled patients between July 1987 and July 1989. During that period, blacks and Hispanics accounted for over 40% of reported AIDS cases in the U.S.[8] In 1996, one of the first studies of a three-drug combination of antiretroviral agents for treatment of HIV disease was published in the New England Journal of Medicine.[9] That study, also completed by the AACTG, included 302 patients who enrolled from March 1993 through July 1993 at ten clinical trial sites around the U.S. Seventy nine percent of subjects in that study were of white race, 11% were blacks, and 9% were Hispanics. During that period, blacks and Hispanics accounted for over 49% of reported AIDS cases in the U.S.[10]

However, there has been progress. AACTG a5095 was a multicenter clinical trial examining a triple nucleoside regimen versus two different efavirenz-containing regimens in the treatment of naïve HIV-infected individuals.[11] This study enrolled 1,147 patients between March 2001 and November 2002. Blacks represented 36% of the study population while non-Hispanic whites were 40% and Hispanics were 21%. Importantly the substantial numbers of blacks and Hispanics in this trial allowed the study to identify several important differences in treatment response among the different racial groups (these are discussed in detail in the chapter on HIV treatment). Similar findings have been suggested by earlier trials but could not be confirmed as a result of lower enrollment of blacks and Hispanics in those studies.[12] Most recently, AACTG a5142 compared preferred agents for initial therapy

Table 1 Clinical trial

Clinical trial	No. of participants	% Black	% Hispanic	% White
Gilead 903	600 tx naïve	21	7	64
Gilead 934	509 tx naïve	23	16	59
Abbott MO5–730	664 tx naïve	18	n/a	78
Glaxosmithkline–KLEAN	878 tx naïve	31	8	58
Glaxosmithkline–HEAT	688 tx naïve	36	n/a	51
Glaxosmithkline–ALERT	106 tx naïve	40	n/a	56
Tibotec–POWER 3	327 tx exp	n/a	n/a	75
MERCK–BenchMrk 1	350 tx exp	n/a	n/a	77
Pfizer–MOTIVATE	585 tx exp	n/a	n/a	84

LPV/r and efavirenz, both in combination with two nucleoside reverse transcriptase inhibitors in treatment-naïve patients. A third arm of that study examined LPV/r plus efavirenz without NRTIs.[13] This study enrolled patients from January of 2003 to May of 2004. Blacks comprised 42% of study participants and Hispanics comprised 19%. Thus, finally these studies have come close to enrolling subjects at proportions approaching the racial distribution of the U.S. HIV-infected population. It should be noted that some ACTG sites outside of the U.S. contributed black and Hispanic subjects to this trial although the numbers were not substantial. While AACTG studies have shown progressive increases in the proportion of black and Hispanic subjects in naive trials, industry studies have generally lagged behind. Many recent industry sponsored trials of treatment-naïve HIV-infected patients have enrolled less than 30% black and less than 10% Hispanic patients (Table 1).[14–19] These studies enrolled patients in 2000 or later. Since 2000, blacks and Hispanics have comprised over 65% of the AIDS cases within the U.S. and roughly 80% of the new HIV cases diagnosed each year. Thus, there remains need for improvement. Studies of treatment-experienced patients have performed even more poorly, often enrolling fewer than 20% minorities.[20–22] Recently the FDA has imposed new mandates that encourage pharmaceutical companies to include minorities and women at rates comparable with the rates of HIV/AIDS in the U.S. population. These new mandates may lead to better understanding of the use of newer agents in diverse populations.

Comparison to Other Research Areas

Low rate of participation in HIV-related clinical trials among African Americans (AA) and Hispanics is well documented but it is not unique to HIV clinical trials. Communities of color historically have low participation in clinical trials in many research areas even when minorities are disproportionally impacted by the clinical disease. One of the best examples is in the area of cancer research. Between 1998 and 2002 the all-sites cancer incidence for AA males was 23% higher than that for whites; colon and rectal cancers were 18% higher for AA males and 24% higher for AA females; lung cancers were 49% higher in AA males than in white males.[23] Even more striking is the fact that all-site cancer death rates were 40% higher for AA males and 18% higher for AA females. This includes twofold higher rate of death from cervical and prostate cancers in AA than in whites.[23] Despite the fact that AA have the highest cancer mortality rates and the poorest survival from cancer, AA traditionally have low rates of participation in cancer research trials.

A review of NCI-sponsored cooperative group nonsurgical treatment trials for breast, lung, colorectal, and prostate cancers including over 75,000 participants found that approximately 3.1% of trial participants were Hispanics, 85.6% were whites, 9.2% were blacks, 1.9% were Asian/Pacific Islanders, and 0.3% were American Indian/Alaskan Natives.[24] When all four cancer types were considered together, Hispanics and blacks were underrepresented. Compared with the 1.8% enrollment fraction for whites, only 1.3% of Hispanic cancer patients and 1.3% of black cancer patients participated in trials, thus Hispanics and blacks were roughly 30% less likely to participate in trials than whites. Enrollment varied by type of cancer. Black patients with breast, colorectal, or lung cancers were significantly less likely to participate in clinical trials than whites, while blacks with prostate CA were nearly 20% more likely to participate than whites. Hispanic patients were less likely to enroll in trials of all four cancer types than whites. Importantly despite recognition of the problem there has been no improvement over time. In the period from 1996 to 2002, the percentage of racial and ethnic minorities participating in clinical trials decreased from 3.7% in 1996 to 3.0% in 2002 for Hispanics and from 11% to 7.9% for blacks over the same period.[24]

Barriers to Participation

History of African Americans and the U.S. Medical Establishment: Origins of Mistrust

Historically the interactions between the AA community and the medical establishment have been challenged by racial discrimination, disempowerment, and lack of access. A historical discussion of African Americans and the medical establishment must include events that occurred during the antebellum South. Prior to the adoption of the 13th and 14th Amendment of the Constitution and the first and second Civil Rights Acts, the status of African Americans was that of chattels. The main purpose of a chattel from the slave owner's perspective was to provide the maximum daily work. If an owner's livestock or chattel were ill, the owners would try to initiate care themselves; only when the illness was serious were chattel physicians brought in to provide care.

Harriet Washington wrote that the care provided was reflective of both the medical knowledge and the pervasive racism at that time. For example, surgical procedures such as bloodletting, the lack of sterile technique or anesthesia in surgery, and trephination (therapeutic holes drilled in skulls) were coupled with beliefs that AA had higher threshold of pain, or that infection was because of AAs' innate inferior biological systems rather than unsterile medical conditions.[25] These commonly held distinctions among others led to slave science and slave medicine with the underlying premise that disease processes occurred differently compared with Caucasians. In fact, Southern physicians had slave-specific diseases such as drapetomania coined by Dr. Samuel Cartwright, the urge to run free from the master.[26] These purported differences led to experiments on slaves.

Experiments on slaves were conducted when slaves were loaned to physicians or physicians purchased slaves for the purpose of experimentation. Analogous to modern day experimentation on animals, surgeries, medical procedures, and the development of surgical instruments were conducted and perfected on African American persons before they were conducted on white persons. Famous examples include ovarian tumor removal (Dr. McDowell); urinary bladder stone removal (Dr. P.C. Spencer); vesico-vaginal fistula repair, and speculum development (Dr. Marion Sims, the father of gynecology).[25, 27, 28] Two hundred slaves of Thomas Jefferson were inoculated with smallpox before Jefferson allowed the vaccine to be distributed to family. Often, studies were performed based on empirical design rather than on scientific rigor. Examples include empirical studies for typhoid and for heat exposure. Slaves were subjected to being buried up to their necks in open-pit ovens to discover solutions to heat exposure.[27]

The exploitation of differences between AA and Caucasians evolved into display of AA persons in circuses and freak shows. The Hottentot women and individuals from the pygmy tribes were dressed in stereotypical displays to overemphasize anatomical differences between AA and Caucasians and to emphasize supposed similarities between AA and animals.[25] Death was not a respite from exploitation as graves were desecrated by night raiders who dug up bodies or parts in response to the growing need of bodies for anatomy lessons in medical schools.

The evolution of medical education in America in the late 1800s involved the incorporation of German and French scientific techniques and disciplines. Competition among medical schools for medical students was often decided by the rates of medical and surgical procedures and the availability of autopsies for education. Both the indigent and slaves were highly sought after as patients for surgical demonstrations and for highly prized autopsies.[25, 27] The desecration of graves by so called "night raiders" also became a tool of fear for newly freed African Americans used in the postbellum South to prevent leaving. The health of African Americans was not entirely dependent upon the slaves' doctors. The skill set of AA traditional healers was notable. Onesimus is attributed to teaching Dr. Jennings about variolation for treatment of smallpox disease.[29] Limited numbers of AA in the North were able to be educated and attended medical schools such as University of Pennsylvania, Harvard Medical School, and Chicago Medical School. In 1890, Dr. Daniel Hale Williams, a graduate from Chicago Medical School, established one of the first Black private hospitals, Provident Hospital, in response to the segregation of nursing and medical education.[29] Other Black graduates followed suit and post-Civil War established Black Hospitals and schools of nursing and medicine. In fact by 1910, there were over 20 African American medical schools and 40 Black-established Hospitals. By 1923, the number of Black private hospitals increased to approximately 200.[29, 30]

African American medical schools and other programs came under strict scrutiny by the Carnegie Foundation, and the American Medical Association (AMA) commissioned report, commonly referred to as the "Flexner Report."[29, 31] The AMA had become concerned at the decreasing reputation of physicians coupled with the increase in proprietary medical schools and the practice of medicine by nonphysicians. The purpose of the study was to observe and rate the 147 medical schools. Flexner used the template of John Hopkins Medical School and schools in Germany to determine what was considered a rigorous medical education. Flexner's report was particularly stringent and harsh to African American medical schools, giving poor ratings to all but Meharry and Howard. Flexner's future plans for these specific two schools were to improve their curricula and infrastructure but only so that AA physicians can serve as hygienists and prevent the spread of disease to white communities.[29, 31] Howard and Meharry were the source of medical education for the majority of AA physicians until medical school and hospital desegregation in the 1960s.

One of the most well-known examples of racial discrimination and exploitation imposed on AA is the Tuskegee Syphilis study, now referred to as the U.S. Public Health Service Syphilis Study, which was a Public Health Service sponsored study of syphilis that ran from 1932 to 1972. A study of untreated syphilis in Oslo, Norway prompted the "scientific hypothesis" that the symptoms of tertiary syphilis in White men would be different (mainly neurological) from that in African American men (cardiovascular).[29, 30, 32] Four-hundred thirty-one African American men with syphilis and at a second stage, 200 controls were recruited to participate in this study of the natural history of syphilis.[32, 33] "Compensation" for participation included $25 for clinic visits and $50 for burial insurance. Subjects underwent multiple biopsies, blood draws, and lumbar punctures as part of the study.[33] The lumbar punctures were disguised as treatment or spinal shots for the "Bad Blood" that the men were told they were ill from. In 1941, penicillin became readily available for treatment of syphilis. Participants in the study were not supplied with penicillin and were actively discouraged from seeking treatment elsewhere. Despite the discovery of penicillin as a cure and the introduction of federal legislation requiring testing and treatment of veneral disease in 1943 and the Helsenki Code in 1964, requiring informed consent for research subjects, the experiment continued unfettered.

As the goal was to elicit information at the terminal stage of syphilis through autopsies, a credited quote by one of the study doctors, "As I see it, we have no further use of these patients until they die."[32] As a result, they suffered the consequences of untreated syphilis, which included blindness, paralysis, dementia, cardiac disease, and death. It is estimated that as many as 28 men died directly from syphilis; 100 men died from complications of syphilis; and 40 wives and 19 children became infected from sexual and vertical transmission.[32, 34]

In 1973, Fred Gray, an AA civil rights attorney litigated a $1.8 billion class action suit, "Pollard vs. the United States" on behalf of Mr. Charlie Pollard and other survivors. Gray negotiated an out-of-court settlement for ten million dollars ($37,500 to each survivor and 15,000 to families of the deceased). The settlement was to be used to create a Federal program specifically to supply lifetime medical and burial benefits for survivors and later their wives and children.[35] In 1997, President Bill Clinton after negotiations by Dr. Vanessa Gamble, MD, PhD, chairwoman of the Tuskegee Syphilis Legacy Committee[36] made an official apology to black men for the shameful U.S. experiment in which their syphilis went untreated by government doctors.[31] The Tuskegee University National Center for Bioethics was created as a response to the Presidential apology.[30,32] Knowledge of the Tuskegee study is very pervasive in the AA community and as is often the case with oral histories, the true history is often distorted or exaggerated to the degree that some AA believe that black men were intentionally infected with syphilis by the U.S. government as a part of this study. A survey of AA patients seeking outpatient medical care at an urban public hospital revealed that all of the 33 individuals surveyed had some knowledge of the study but few could describe the specific details.[37] Even if individuals are not certain about the details of the study, most are certain that blacks were harmed at the hands of the U.S. government. In the acclaimed book "Bad Blood: The Tuskegee syphilis Experiment," Jones wrote "For many blacks the Tuskegee study became a symbol of their mistreatment by the medical establishment, a metaphor for deceit, conspiracy, malpractice, and neglect, if not outright racial genocide."[34] Thus, it is not difficult to understand why certain myths regarding HIV remain commonly held beliefs in some parts of the black community; these myths have a basis in historical injustices imparted on the black community. Further trusted institutions and individuals in the black community have promoted some of these myths. For example, The Nation of Islam has disseminated literature that describes AIDS as a form of genocide against blacks.[38] Essence magazine, a popular black womens' magazine, published an article entitled "AIDS: Is It Genocide," in which a prominent black New York physician stated that "there is a possibility that the virus was produced to limit the number of African people and people of color in the world who are no longer needed."[39] Most recently, Reverend Jeremiah Wright, a nationally renowned black minister from Chicago, stated on national television that it was possible that the HIV virus was created by the U.S. government and Kanye West, an award winning popular rap artist and sought-after musical producer has stated governmental involvement in the production of AIDS in America and Africa in his rhymes and in concert. In his hit single "Heard 'Em Say," he raps "So this is in the name of love like Robert say/Before you ask me to go get a job today/Can I at least get a raise from minimum wage?/And I know the government administered AIDS/So I guess we just pray like the government say."[40]

Bogart et al. surveyed 500 African Americans regarding beliefs and perceptions related to HIV/AIDS.[41] Twenty-six percent of the group believed that "AIDS is a man-made disease created in a U.S. government lab"; 56% thought that "There is a cure for AIDS but it is being withheld from the poor," and 58% believed that "People who take the new medicines for HIV are human guinea pigs for the government"

Table 2 Myths and conspiracy beliefs about HIV/AIDS: survey of 500 African Americans

	Agree somewhat or strongly (%)		
	Overall	Men ($n = 174$)	Women ($n = 326$)
AIDS is a man-made virus created in a government lab	26.6	30.5	24.5
There is a cure for AIDS but it is being withheld from the poor	53.4	55.2	52.5
People who take the new medicines for HIV are human guinea pigs for the government	43.6	43.7	43.6
A lot of information about AIDS is being held back from the public	58.8	62.6	56.8
The medicines used to treat HIV cause AIDS	6.0	7.5	5.2

Adapted from Bogart et al.[41]

(Table 2). With such myths being frequently held or heard about in the AA community it is not surprising that AA fear the medical establishment and, in particular, fear clinical trials. The medical and health service literature has extensive articles that outline AA medical mistrust or distrust. A Medline search of mistrust or distrust and African Americans reveals 109 and 90 articles, respectively. A telephone survey of 527 AA and 382 white respondents from across the U.S. found that AA were more likely than whites not to trust that their physician would fully explain research participation (41.7% vs. 23.4%, $p < 0.01$) and to state that they believed their physicians exposed them to unnecessary risks (45.5% vs. 34.8%, $p < 0.01$). After controlling for SES (socioeconomic status) in a logistic regression model, race remained strongly associated with higher distrust.[42]

Access to Care/Access to Research

The Commonwealth Fund interviewed 6,722 persons regarding disparities in quality of health care.[43] Of the 6,722, 1,037 were AA and 1,153 were Hispanics. African Americans and Hispanics in the sample had higher percentages of people who rated their health as fair or poor, did not have a regular doctor, and reported communication problems with their physicians. Also concerning was the impact of race on attitudes toward health care; AA and Hispanics had higher rates of respondents who felt that they would receive better care if they were of a different race or ethnicity and they were less confident of receiving quality health care in the future. Access to research requires at a minimum access to quality health care. Variables that impact access to both include socioeconomic status, age, education, employment, geographic region, and health status.

Poverty disproportionately impacts racial and ethnic minorities, and SES has consistently correlated with clinical trial participation in the U.S. Persons living with HIV have a high incidence of poverty. At least 15% of participant in the SHAS project reported annual income $<10,000$ per year.[6] The median household income of women who participate in the Women's Interagency HIV Study (WIHS), the largest cohort study of HIV-infected women in the U.S., is $4,500 per year.[44] Low SES results in lower access to health care, lower and later HIV screening, limited access to research institutions, less access to private health insurance, and more dependence on Medicare and Medicaid. In addition, the costs associated with research participation (travel, child-care, absence from work) are often not covered by clinical trials. This added financial burden for individuals who may live with constant concerns related to economic survival undoubtedly serves to further deter clinical trial participation.[45]

Cunningham et al. in the HIV Cost and Services Utilization Study (HCSUS) reported that competing needs such as need for money for food, housing, clothing, or need for transportation impacted participant access to care.[46] These same factors have been included along with the need for child care and compensation for missed work as reasons why there are lower clinical trial participation rates among minorities and minority women.[47]

Lack of education further limits the potential for participation in clinical trials. Educational level can be a proxy for the ability to read and comprehend study protocol and documents. For true informed consent, the participant has to be able to read the informed consent forms to understand what is being required of him or her. Current recommendations are written at a sixth grade reading level to maximize comprehension. Focus group discussions have shown that being unable to read or understand the informed consent forms or the concept of informed consent encourages distrust of clinical research and academic medical establishments. Furthermore, the use of research terminology can be confusing and studies have demonstrated that African Americans may not recognize certain terms to describe research. For example, King et al. focus groups of 60 HIV-positive AA men and women; several AA stated that they would participate in a "study" but did not want to participate in a "trial." Additionally, clinical trials are usually conducted within academic medical centers and tertiary care hospitals. This can limit access due to geography, often requiring individuals to travel outside their communities. Further major medical centers can be intimidating to individuals who are unfamiliar with them.[48]

Investigator/Provider Barriers

Historical injustices imparted on minority and other communities led to vigorous efforts to improve the protection of human subjects. The Declaration of Helsinki and the Belmont report by the National Commission for the Protection of Human

Subjects of Biomedical and behavioral research established standards for human subject protection, and institutional review boards (IRBs) were established. These regulations had tremendous positive effects in improving protection of human subjects; however, a consequence of heightened awareness of vulnerable populations may have contributed to exclusion of minority populations from clinical trials. Researchers feared the perception of exploitation of vulnerable populations and thus avoided the issue. In the early 1990s, the research community became increasingly concerned that research that was not inclusive of women and minorities may not be widely applicable to the public and that is was unjust to exclude certain populations from the benefit (and risks) of participation in research.[42] These concerns led to the NIH Revitalization ACT of 1993.[49] NIH research guidelines were revised in response to this law and mandated the inclusion of women and racial/ethnic minorities in federally funded research and that for phase II clinical trials, sufficient numbers of women and minorities be included to allow valid analyses of differences in the effect of interventions on these populations.[50] Despite this mandate, participation in clinical trials among women and minorities remains low. Of the 4,739 black participants of the SHAS project, only 15% ever participated in a clinical trial. For men in this study, the most common reason for not participating in clinical research was lack of information about research/not being offered enrollment; this accounted for 75% of all nonparticipants. Among women, the most common reasons for nonparticipation were lack of information about research/not being offered enrollment (75%), not wanting to be a "guinea pig" (10%), and not qualifying.[6] These findings are very similar to those of Stone et al. more than 10 years earlier.[51]

While the government mandate was a step in the right direction, such encouragement by itself cannot overcome the many barriers to increasing minority clinical trial participation. Potential participants can only enter clinical trials once they become aware that they are available and of what they might offer. Outside of direct and passive recruitment by clinical trial team members, participants are introduced to clinical trials by their physicians. Therefore, investigative team and participant providers are potential gatekeepers to participants; their impact on such participation is determined by their awareness and attitudes regarding clinical trial research. We performed an anonymous computer-based survey of study coordinators and research nurses from the AACTG clinical trials units in order to assess their attitudes and perceptions regarding recruitment and enrollment of women, IVDUs, and minorities (targeted populations) in ACTG clinical trials.[52] Most participants ranked white men as being the most interested in clinical trials compared with members of the targeted populations. They also stated that their interactions were the most effective with white men than with other persons. Clinical scenarios revealed that site personnel felt that they were less likely to enroll individuals who had missed previous clinical appointments, and who did not speak English. It is clear that these perceptions among research personnel that IDUs, Hispanics, blacks and, to a lesser extent, women had less interest in participation in clinical trials than white males can significantly affect recruitment of the targeted populations.

Researcher and medical providers must seek to overcome their own perceptions, biases, and stereotypes in addition to the challenges posed by higher prevalence of mistrust among some AA. The role of the community based or academic provider can be as a gatekeeper and either facilitate or prevent enrollment within clinical trials. Of note, Gifford's study revealed that participants who had positive attitudes toward HIV medications and trust in their HIV provider were more likely to have a positive attitude toward research.[4] In other words, it appears that access to HIV care and trust can impact attitudes toward research.

A study of 200 HIV-infected AA receiving HIV care at the Pittsburgh AIDS Center for Treatment found that only 57% of survey participants had ever been asked to participate in an HIV treatment trial but of those who were asked, 86% agreed to participate.[53] Of the 98 patients who agreed to participate, 82% actually enrolled in clinical trials and 86% of those completed their study. Contrary to other studies these researchers found that distrust of the medical establishment was *not* associated with participation in trials or willingness to participate in future studies. Another study evaluated 286 urban HIV-infected persons (55% AA, 34% Latino) regarding attitudes toward AIDS clinical trials.[53] This study found that despite low knowledge of clinical trials and lower SES, 87% of those surveyed were somewhat or very willing to participate in AIDS clinical trials. Eighty-five percent of participants were willing to participate if the trials "helps cure AIDS"; 82% would participate if the study would "help lower the number of HIV infections in the community," and 90% would participate if "their primary doctor recommended it." Thus, it is clear that minority patients are willing to participate and the relationships with a primary provider can help overcome distrust issues. For males in this study greater understanding of clinical trials and the benefit of free health care positively impacts willingness to participate, while distrust of researchers impacted negatively. Meanwhile, women in this study placed a high importance on the benefit of the research to others. Studies at a major public hospital AACTG site found that providers perceived that minority patients were less interested in clinical trials and were less likely to inform minority patients about available trials because of these perceptions. And, in fact, this site had a history of enrolling fewer minorities in clinical trials, but once all patients were consistently informed about clinical trials and provided the same information about clinical trials, enrollment became equal by race/ethnicity.[54–56]

These studies demonstrate multiple important points: first AA are willing to participate in clinical trials, and they can successfully enroll and complete trials. Efforts to provide education about clinical trials can overcome distrust of researchers. Indeed when survey participants were asked how AA enrollment in clinical trials might be improved, AA survey participants expressed the need for more honest and respectful communication with researchers and the importance of providing complete information regarding the goals, risks, and benefits of the research.[37] Further, despite some individuals' concerns that the benefits of research do not reach AA and the poor, many AAs' willingness to participate is driven as much by altruism as by self-benefit. Finally, it is clear that provider recommendation and invitation to participate play a critical role in patients' decision making.

Study-Related Barriers

An additional potential barrier to AA participation in clinical trials is the design of the study. A review of the eligibility criteria of 32 seminal HIV treatment randomized clinical trials in the ACTG and Community Programs for Clinical Research on AIDS (CPCRA) revealed that as many as 67% (median 42%) of participants in the WIHS observational cohort would have been excluded from participation in those protocols on the basis of clinical (including pregnancy), laboratory, or concomitant medication criteria.[57] While it cannot be questioned that inclusion/exclusion criteria are necessary for the conduct of clinical trials, one has to consider the disproportional impact some criteria may have in excluding specific populations. For example, exclusion based upon active or historical substance abuse disproportionately excludes AA who have higher rates of HIV acquired from IVDU. AA also have more comorbid conditions such as hepatitis C, renal insufficiency, and hypertension. Exclusions on the basis of these criteria disproportionately exclude AA. The fact that most of the women in the WIHS cohort would be excluded from the major NIH-sponsored clinical trials raises serious concerns regarding the applicability of those study findings to the population of HIV-infected women. Moreover, it runs counter to the NIH-stated goals of wider inclusion of women and minorities. The review also pointed out that 83% of CPCRA studies and 40% of ACTG studies included subjective investigator-dependent eligibility criteria that could subject to investigator biases.[57] Examples of these are "Any medical or social condition which would adversely affect participation in or compliance with this study," or "Any disease that in the opinion of the investigator or study chair would interfere with the evaluation of the patient" or, "Subjects that the local investigator judges may not adhere to the requirements of this protocol." Such vague exclusion/inclusion criteria have the potential to introduce investigator bias into the selection of who is deemed appropriate for the study.

Strategies to Improve Participation

1. Active not exclusive recruitment: Offering recruitment to all persons within the catchment area would counter observations that AA were not aware of clinical trials being offered nor referred to clinical trials. Although fear and mistrust are important predisposing factors to participation, making clinical trial referrals more routine could begin to decrease suspicions among potential study participants and decrease the influence of investigator/provider bias.
2. Community oriented research: The involvement of the community as a partner from the study protocol development, inception and implementation is important in establishing trust and community buy-in. Involving the community at the early stage of development can be useful in obtaining consultation on language, translation, site location, and the importance of research question to the community.

3. Increase diversity of investigators: Currently there are low numbers of African American physicians in academic medicine. Mentorship, research-oriented fellowships of AA community-based physicians or physicians facing retirement may be methods in order to increase the supply.
4. Honoraria: Although altruism is listed as a reason for participating, many low-income clinical trial participants enroll because of the supplemental income that honoraria provide. Providing meals, transportation in the form of taxi or bus tokens, and grocery vouchers have been useful mechanisms in conjunction with minimum cash payments.[48] Transparency in the amount to be paid for which services and when that amount will be paid should be clear to the participant during the informed consent process. Any expenses that could accrue, parking and insurance costs for laboratory expenses must be divulged to the potential participant.
5. Participants need to be educated about the value of research and the potential impact research can have on one's health. Community forums with clear language, providing time for questions and answers, and being cognizant of suspicion. Culturally relevant pamphlets defining terms and procedures can be displayed in physician offices and waiting rooms.
6. Community-based providers need to be educated about the societal, academic, and financial value of conducting research. Fears about losing patients to academic medical centers should be respected and addressed. Realistic and pragmatic discussions about the implementation of research in the private office can be conducted in the medical office or in conjunction with local medical societies.
7. Academic medical researchers and teams need to create partnerships with community organizations and providers. Partnerships will extend beyond treating community organizations and providers as recruiting bins, rather, there will be mutual learning and teaching in preparation of the study. The community partner will bring in expertise regarding cultural nuances or lexicons while protecting against unintentional or direct biases and stereotypes of academic medical research teams. Shared resources can potentially eliminate funding prohibitions on certain items of necessity for study participants. Shared resources can also translate into the use of the research team's assistance in data collection in preparation for community monthly reports or grant writing.

References

1. CDC: AIDS Surveillance Report. 2008
2. Medline Search. July 1, 2008
3. Mackenzie S. Scientific silence: AIDS and African Americans in the medical literature. American Journal of Public Health. July 2000, 90(7):1145–1146
4. Gifford AL, et al. Participation in research and access to experimental treatments by HIV-infected patients. New England Journal of Medicine. May 2002, 346(18):1373–82
5. AIDS Clinical Trials Group Annual Report 2002

6. Sullivan PS, McNaghten AD, Begley E, Hutchinson A, Cargill VA. Enrollment of racial/ethnic minorities and women with HIV in clinical research studies of HIV medicines. Journal of the National Medical Association. March 2007, 99(3):242–50

7. Volberding PA, Lagakos SW, Grimes JM, Stein DS, Rooney J, Meng TC, Fischl MA, Collier AC, Phair JP, Hirsch MS, et al. A comparison of immediate with deferred zidovudine therapy for asymptomatic HIV-infected adults with CD4 cell counts of 500 or more per cubic millimeter. New England Journal of Medicine. 1995 August 17, 333(7):401–7

8. CDC HIV/AIDS Surveillance Report, 1988

9. Collier AC, Coombs RW, Schoenfeld DA, Bassett RL, Timpone J, Baruch A, Jones M, Facey K, Whitacre C, McAuliffe VJ, Friedman HM, Merigan TC, Reichman RC, Hooper C, Corey L. Treatment of human immunodeficiency virus infection with saquinavir, zidovudine, and zalcitabine. AIDS Clinical Trials Group. New England Journal of Medicine. April 1996 18, 334(16):1011–7

10. CDC HIV/AIDS Surveillance Report, 1993

11. Gulick RM, Ribaudo HJ, Shikuma CM, et al. Triple-nucleoside regimens versus efavirenz-containing regimens for the initial treatment of HIV-1 Infection. New England Journal of Medicine. 2004, 350:1850–1861

12. Wegner S, Vahey M, Dolan M, et al. Racial differences in clinical efficacy of efavirenz-based antiretroviral therapy. In: Program and Abstracts of the 9th Conference on Retroviruses and Opportunistic Infections. Seattle, Washington, DC. February 24–28, 2002. Abstract 428

13. Riddler SA, Haubrich R, DiRienzo AG, Peeples L, Powderly WG, Klingman KL, Garren KW, George T, Rooney JF, Brizz B, Lalloo UG, Murphy RL, Swindells S, Havlir D, Mellors JW. The AIDS Clinical Trials Group Study A5142 Team. Class-Sparing Regimens for Initial Treatment of HIV-1 Infection. New England Journal of Medicine. 2008, 358:2095–2106

14. Gallant JE, Staszewski S, Pozniak AL, et al. Efficacy and safety of tenofovir DF vs stavudine in combination therapy in antiretroviral-naïve patients: a 3-year randomized trial. JAMA. 2004, 292:191–201

15. Gallant JE, DeJesus E, Arribas JR, Pozniak AL, Gazzard B, Campo RE, Lu B, McColl D, Chuck S, Enejosa J, Toole JJ, Cheng AK, the Study 934 Group. Tenofovir DF, Emtricitabine, and Efavirenz vs. Zidovudine, Lamivudine, and Efavirenz for HIV. New England Journal of Medicine. 2006, 354:251–260

16. Eron J Jr, Yeni P, Gathe J Jr, Estrada V, DeJesus E, Staszewski S, Lackey P, Katlama C, Young B, Yau L, Sutherland-Phillips D, Wannamaker P, Vavro C, Patel L, Yeo J, Shaefer M, KLEAN study team. The KLEAN study of fosamprenavir-ritonavir versus lopinavir-ritonavir, each in combination with abacavir-lamivudine, for initial treatment of HIV infection over 48 weeks: a randomised non-inferiority trial. Lancet. August 2006 5, 368(9534):476–82

17. Smith K, et al. Program and abstracts of the 15th Conference on Retroviruses and Opportunistic Infections, 2008: Poster 774

18. Smith KY, Weinberg WG, Dejesus E, Fischl MA, Liao Q, Ross LL, Pakes GE, Pappa KA, Lancaster CT, the ALERT (COL103952) Study Team. Fosamprenavir or atazanavir once daily boosted with ritonavir 100 mg, plus tenofovir/emtricitabine, for the initial treatment of HIV infection: 48-week results of ALERT. AIDS Research and Therapy. 28 March 2008, 5(1):5

19. Gathe J, da Silva B, Loutfy M, and others. Study M05–730 primary efficacy results at week 48: phase 3, randomized, open-label study of lopinavir/ritonavir tablets once daily vs twice daily, co-administered with tenofovir DF + emtricitabine in ARV-naive HIV-1-infected subjects. In: 15th Conference on Retroviruses and Opportunistic Infections (CROI 2008). Boston, MA. February 3–6, 2008. Abstract 775

20. Molina JM, Cohen C, Katlama C, et al. TMC114/r in treatment-experienced HIV patients in POWER 3: 24-week efficacy and safety analysis. In: Program and abstracts of the XVI International AIDS Conference. Toronto, Canada. August 13–18, 2006. Abstract TUPE0060

21. Cooper D, Gatell J, Rockstroh J, et al. For the BENCHMRK-1 Study Group. Results of BENCHMRK-1, a phase III study evaluating the efficacy and safety of MK-0518, a novel HIV-1 integrase inhibitor, in patients with triple-class resistant virus. In: Program and abstracts of the 14th Conference on Retroviruses and Opportunistic Infections. Los Angeles, CA. February 25–28, 2007. Abstract 105aLB

22. Lalezari J, Goodrich J, DeJesus E, et al. Efficacy and safety of maraviroc plus optimized background therapy in viremic ART-experienced patients infected with CCR5-tropic HIV-1: 24-week results of a phase 2b/3 study in the U.S. and Canada. In: Program and Abstracts of the 14th Conference on Retroviruses and Opportunistic Infections. Los Angeles, CA. February 25–28, 2007. Abstract 104bLB

23. Jemal A, Siegel R, Ward E, Murray T, Xu J, Smigal C, Thun MJ. Cancer Statistics, 2006. CA: A Cancer Journal for Clinicians. 2006, 56:106–130

24. Murthy VH, Krumholz HM, Cary P. Gross participation in cancer clinical trials: Race-, sex-, and age-based disparities. JAMA. 2004, 291(22):2720–2726

25. Washington HA. Medical Apartheid. Copyright © 2007 Harlem Moon, a division of Random House, Inc

26. Dictionary of Psychology 2001, Originally Published by Oxford University Press 2001

27. Randall VR. Slavery, segregation and racism: trusting the health care system ain't always easy! An African American perspective on bioethics. St Louis Univ Public Law Rev. 1996, 15(2):191–235

28. Savitt TL. Race and Medicine in Nineteenth and Early Twentieth-Century America. Kent, Ohio: Kent State University Press, 2007

29. Morais HM. The History of the Negro in Medicine (International Library of Negro Life and History). New York, Publishers Company. 1967

30. Africana: The Encyclopedia of the African and African American Experience. Kwame Anthony Appiah and Henry Louis Gates, Jr., Editors. New York, NY: Basic Civitas Books

31. Andrew HB. The Flexner report and the standardization of American medical education. JAMA. 2004, 291(17):2139–2140

32. Brunner, B. The Tuskegee Syphilis Study. http://www.tuskegee.edu/Global/Story.asp?s$= $1207586 (last accessed July 10th, 2008)

33. Thomas SB, Quinn SC. The Tuskegee Syphilis Study, 1932 to 1972: implications for HIV education and AIDS risk education programs in the black community. American Journal of Public Health. 1991, 81:1498–1505

34. Jones JH. Bad Blood: The Tuskegee Syphilis Experiment. New York: Free Press, January 1993

35. Gray F. Tuskegee Syphilis Study: The Real Story and Beyond. Montgomery, Alabama: River City Publisher, 1998

36. Baker S, Brawley O, Marks L. Effects of untreated syphilis in the negro male, 1932 to 1972: A closure comes to the Tuskegee study. Urology. 2004, 65(6):1259–1262

37. Corbie-Smith G, Thomas SB, Williams MV, Moody-Ayers S. Attitudes and beliefs of African Americans toward participation in medical research. Journal of General Internal Medicine. September 1999, 14(9):537–546(10)

38. Smith R. Muhammad warns Blacks to beware: social AIDS. Eclipse: The Black Student News Magazine of the University of Maryland. November 23 1988, 21:6

39. Bates K. AIDS: Is it genocide? Essence. September 1990, 21:77–116

40. West K. (Feat. Adam Levine of Maroon 5) Song. Heard 'Em Say. Album: Late Registration (2005)

41. Bogart LM, Thorburn S. Are HIV/AIDS conspiracy beliefs a barrier to HIV prevention among African Americans? Journal of Acquired Immune Deficiency Syndrome. 2005, 38:213–218

42. Corbie-Smith G, Thomas SB, St. George DM. Distrust, race, and research. Archives of Internal Medicine. 2002, 162(21):2458–2463

43. Collins KC, Hughes DL, Doty MM, Ives BL, Edwards JN, Tenney K. Diverse Communities, Americans. The Commonwealth Fund, March 2002

44. French A, et al. Program and Abstracts of the 44th Annual Meeting of the Infectious Diseases Society of America. 2006. Abstract. 935

45. Giuliano AR, Mokuau N, Hughes C, Tortolero-Luna G, Risendal B, Ho RCS, Prewitt TE, McCaskill-Stevens WJ. Participation of minorities in cancer research: the influence of structural, cultural, and linguistic factors. Annals of Epidemiology. 2000 November, 10(8 Suppl):S22–34

46. Cunningham WE, Andersen RM, Katz MH, Stein MD, Turner BJ, Crystal S, Zierler S, Kuromiya K, Morton SC, St Clair P, Bozzette SA, Shapiro MF. The impact of competing subsistence needs and barriers on access to medical care for persons with human immunodeficiency virus receiving care in the United States. Medical Care. 1999 December, 37(12):1270–81

47. Advani AS, Atkeson B, Brown CL, Peterson BL, Fish L, Johnson JL, Gockerman JP, Gautier M. Barriers to the participation of African American patients with cancer in clinical trials. Cancer. 2003, 97(6):1499–1506

48. King WD, Ramey R, Jones, S, Clemons K, Wyatt G. Assessing the Attitudes of HIV Seropositive Black Men and Women Towards Participation in HIV Clinical Trials. The 3rd IAS Conference on HIV Pathogenesis and Treatment Abstract no WePe13.13P12

49. National Institutes of Health Revitalization Act of 1993. http://thomas.loc.gov/cgi-bn/query/ Dc103.5./temp/$\sim$c1039LS2u1.

50. National Institutes of Health (2001). NIH policy and guidelines on the inclusion of women and minorities as subjects in clinical research. http://grants.nih.gov/grants/funding/women_min/ guidelines_amendment_10_2001.htm.

51. Stone VE, Mauch MY, Steger K, Craven DE. Race, gender, drug use and participation in AIDS clinical trials. Journal of General Internal Medicine 1997, 12:150–57

52. King WD, Defreiitas D, Smith K, Andersen J, Perry LP, Adeyemi T, Mitty J, Fritsche J, Jeffries C, Littles M, Fischl M, Pavlov G, Mildvan D. For the Underrepresented Populations Committee of the Adult AIDS Clinical Trial Group (AACTG) Attitudes and perceptions of AIDS clinical trials group site coordinators on HIV clinical trial recruitment and retention: a descriptive study. AIDS Patient Care STDS. August 2007, 21(8):551–63

53. Garber M, Hanusa BH, Switzer GE, Mellors J, Arnold RM. HIV-infected African Americans are willing to participate in HIV treatment trials. Journal of General Internal Medicine. January 2007, 22(1):17–42

54. Stone VE, Mauch MY, Steger K, Craven DE. Race, gender, drug use and participation in AIDS clinical trials. Journal of General Internal Medicine 1997, 12:150–57

55. Stone VE, Mauch MY, Steger KA. Provider attitudes regarding the participation of women and persons of color in AIDS clinical trials. Journal of Acquired Immune Deficiency Syndrome. 1998, 19:245–53

56. Freedberg KA, Sullivan L, Georgakis A, Savetsky J, Stone VE, Samet JH. Improving participation in clinical trials: Impact of a brief intervention. HIV Clinical Trials. 2001, 2(3):205–212

57. Gwadz MV, Leonard NR, Nakagawa A, Cylar K, Finkelstein M, Herzog N, Tharaken M, Mildvan D. Gender differences in attitudes toward AIDS clinical trials among urban HIV-infected individuals from racial and ethnic minority backgrounds. AIDS Care. October 2006, 18(7):786–794(9)

The Impact of HIV Policies and Politics on Communities of Color

M. Keith Rawlings and Deborah Parham Hopson

Medicaid, Medicare, and the Ryan White HIV/AIDS Program are the three primary public payers of HIV/AIDS care in the U.S. today (see Fig. 1). Though far from flawless, they create access to services for scores of underserved minority people living with HIV/AIDS (PLWHA). These programs are key to scaling back the ominous and disproportionate presence of HIV/AIDS among underserved people of color.

In 2005,[*] this presence was visible in the demographics of PLWHA (see Fig. 2):

- Approximately half of the people who developed HIV/AIDS were blacks[†] and one-fifth were Hispanics.[1]
- African American men were nearly eight times more likely to have AIDS than non-Hispanic white men, and Hispanic men were nearly three times more likely to have AIDS than non-Hispanic white men.[2]
- African American women were nearly 23 times more likely to have AIDS than non-Hispanic white women, and Hispanic women were five times more likely to have AIDS than non-Hispanic white women.[3]
- American Indian and Alaska Natives were more than twice likely to have AIDS than non-Hispanic whites.[2]

In addition to disproportionate rates of HIV/AIDS, health disparities and poor access to health care among minorities living with HIV are well documented in the literature.[4] Public health programs must work with increasing effectiveness to mitigate those problems. This imperative is made more difficult by interrelated problems such as disproportionate rates of poverty; lack of health insurance; and a shortage

---

[*] At the time of publication, 2005 was the most recent year for which HIV/AIDS statistics were made available by the Centers for Disease Control and Prevention.

[†] "Black" is used by the U.S. Census Bureau.

M.K. Rawlings (✉)
Peabody Health Center, AIDS Arms, Inc., Dallas, TX, U.S.
E-mail: Krawlings@aidsarms.org

V. Stone et al. (eds.), *HIV/AIDS in U.S. Communities of Color*.
DOI: 10.1007/978-0-387-98152-9_14, © Springer Science + Business Media, LLC 2009

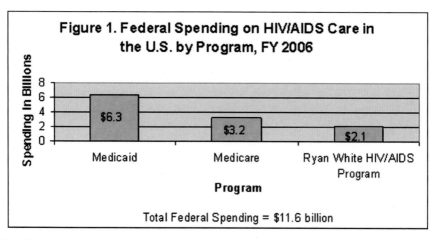

Fig. 1 Federal Spending on HIV/AIDS Care in the U.S. by Program, FY 2006 (Henry J. Kaiser Foundation - KFF)

Figure 2. AIDS Rate by Race/Ethnicity and Gender, 2005 (per 100,000 population)			
Race/Ethnicity	Males	Females	Total
White, non-Hispanic	12.1	2.0	6.9
Black, non-Hispanic	95.1	45.5	68.7
Hispanic	36.0	11.2	24.0
Asian/Pacific Islander	7.2	1.6	4.3
American Indian/Alaska Native	14.3	4.4	9.3
Total	24.9	8.6	16.6

Fig. 2 AIDS Rate by Race/Ethnicity and Gender, 2005 (per 100,000 population) (CDC)

of indigenous, high-quality health care providers in many communities of color.[5–10] Moreover, some communities of color are palpably wary about the "government" aspect of public health care programs and thus hesitate before engaging the health care system. Each of those barriers must be overcome for the promise of Medicaid, Medicare, and the Ryan White HIV/AIDS Program to be realized among PLWHA of color.

The roles of the nation's public health programs are complementary and critical to addressing HIV/AIDS. The two largest programs in terms of public investment are Medicaid and Medicare, but they leave gaps in coverage in terms of both program eligibility and services covered. The mission of the comparatively small Ryan White HIV/AIDS Program is to fill those gaps, which it currently does for approximately 531,000 PLWHA per year – between two and three times as many PLWHA as are covered by Medicaid.[11]

Understanding the relationship among the large federal programs serving underserved PLWHA of color is necessary if our nation is to stem the tide of the HIV/AIDS epidemic among minorities. With that understanding, health disparities among minorities – including the disproportionate impact of HIV/AIDS – can be addressed.

Medicaid

Medicaid is the largest public health care program in the nation and is the largest payer of care for PLWHA by far.[12] At $6.3 billion, Medicaid accounted for 51% of all federal HIV/AIDS spending in fiscal year 2006, with more than 200,000 PLWHA enrolled in the program.[13] No other public or private insurance plan or assistance program covers such a comprehensive range of services (see Table 1).[14]

Medicaid is a federal–state (and territory) partnership. Each state and territory operates its own Medicaid program. The federal government matches state spending on Medicaid on an unlimited basis. States maintain significant discretion in designing and administering Medicaid programs, but federal law sets minimum eligibility requirements for mandatory populations, including the following:

- All pregnant women, regardless of age or family circumstances, if their incomes are at or below 133% of the federal poverty level (FPL)
- Children under age 6 with family incomes totaling less than 133% of the FPL ($1,737 per month in 2004 for a family of three) and older children (ages 6–18)

Table 1 Medicaid Summary, 2004, The Henry J. Kaiser Family Foundation (KFF)

Who is eligible	What it covers	Administrator	Total served	PLWHA served
Low-income children and parents, people with disabilities, and seniors (age 65 and older)	Physician and hospital care; laboratory and diagnostic services; nursing home care; and at State option, a comprehensive array of acute care and long-term services (e.g., personal assistance with activities of daily living)	States, subject to oversight by the Centers for Medicare and Medicaid Services	58,420,500	>200,000

Source: The Henry J. Kaiser Family Foundation Total Medicaid enrollment, FY 2004. Available at: www.statehealthfacts.org/comparemaptable.jsp?ind=198&cat=4. Accessed December 14, 2007

with family incomes totaling less than 100% of FPL ($1,306 per month in 2004 for a family of three)
- Some low-income parents of minors [parents' Medicaid eligibility standard is usually tied to the standard used in a State's Temporary Assistance to Needy Families (TANF) program instead of to the FPL and tends to be considerably lower than the 133% of the FPL used for pregnant women]
- Low-income people with disabilities and the elderly who qualify for the Supplemental Security Income (SSI) program or meet similar state-set income requirements (SSI guarantees benefits only up to 74% of the FPL; approximately 78% of Medicaid beneficiaries with disabilities qualify on the basis of their SSI eligibility); a person is defined as disabled under Social Security when he or she is unable to work because of a medical condition and his or her medical condition is expected to last at least 1 year or to result in death.[15]

The eligibility criteria help open doors to health care that might otherwise be closed for many minority PLWHA. States can go beyond these federal minimum eligibility standards to ensure even greater access to care. For example, many states choose to extend Medicaid to people with disabilities who have income up to 100% of FPL instead of up to the federal threshold of 74%.

Of the more than 200,000 PLWHA with Medicaid insurance in the U.S. today, most qualify on the basis of disability and eligibility for SSI benefits. A second major eligibility pathway for PLWHA is "optional coverage for the medically needy," offered by 36 states and the District of Columbia. This coverage permits people in a Medicaid eligibility category with income above the income standard to qualify if medical expenses subtracted from income leave a dollar amount below the state-established medically needy limit. In some cases, people must spend down to very low income levels to qualify as medically needy. In one study, the median medically needy income limit was 55% of the FPL.[16]

Medicaid: Reaching PLWHA of Color

Medicaid has provided access to services for tens of thousands of PLWHA of color. Several components of the program ensure its relevance to eligible PLWHA.

Guaranteed coverage. Unlike the Ryan White HIV/AIDS Program, Medicaid is an entitlement program with defined sets of benefits. All people who meet the program eligibility requirements have an enforceable right to enroll in Medicaid and to receive services on a timely basis. Eligible people cannot be denied Medicaid.

Mandatory services. Just as federal law requires that Medicaid cover specific populations, it also stipulates mandatory services that states must cover. Mandatory services include core services such as ambulatory and inpatient care, laboratory services, and nursing home care. States can also offer additional "optional services" to meet the needs of the Medicaid population. Optional services include prescription drug coverage (which is currently provided by all Medicaid programs), physical and occupational therapy, personal care, and rehabilitation services.

Obligatory coverage of children. Minorities account for the vast majority of AIDS cases diagnosed among people under 19 years of age in the U.S.[17,18] For example, among reported AIDS diagnoses in 2005, only 17% of adolescents 13–19 years of age were black, yet they accounted for 69% of reported HIV/AIDS cases.[19] In the same year, 86% of babies born with HIV/AIDS in 2005 belonged to minority groups.[20] All children who are U.S. citizens with family incomes below the poverty level are eligible for Medicaid. Medicaid's Early and Periodic, Screening, Diagnosis, and Treatment (EPSDT) benefit guarantees coverage for beneficiaries under age 21 for all mandatory and optional Medicaid services when medically necessary. People in this group cannot be denied a Medicaid-covered service because a state has chosen not to provide it to adults. Additionally, people in this group are not subject to coverage limits that may apply to adults.

Safeguards against discrimination and long waiting periods. Federal law extends several consumer protections to Medicaid beneficiaries. Services must be provided statewide; benefits must be comparable among different groups of Medicaid beneficiaries, and benefits must be adequate in amount, duration, and scope to reasonably achieve their purpose. Medicaid must also provide benefits with reasonable promptness. States cannot determine that a beneficiary needs a service and then impose a waiting period.

Beneficiaries cannot be denied service because of an inability to pay. States can impose cost sharing for Medicaid coverage for people with incomes below the FPL, though cost is typically less than $3 per service unit. States with cost-sharing provisions must ensure that beneficiaries living below the FPL are not denied care because of an inability to pay. If coverage for a prescription drug is in doubt, pharmacists are required by law to dispense a temporary supply in emergency situations (i.e., where drugs are necessary to prevent death or serious harm to health) in which payment authorization is initially denied. Medicare, on the other hand, does not have such a requirement.[21]

Medicaid: Recognizing the Shortcomings

Although Medicaid creates access to care for eligible PLWHA, it is not without its flaws and can, in some circumstances, limit coverage to those in need. Such limitations create the need for other public interventions, such as the Ryan White HIV/AIDS Program and Medicare. They also illuminate why Medicaid works for some minority PLWHA but for not all.

Onerous application process. Applying for Medicaid can prove problematic. In some states, the application itself can be around 20 pages in length – not a trivial issue for minority PLWHA with low literacy and daily functioning levels.[22,23] Applicants must provide detailed financial documentation to prove that their income and resources (e.g., savings) are below Medicaid limits. This requirement seems straightforward, but it poses difficulties for people who have never had a bank account or a steady job. In addition, a citizenship documentation requirement established by the 2005 Deficit Reduction Act can create unintended difficulties for U.S. citizens who do not have a passport or a birth certificate to prove their citizenship.

Restrictive and inadequate definition of disability. Several features of Medicaid's disability requirement can penalize PLWHA. Most PLWHA become eligible for Medicaid because they have been determined "disabled" and meet SSI income standards. Currently, PLWHA who do not have an AIDS diagnosis cannot be determined disabled. Moreover, people deemed disabled must be unable to engage in any "substantial gainful activity" as a result of a medically determinable impairment that has lasted or is expected to last for a period of at least 12 months or to result in death.[27]

Not all physical and mental impairments are considered to be markers of disability. For example, drug addiction and alcoholism are specifically excluded as primary disabling conditions, even if they prevent a person from working.[24] Because those conditions are linked with higher rates of HIV in communities of color, such restrictions may limit access to Medicaid insurance for minority PLWHA.

Low provider reimbursement rates. States have considerable latitude in establishing service reimbursement rates. States can make service provision to Medicaid-insured minority PLWHA unaffordable when reimbursement rates are inadequate for covering provider costs. Low reimbursement rates for HIV specialists and dental and mental health care providers have been persistent problems in some States.

Limited autonomy in choosing a care provider. Many Medicaid programs have moved or are moving to managed care arrangements for beneficiaries. Managed care typically requires beneficiaries to enroll with a specific primary care provider who, by contract with the Medicaid agency, accepts certain responsibilities for providing and authorizing needed medical care. Providers who are not in the managed care network or who are not referred by the primary care provider in a Primary Care Case Management (PCCM) system may not be able to be reimbursed for services provided to Medicaid beneficiaries.[25] Thus, Medicaid-managed care programs can limit the access of a person living with HIV/AIDS to his or her provider of choice.

The requirements are not aligned with the nature of HIV/AIDS in the age of highly active antiretroviral therapy or with the need for Medicaid coverage among PLWHA of color in whom HIV disease may not yet have progressed to AIDS. The requirements do not take into consideration that someone who is disabled today may not be disabled tomorrow, thanks to effective treatment tools like highly active antiretroviral therapy (HAART), and they penalize those who are capable of maintaining employment but who, nevertheless, struggle with the costs of treatment.

Because eligibility for Medicaid and Medicare on the basis of disability cannot be established without an AIDS diagnosis, many PLWHA are left without insurance. This lack of coverage works as a disincentive to stay in care and promotes the use of emergency rooms for ambulatory medical care. The result is more opportunistic infections, accelerated disease progression, and higher rates of comorbidity and mortality among the uninsured.

Policy makers are considering proposed legislation to permit states to extend Medicaid to a new optional population: predisabled people living with HIV.[26] At the present time, only a small number of states cover predisabled people with HIV through waiver programs.

Medicare

Medicaid is largely a program serving groups of low-income people (i.e., poor children, parents, seniors, and people with disabilities), whereas Medicare is a health insurance program for workers who pay into Social Security and their spouses and dependents. People pay to the Medicare system throughout their work lives. They become eligible for Medicare coverage

- Once they reach age 65 or
- If they are under age 65, once they have been determined to have a disability and have satisfied the Medicare waiting period [no waiting period exists for people with amyotrophic lateral sclerosis (ALS), also known as Lou Gehrig's disease]

Medicare currently covers 41 million people, approximately 35 million of whom are over 65 years of age.[27] At least one-third of Medicare beneficiaries of all ages have disabilities or a long-term illness such as HIV/AIDS that limits their independence.

Medicare is the nation's second largest source of financing for HIV/AIDS health care services; it accounts for approximately one-fourth of federal spending on HIV/AIDS care in the U.S.[28] An estimated 100,000 PLWHA currently receive Medicare benefits.[28] Most PLWHA who receive Medicare benefits are under age 65 and qualify as a result of their disability status.[29]

Medicare helps pay for a broad array of services that are relevant to the care and treatment of HIV/AIDS (see Table 2). Medicare's coverage of long-term care is limited to postacute care through its skilled nursing facility benefit and home health care benefit.

Medicare: Benefits for PLWHA of Color

Wide choice of providers. The Medicare program generally offers higher reimbursement rates to providers than Medicaid does, which makes Medicare more attractive to providers. The result is greater choice for minority PLWHA who often live in underserved communities of color where medical care may be scarce.

Access to prescription drugs. The Medicare Prescription Drug, Improvement, and Modernization Act (Part D) of 2003 created a right for Medicare beneficiaries to purchase prescription drug coverage and established subsidies for low-income people. Part D gives prescription drug coverage to roughly 42 million Medicare beneficiaries, including an estimated 100,000 PLWHA who are receiving Medicare benefits.[30] Under the Part D program, Medicare beneficiaries choose coverage to purchase from a selection of competing private plans.[30]

Table 2 Medicare Summary, 2005, The Henry J. Kaiser Family Foundations (KFF)

Who is eligible	What it covers	Administrator	Total served	PLWHA served
• People age 65 and older • Workers, spouses, and adult dependents under age 65 who have disabilities • People with end-stage renal disease (i.e., permanent kidney failure requiring dialysis or a transplant)	Broad array of routine, acute, and preventive care services, including: • Physician services • Hospital services • Rehabilitation and home health services • Medical equipment essential to the health and independence of beneficiaries	Centers for Medicare and Medicaid Services	Total of 41 million are served: • 35 million age 65 or older • 6 million under age 65 with physical or mental disabilities that will prevent work for at least a year or that are expected to result in death	100,000

Source: The Henry J. Kaiser Family Foundation Navigating Medicare and Medicaid, 2005: resource guide for people with disabilities, their families, and their advocates. 2005; February. Available at www.kff.org. Accessed January 2, 2008

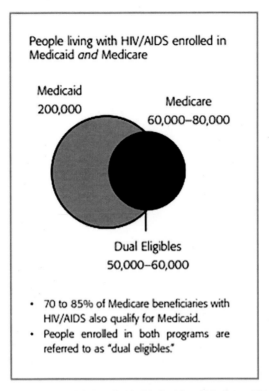

People living with HIV/AIDS enrolled in Medicaid *and* Medicare

Medicaid
200,000

Medicare
60,000–80,000

Dual Eligibles
50,000–60,000

- 70 to 85% of Medicare beneficiaries with HIV/AIDS also qualify for Medicaid.
- People enrolled in both programs are referred to as "dual eligibles."

Fig. 3 People Living With HIV/AIDS Enrolled in Medicaid and Medicare (HRSA)

Because PLWHA are disproportionately poor compared with other Medicare beneficiaries, the majority of Medicare beneficiaries with HIV/AIDS are "dual eligibles" (i.e., eligible for both Medicare and Medicaid) who received comprehensive drug coverage through Medicaid prior to the establishment of the Medicare Part D program (see Fig. 3). Most of those beneficiaries have comparable drug coverage to Medicaid, but in some cases, plan variations and other benefit features have created new gaps in drug coverage.

Although the Part D program may have taken some fiscal pressure off Medicaid programs, high-cost sharing has created new pressures for AIDS drug assistance programs (ADAPs) that have stepped in to protect against gaps in coverage for Medicare beneficiaries with HIV/AIDS. This problem particularly affects low-income PLWHA whose incomes are too high to qualify for the low-income subsidy that provides assistance in paying the Part D premium and cost sharing (available to beneficiaries who qualify based on low incomes capped at 150% of the FPL).[31]

Medicare drug coverage may provide advantages over ADAP for PLWHA of color. Medicare covers many non-AIDS-related treatments that are not covered in many State ADAP formularies. Moreover, because Medicare is an entitlement, those who are enrolled in Part D are guaranteed coverage. State ADAPs can run out of funds entirely, which forces them to create waiting lists for enrollment. Although ADAPs have generally been successful at avoiding total depletion of funds, they have been compelled to limit drug formularies.

Medicare: Problems for PLWHA of Color

Despite Medicare's role as an insurer for many Americans, Medicare policy can create significant eligibility and financial burdens for people of color. This burden arises from the time lapse between determination of a disability and start of Medicare coverage. Additionally, the cost-sharing structure for Medicare benefits is better suited to seniors with higher incomes than most nonelderly people who depend on income assistance from the Social Security Disability Insurance (SSDI) program.

Lengthy enrollment process. Once someone is determined by Social Security to have a disability, workers (or spouses and some adult dependents) apply for SSDI. SSDI provides income assistance to people with a permanent disability, and benefits begin 5 months after Social Security makes a disability determination. Once nonelderly people with disabilities start receiving SSDI, an additional 24-month waiting period exists before Medicare coverage begins.[32] The result is a wait of at least 29 months before beneficiaries can receive benefits through Medicare – a significant gap in coverage. The lowest income people with disabilities can receive Medicaid, which begins right after a disability determination, but many low-income people are "too rich" for Medicaid coverage.

Level of benefits reflects income history rather than current need. SSDI benefits are directly related to the amount of Social Security paid in by the beneficiary, which, in turn, is directly related to income earned. In 2006, the median income for a white, non-Hispanic household was $52,423 compared with $31,969 for a black household and $37,781 for a Hispanic household. People of color are often able to contribute less to Social Security and, thus, receive less SSDI when they need it.[33]

Discourages employment and autonomy. For people under age 65, the Medicare program has historically discouraged or prevented people from working while receiving benefits. In an effort to allow more people to work while receiving Medicare, Congress added several work incentives to the Social Security Act. Now, beneficiaries can receive education, training, and rehabilitation to start a new line of work and keep some or all SSDI or SSI cash benefits, Medicaid coverage, and Medicare coverage while working.

Drug coverage is out of reach for many. Medicare beneficiaries are not guaranteed drug coverage, although the Modernization Act (Part D) has made such coverage available to more beneficiaries. Some beneficiaries, particularly those who are eligible for the Extra Help program, whose resources are less than $11,710 (single) or $23,410 (married) will have minimal costs; others may face significant out-of-pocket expenses. About 30,000 Medicare beneficiaries with HIV/AIDS are not dually eligible for Medicaid and Medicare. Many of those people are believed to face gaps in their prescription drug coverage, sometimes including barriers to accessing antiretroviral therapy. People without drug coverage are more likely to have lower incomes than those who have coverage. Disturbingly, people most likely to need such coverage because of poor health – like PLWHA and people of color – are no more likely to have drug coverage than those with better health.[34] PLWHA who lack Medicare prescription drug coverage often use ADAPs as their primary source for HIV medications.[21]

The Henry J. Kaiser Family Foundation estimates that between 12 and 13% of the hundreds of thousands of PLWHA who are in care are dually enrolled in both Medicare and Medicaid.[29] This group consists of people with disabilities who qualify for Medicare and who, on the basis of their very low incomes, also qualify for Medicaid. Medicaid can supplement gaps left by Medicare coverage, although it cannot pay for prescription drugs that are covered by Medicare.

Ryan White HIV/AIDS Program

The Ryan White HIV/AIDS Program fills gaps in coverage left by Medicaid, Medicare, other insurance programs, and the person's ability to pay. The program is the "payer of last resort" for underserved PLWHA; program funds may not be used to replace other funds.[35] The Ryan White HIV/AIDS Program reaches approximately 531,000 PLWHA and family members per year (see Table 3).

- Of those 75% are from communities of color (52% black, 23% Hispanic).[36]
- 71% of HIV-positive clients and 81% of HIV-affected clients had incomes at or below the FPL in 2004.[36]

Unlike the typical insurance program, the Ryan White HIV/AIDS Program does not distribute funds or insurance cards to HIV-positive consumers. Instead, funds are awarded to providers across the country (approximately 2,300 in 2007) that deliver services to underserved people for whom no other payer exists.

The Ryan White HIV/AIDS Program offers an even greater level of state and local autonomy than Medicaid. This autonomy allows jurisdictions to build

Table 3 Ryan White HIV/AIDS Program Summary, HRSA (HRSA)

Who is eligible	What it covers	Administrator	PLWHA served
Low-income, uninsured, and underinsured men, women, children, and youth with no other way to meet their needs for; medical care and support	Wide array of outpatient medical care services, medications, and essential support services that help bring people into care and keep them in care	Health Resources and Services Administration (HRSA) HIV/AIDS Bureau (HAB)	531,000

Source: HRSA. About the Ryan White HIV/AIDS Program. Available at: www.hab.hrsa.gov/aboutus.htm. Accessed December 13, 2007

programs that address the manifestations of the epidemic that are unique to their specific communities and that reflect the different cultures and populations served.

The Ryan White HIV/AIDS Program: Doing What Others Cannot

The Ryan White HIV/AIDS Program exists to fill the many gaps in service for PLWHA. Ryan White funding is always finite because it is a line-item appropriation rather than an entitlement; therefore, it is essential that all PLWHA who are eligible for Medicaid or Medicare obtain all possible benefits from those programs first.

Ryan White provides health services to both uninsured PLWHA as well as to the underinsured, that is, people who may have some coverage but whose coverage is inadequate for meeting essential needs.

Reaches beyond an AIDS diagnosis. Medicaid and Medicare generally restrict eligibility to PLWHA whose disease has progressed to AIDS; the Ryan White HIV/AIDS Program does not, thus it is the only major safety net for uninsured people living with HIV whose illness has not progressed to AIDS. This difference means that the demographic profile of Ryan White HIV/AIDS Program clients more closely mirrors recent infection patterns than does the demographic profile of Medicaid and Medicare beneficiaries with HIV/AIDS. Therefore, the Ryan White HIV/AIDS Program is particularly important to providing health care services to people of color.

A commitment to reflectiveness and cultural competency. The Health Resources and Services Administration (HRSA) HIV/AIDS Bureau (HAB) administers the Ryan White HIV/AIDS Program. HRSA has ensured that the composition of the program staff reflects the epidemic demographically in terms of age, gender, and race. This composition helps HRSA bring a sense of cultural understanding to policies and programs that address HIV/AIDS among minorities.

HIV/AIDS-funded grantees and providers are required to demonstrate cultural competency. They must also demonstrate that they know where the greatest need in their community lies and that they have a plan for reaching that part of the community. For many grantees, the greatest need lies in communities of color. The funding requirements ensure that organizations are better attuned to the needs of minority PLWHA and develop programs that reduce barriers to access and disparities in health outcomes.

Community and consumer involvement. Community involvement in the service planning and delivery process is a cornerstone of the Ryan White HIV/AIDS Program, particularly of the program's two largest initiatives: Part A, Grants for Eligible Metropolitan Areas and Part B, Grants for States and Territories. Community members ranging from activists to health care providers and from health departments to community-based organizations are actively involved in planning and delivering HIV/AIDS services. This component of the Ryan White HIV/AIDS Program helps to ensure that local Ryan White investment is made where it is most needed. By giving states and metropolitan regions a measure of autonomy, the Ryan White

HIV/AIDS Program develops relevant services for a wide range of settings in a variety of communities.

PLWHAs are also involved in the planning and delivery of services under the Ryan White HIV/AIDS Program. This involvement predates passage of the first Ryan White Comprehensive AIDS Resources Emergency Act (CARE Act) in 1990. Consumers were actively involved in lobbying for a program that reflected the real needs of PLWHA. Over the past 17 years, they have been involved in administering the program at every level.

The legislation did not leave consumer involvement to chance. For example, Part A requires each grantee to have a planning body, and PLWHA must compose at least 33% of that body. Other grant programs have urged, and in some cases required, the creation of consumer advisory boards. Consumers have also worked in a variety of professional capacities, from clinician to case manager, within HIV/AIDS service organizations. As a group, they reflect the local population of underserved communities. Consumer involvement helps align community plans and services with the daily reality confronted by local, underserved, minority PLWHA.

Clinical and technical training. The Ryan White HIV/AIDS Program supports grantees and providers through training. Initiatives such as the AIDS Education and Training Centers (AETCs), which includes a National Minority AETC, build capacity among minority health care professionals and organizations serving communities of color. Such services improve the ability of local organizations to serve minority PLWHA, as do capacity-building and planning grants targeted to underserved communities.

Funds are targeted to areas with greatest need. Several features of the Ryan White HIV/AIDS Program ensure that funds are awarded on the basis of current unmet need. Funds can be redirected as the epidemic evolves from year to year. Because of this flexibility, federal grants were awarded to organizations serving communities of color when the epidemic began spreading rapidly among minorities.

Particularly in the Part A and Part B programs, grantees also have the ability to redirect funds to serve areas where needs have emerged in their jurisdictions. Thus, in communities where need is most significant among white men who have sex with men, grantees may target funds to serve that population. Likewise, if need is greatest among minority heterosexual men, grantees may use funds to meet the needs of that population. If unmet need exists in several subpopulations, as is typically the case, flexibility within the Ryan White HIV/AIDS Program allows and, indeed, mandates that funds be used to meet the needs of all.

The Ryan White HIV/AIDS Program has targeted the needs of minorities from the federal level. Since 1998, the Minority AIDS Initiative (MAI) has provided specific resources to increase the availability of services and access to care for minority PLWHA. The MAI was codified into law by Congress in 2007 as part of the reauthorization of the Ryan White HIV/AIDS Program in the Ryan White HIV/AIDS Treatment Modernization Act. Throughout the history of the Ryan White HIV/AIDS Program, a number of special initiatives have also helped to improve access to care for minorities. Examples are the Part D African American Children's Initiative and the Special Projects of National Significance that address HIV/AIDS along the

U.S.–Mexico Border, among young MSM of color, and among American Indians and Alaska Natives.[?,37]

Ryan White: The Other Side

The extraordinary success with which the Ryan White HIV/AIDS Program has adapted and grown to meet the needs of minorities raises an important question: Do Medicaid, Medicare, and the Ryan White HIV/AIDS Program collectively provide a sound safety net for all PLWHA of color? The answer, unfortunately, is no.

Ryan White funds are limited. Ryan White HIV/AIDS Program spending is a "discretionary" item in each fiscal year's federal budget. Funding levels often do not – and have not in the past – equal the level of need among underserved PLWHA. Moreover, because Ryan White is not an entitlement, eligible people are not guaranteed access to Ryan White-funded services. When an organization's Ryan White funds have been exhausted, few options exist besides providing uncompensated care.

Unintended impact on personal choice. Ryan White funds are awarded to organizations rather than to individuals. Given the limited nature of Ryan White funds, typically only a few organizations within a region receive funding. In some suburban, exurban, and rural areas, only one organization may be funded – or none at all. This limitation restricts access to care through logistical and transportation barriers as well as through barriers associated with cultural competency.

Technical requirements may favor heavily resourced organizations. The technical process surrounding application for a Ryan White HIV/AIDS Program grant can favor large, heavily resourced organizations. Grant writing and proposal preparation require a high level of technical knowledge, business acumen, and writing expertise, and award conditions carry significant administrative requirements related to issues such as quality management. Such demands can put small, cash-strapped organizations that serve minorities at a disadvantage when competing with larger entities for funds.

Needle Exchange

HIV and Injected Drug Use in Communities of Color

Since the beginning of the epidemic, injected drug use (IDU) has directly or indirectly accounted for one-third of the AIDS cases in this country.[38] In 2005, injected drugs use accounted for 14% of all new HIV infections.[39] Of the cumulative AIDS cases diagnosed through 2005 attributed to injected drug use, over 50% of the cases were black, non-Hispanic and 26% Hispanic compared with 20% white, non-Hispanic individuals. These statistics confirm IDU as an ongoing significant factor in the spread of HIV in communities of color.

The high association of HIV transmission with injected drugs led activists and clinicians to seek interventions to reduce risk. One such intervention is needle exchange programs (NEPs). Formal needle exchange programs date back to the early 1980s in Amsterdam when the first program was formed in response to a concern for a Hepatitis C virus (HCV) outbreak among injected drug users. The first NEPs specifically directed toward the prevention of HIV began in Britain soon after and other European countries developed their own NEPs. After learning about the success of European needle exchange programs, similar programs, both legal and illegal, began to form around the U.S.

Most NEPs are based on the principles of harm reduction. The premise of harm reduction theory is to reduce negative consequences of individual behaviors by leading one to safer behavior that will ultimately lead to abstinence of such behavior.[40] Thus with IDU, the harm reduction philosophy behind NEPs provides not only direct benefits but also indirect benefits. Although the initial focus of NEPs is to exchange clean needles and/or syringes for used ones, the intention of many programs is to provide a linkage point for IDUs to access drug rehabilitation and treatment services. Several studies have shown that needle exchange programs significantly decrease the transmission of HIV.[41]

Ban on Federal Funding for Needle Exchange Programs

Despite the supporting evidence of NEPs as an effective prevention tool, the use of federal funding for needle exchange programs has been banned by Congress since 1988. The rationale for this ban is tied to the notion that governmental support of such programs would directly conflict the government's stance on the war on drugs. Some have suggested that injected drug use and crime would increase. Despite the evidence that needle exchange programs are effective in combating the spread of the virus, the federal ban on needle exchange continues to stand. Various medical organizations including the American Medical Association and World Health Organization along with civil rights groups such as the National Association for the Advancement of Colored People and the National Urban League have identified needle exchange as an effective prevention method for combating HIV.

Over 200 needle exchange programs exist in over 36 states, including the District of Columbia, but each program has its own distinct funding source. These differences in funding policies and regulations impact the effect these programs have against transmission of the infection.[42] With the lack of a national policy on such programs and the continued federal ban on funding of NEPs, the virus will continue to spread not only among IDUs, but to their families and the broader community. Because of the fact that racial and ethnic minorities compose a large percentage of IDUs (or are indirectly affected by IDU) and access to care is low among this population, NEPs appear to provide a crucial linkage point to medical services. The policy of banning funding for needle exchange programs needs to be reevaluated in the context of current demographic shifts in order to address the racial disparities in HIV transmission.

Implications of New CDC Testing Recommendations

Description of CDC Testing Recommendations

Currently, approximately 25% of the estimated 1,039,000–1,185,000 persons in the U.S. living with HIV are undiagnosed and 40% of those newly diagnosed develop AIDS within 1 year of diagnosis.[43] In response to these statistics, in 2003, the Center for Disease Control (CDC) launched the *Advancing HIV Prevention Initiative* to "reduce barriers to early diagnosis of HIV infection and increase access to quality medical care, treatment, and ongoing prevention services for HIV-positive persons and their partners."[44] The findings from this initiative revealed that testing of high-risk individuals in acute care settings, such as emergency department, remained low.[45]

Previous CDC guidelines have recommended routine HIV testing for inpatients and outpatients in acute-care hospital settings.[46] The 2001 guidelines were amended to add routine testing in health care settings with $\geq 1\%$ HIV prevalence and recommended targeted testing based on risk factors in health care settings with lower HIV prevalence rates, and routine testing for all persons seeking treatment for sexually transmitted diseases.[47]

In September 2006, the CDC released its Revised Recommendations for HIV Testing of Adults, Adolescents, and Pregnant Women in Health-Care Settings to provide for health care settings to incorporate HIV testing into normal medical care.[6] The four points of the recommendations are to advocate for voluntary "opt-out" screening in health care settings rather than "op-in" screening, no requirement for a separate written consent for HIV testing, annual retesting for high-risk individuals, and rescreening of pregnant women in their third trimester.[6] Overall, the new testing policy has been received with much agreement and enthusiasm by the medical community especially with respect to increasing the testing capabilities. Despite the wide acceptance, some patient advocacy and social justice organizations have expressed concern over the informed consent process and lack of counseling involved with testing.[48]

How the New Recommendations Affect Communities of Color

With the removal of barriers from previous recommendations, the new guidelines are designed to increase efforts to diagnose those with HIV and link infected patients into care. Although the CDC's revised recommendations increase testing access to minorities that utilize the health care system, there still exists a marginalized and hard to reach population that does not utilize the healthcare system.[49] This marginalized population is largely composed of racial and ethnic minorities, substance users, and the poor where the epidemic is rapidly spreading.[10] Grass roots organizations and community-based outreach programs that directly target this group are effective forces in reaching this group.

Provider Training and Access to Care

Healthcare disparities continue to exist within communities of color.[50] The disparities are more profound in HIV care. Many factors contribute to these disparities and lead to differences in the provision of care and treatment.

A significant portion of blacks and Hispanics present to care at a later stage than their white counterparts.[51] Once these patients receive care, their receipt of antiretroviral therapy and other therapeutic drugs is less likely than other HIV patients, which reveals differences in quality of care.

As noted in the previous section on Medicaid and Medicare, health insurance status is a significant factor in the access to care for communities of color. Black and Hispanic HIV/AIDS infected patients are more likely to have Medicaid or be uninsured than white HIV/AIDS infected patients.[52] Although insurance status is critical, the Institute of Medicine report indicated that regardless of insurance coverage, racial and ethnic minorities with HIV had worse access to care than whites.[53] This leads to the conclusion that access to adequate providers with HIV-related experience is a serious consideration in access to care for minority HIV patients.

Demographic data shows that the HIV epidemic is spreading rapidly in communities in the Southern part of the country where 55% of the black population and 33% of Hispanic population are located.[54,55] Unfortunately, the majority of providers with HIV experience are not located in those geographic areas.[56] Not only is the geographic distribution of medical providers that care for HIV/AIDS patients not consistent with the distribution of new cases of HIV, but there are few medical personnel who reflect the same racial and ethnic background as the groups most affected by the epidemic. Racial concordance is cited as another critical indicator of improved access and quality to HIV care.[12]

Additionally, there is no clear agreement in the medical community of the types of providers and training suited to care for HIV-infected patients.[57] This lack of consensus creates an additional barrier to comprehensive care and has a deleterious impact on communities of color.

Discussion

Medicaid, Medicare, and the Ryan White HIV/AIDS Program play important roles in extending health care to minority PLWHA. Without those programs, many PLWHA who receive ambulatory care today would be forced out of outpatient care and back into emergency rooms. AIDS morbidity and mortality would increase, as would the suffering of PLWHA and their families.

Despite the benefits, the shortcomings of the three largest public payers of HIV/AIDS care must be addressed. The patchwork system of public health coverage in the U.S. currently leaves many PLWHA of color – and many Americans – uncovered.

Significant barriers to enrollment and care in these programs exist for PLWHA of color. Many people who meet Medicaid and Medicare enrollment requirements and who are eligible for Ryan White HIV/AIDS Program services are unaware that they are eligible for support. Moreover, navigating the technical attributes of the programs can be daunting, even for health care professionals, and can prove insurmountable for many eligible people.

Like most insurance programs in the U.S., whether public or private, Medicaid, Medicare, and the Ryan White HIV/AIDS Program lack adequate preventive care components. The Ryan White HIV/AIDS Program was developed for people already living with an HIV/AIDS diagnosis; however, Medicaid and Medicare were not. Many eligible PLWHA of color become enrolled in Medicaid and Medicare only after they have tested positive for HIV and are provided enrollment assistance by a Ryan White-supported case manager or entitlements counselor. Ultimately, the costs to people of color are paid in wholly unnecessary and preventable morbidity for a host of acute and chronic conditions.

Potentially hundreds of thousands of PWLHA in the U.S. are not in care, and Medicaid and Medicare do not generally cover the kinds of outreach programs that could help reach those people. The Ryan White HIV/AIDS Program does outreach to a diminishing extent given its increased focus on medical care and reduced spending on support services such as outreach. Current federal policy tasks the Centers for Disease Control and Prevention's HIV prevention programs with reaching PLWHA who are not in care.

The discussion of federal health policy that more adequately responds to the needs of PLWHA of color is taking place in the context of a national conversation about how to improve health care for all Americans. Given the technical and political issues at stake, it is not likely that this conversation will be brief or that the barriers to care for those not receiving it will be resolved in the near term. Thus, everyone concerned with serving PLWHA of color must understand how the principal programs in place today – Medicaid, Medicare, and the Ryan White HIV/AIDS Program – work independently and together to improve access to care for underserved people. Because only with this understanding can improve the health and lives of underserved people and to stem the tide of HIV/AIDS among communities of color.

A national policy addressing the access to care and training issue is critical to combating the spread of this infection and is sorely needed. There is a high probability that the new testing guidelines will identify more people who are HIV infected. However, like the current demographic of recently diagnosed individuals, they will be poor, minority, and live in the southern U.S. This population will greatly strain existing resources particularly in the public sector. National policies that address the geographic maldistribution of providers provide incentives for clinicians to enter (and remain) in HIV care, and standardized HIV training at the pre and postgraduate level is needed. Failure to do so will most assuredly lead to an exacerbation of the current disproportionate impact of HIV on communities of color.

References

1. Centers for Disease Control and Prevention (CDC). HIV/AIDS and African Americans. Available at: www.cdc.gov/hiv/topics/aa/index.htm. Updated June 28, 2007. Accessed December 12, 2007
2. CDC. 2005 HIV/AIDS Surveillance Report, Vol. 17. Available at: www.cdc.gov/hiv/topics/surveillance/resources/reports/2005report/pdf/2005SurveillanceReport.pdf. Revised June 2007. Accessed January 2, 2008
3. The Office of Minority Health (OMH). HIV/AIDS Data Statistics. Available at: www.omhrc.gov/templates/browse.aspx?lvl=2&lvlID=22. Accessed December 13, 2007
4. Diaz T, Chu S, Buehler J, et al. Socioeconomic differences among people with AIDS: results from a multistate surveillance project. Am J Prev Med. 1994; 10: 217–222
5. U.S. Census Bureau. Poverty: 1999. Census 2000 Brief. Available at: http://www.census.gov/prod/2003pubs/c2kbr-19.pdf. Updated May 2003. Accessed December 12, 2007
6. Health Resources and Services Administration (HRSA) HIV/AIDS Bureau. American Indians, Alaska Natives, and HIV/AIDS in the United States, 2006. Available at: http://hab.hrsa.gov/history/AmIndiansAlaskaNatives/. Accessed December 14, 2007
7. U.S. Census Bureau News. Income Climbs, Poverty Stabilizes, Uninsured Rate Increases [Press Release]. August 29, 2006. Available at: www.census.gov/Press-Release/www/releases/archives/income_wealth/007419.html. Accessed January 2, 2008
8. Families U.S. Improving Health Coverage and Access for African Americans. Minority Health Initiatives. January, 2006. Available at: www.familiesusa.org/assets/pdfs/minority-health-tool-kit/AfrAm-fact-sheet.pdf. Accessed December 13, 2007
9. Families U.S. Improving Health Coverage and Access for Latinos. Minority Health Initiatives. January, 2006. Available at: www.familiesusa.org/assets/pdfs/minority-health-tool-kit/Latino-fact-sheet.pdf. Accessed December 12, 2007
10. U.S. Census Bureau. Income, Poverty, and Health Insurance in the United States: 2006. Washington, DC; U.S. Government Printing Office 2007:22. (Available at: www.census.gov/prod/2007pubs/p60-233.pdf)
11. HRSA HIV/AIDS Bureau. About the Ryan White HIV/AIDS Program. Available at: www.hab.hrsa.gov/aboutus.htm. Accessed January 8, 2008
12. The Henry J. Kaiser Family Foundation (KFF). Navigating Medicare and Medicaid, 2005a: Medicaid. Available at: www.kff.org/medicare/7240/medicaid.cfm#a1. Accessed December 12, 2007
13. KFF. Medicare and HIV/AIDS [Fact Sheet]. Available at: www.kff.org/hivaids/7171.cfm. Accessed December 12, 2007
14. For more information about Medicaid, please see Navigating Medicare and Medicaid, 2005: Medicaid. Available at: www.kff.org/medicare/7240/medicaid.cfm#a1

15. Centers for Medicare and Medicaid Services (CMS), Mandatory Eligibility Groups. Available at: www.cms.hhs.gov/MedicaidEligibility/03_MandatoryEligibilityGroups.asp#TopOfPage. Accessed December 12, 2007

16. Crowley J. Medicaid Medically Needy Programs: An Important Source of Medicaid Coverage. Washington, DC: Kaiser Commission on Medicaid and the Uninsured. 2003 January. Available at: http://www.kff.org/medicaid/loader.cfm?url=/commonspot/security/getfile.cfm&PageID=14325. Accessed January 24, 2008

17. CDC. Proportion of HIV/AIDS Cases and Population Among Young Adults 13 to 19 Years of Age, by Race/Ethnicity Diagnosed in 2005 – 33 states. Available at: www.cdc.gov/hiv/topics/surveillance/resources/slides/adolescents/slides/Adolescents_1.pdf. Accessed January 9, 2008

18. National Institutes for Allergies and Infectious Diseases. HIV Infection in Infants and Children [Fact Sheet]. 2004 July. Available at: www.niaid.nih.gov/factsheets/hivchildren.htm. Accessed January 8, 2008

19. CDC. 2005. HIV/AIDS Surveillance Report, Vol. 17. Available at: www.cdc.gov/hiv/topics/surveillance/resources/reports/2005report/pdf/2005SurveillanceReport.pdf. Revised June 2007. Accessed January 2, 2008

20. The Office of Minority Health, U.S. Department of Health and Human Services. HIV/AIDS Data/Statistics: 2009. Washington, DC. (Available at: www.omhrc.gov/templates/browse.aspx?lvl=3&lvlid=70)

21. HRSA HIV/AIDS Bureau. The new Medicare drug plan: implications for people living with HIV/AIDS. Available at: http://hab.hrsa.gov/publications/october2005/#a3. Updated October 2005. Accessed December 13, 2007

22. Settles SB. Low Literacy: A Health Care Quality Issue. Washington, DC: U.S. Department of Health and Human Services Office of Minority Health Resource Center. 2003 January/February. Available at: www.omhrc.gov/assets/pdf/checked/Low%20Literacy–A%20Health%20Care%20Quality%20Issue.pdf. Accessed January 8, 2008

23. Kalichman SC, Ramachandran B, Catz S. Adherence to combination antiretroviral therapies in HIV patients of low health literacy. J Gen Intern Med. 1999; 14(5): 267–273. Available at: www.pubmedcentral.nih.gov/articlerender.fcgi?artid=1496573. Accessed January 8, 2008

24. National Endowment for Financial Education (NEFE). Medicare and Medicaid: A Health Care Safety Net for People with Serious Disabilities and Chronic Conditions, Vol. 2. Managing Medical Bills: Strategies for Navigating the Health Care System. 2006

25. HRSA. Opportunities to Use Medicaid in Support of Access to Health Care Services. HRSA Medicaid Primer. Available at: http://www.hrsa.gov/medicaidprimer/default.htm. Accessed December 13, 2007

26. Interview with Jeffrey S. Crowley, Health Policy Institute, Georgetown University. December 4, 2007

27. Kaiser Family Foundation. Navigating Medicare and Medicaid, 2005b: A Resource Guide for People with Disabilities, Their Families, and Their Advocates. Available at: www.kff.org/medicare/7240.cfm. Updated February 2005. Accessed January 8, 2007

28. Kaiser Family Foundation. Medicare and HIV/AIDS [fact sheet]. October 2006. Available at: www.kff.org/hivaids/ upload/7171–03.pdf. Accessed December 12, 2007

29. Kaiser Family Foundation. Financing HIV/AIDS Care: A Quilt with Many Holes. HIV/AIDS policy brief. May 2004. Available at: www.kff.org/hivaids/upload/Financing-HIV-AIDS-Care-A-Quilt-with-Many-Holes.pdf. Accessed December 12, 2007

30. HRSA. HIV/AIDS Bureau. Medicare Prescription Drug Benefit and Ryan White Grantees. Available at: www.hrsa.gov/medicare/HIV/about.htm. Accessed January 8, 2008

31. Kaiser Family Foundation. Low-Income Subsidies for the Medicare Prescription Drug Benefit: the impact of the asset test. April 2005. Available at: www.kff.org/medicare/loader.cfm?url=/commonspot/security/getfile.cfm&PageID=52270. Accessed January 9, 2008

32. HRSA HIV/AIDS Bureau. African Americans and HIV/AIDS in the United States. Available at: http://hab.hrsa.gov/history/AfricanAmericans/. Accessed December 14, 2007

33. DeNavas-Walt C, Proctor BD, Smith J. Income, Poverty, and Health Insurance Coverage in the United States, 2006. Washington, DC: U.S. Census Bureau; August 2007. Available at: www.census.gov/prod/2007pubs/p60–233.pdf. Accessed December 12, 2007

34. Gross D, Brangan N. Medicare beneficiaries and prescription drug coverage: gaps and barriers [research report]. Washington, DC American Association of Retired People (AARP); June 1999. Available at: www.aarp.org/research/medicare/drugs/aresearch-import-717-IB39.html. Accessed December 12, 2007

35. HRSA. HIV/AIDS Bureau. ADAP Manual: 2003 Version. Available at: http://hab.hrsa.gov/tools/adap/adapSecIIIChap1.htm. Accessed January 8, 2008

36. HRSA HIV/AIDS Bureau. 2004 Ryan White CARE Act Annual Data Summary. Available at: http://hab.hrsa.gov/reports/2004_Data_Summary/page2.htm. Accessed December 13, 2007

37. HRSA. HIV/AIDS Bureau. Special Initiatives: SPNS Products. Available at: http://hab.hrsa.gov/special/products2g.htm. Accessed January 8, 2008

38. Centers for Disease Control (CDC), Drug-Associated HIV Transmission Continues in the United States, May 2002. http://www.cdc.gov/hiv/resources/factsheets/idu.htm, accessed February 2008

39. CDC Cases of HIV Infections and AIDS in United States, 2005. http://www.cdc.gov/hiv/topics/surveillance/resources/reports/2005report/, accessed February 2008

40. Harm Reduction Coalition. "Principles of Harm Reduction." http://www.harmreduction.org/article.php?list=type&type=62. Accessed March 2008

41. Stancliff S, Agins B, Rich JD, Burris S. Syringe access for the prevention of blood borne infections among injection drug users. BMC Public Health 2003; 3: 37

42. Bastos FI, Strathdee SA. Evaluating effectiveness of needle exchange programmes: current issues and future prospects. Soc Sci Med. 2000; 51(12): 1771–1782

43. Fleming P, Byers RH, Sweeney PA, Daniels D, Karon JM, Janssen RS. HIV prevalence in the United States, 2000 [Abstract]. In: Program and Abstracts of the 9th Conference on Retroviruses and Opportunistic Infections; Seattle, Washington; February 24–28, 2002

44. Advancing HIV Prevention: Progress Summary, April 2003 – September 2005, http://www.cdc.gov/hiv/topics/prev_prog/AHP/resources/factsheets/progress_2005.htm, accessed February 2008

45. CDC. Revised Recommendations for HIV testing of adults, adolescents, and pregnant women in health-care settings. MMWR Recomm Rep. 2006; 55(RR14): 1–17

46. CDC. Recommendations for HIV testing services for inpatients and outpatients in acute – care hospital settings. MMWR Morb Mortal Wkly Rep. 1993; 42: 1–10

47. CDC. Revised Guidelines for HIV counseling, testing, and referral. MMWR Morb Mortal Wkly Rep. 2001; 50: 1–62

48. Holtgrave DR. Costs and consequences of the U.S. centers for disease control and prevention's recommendations for Opt-Out HIV testing. PLoS Med. 2007; 4(6): e194

49. Cunningham WE, Sohler NL, Tobias C, et al. Health services utilization for people with HIV infection: comparison of a population targeted for outreach with the U.S. population in care. Med Care. 2006; 44(11): 1038–1047

50. U.S. Department of Health and Human Services, Agency for Healthcare Research and Quality. National Healthcare Disparities Report, 2006. http://www.ahrq.gov/QUAL/nhdr06/report/Index.htm. Accessed March 2008

51. Cargill VA, Stone VE. HIV/AIDS: a minority health issue. Med Clin North Am. 2005; 89(4): 895–912

52. Kaiser Foundation. Key Facts: African Americans and HIV/AIDS. 2003

53. Heslin KC, Anderson RM, Ettner SL, Cunningham WE. Racial and ethnic disparities in access to physicians with HIV-related expertise. J Gen Intern Med. 2005; 20: 283–289

54. U.S. Department of Commerce, Economics and Statistics Administration. U.S. Census Bureau. The Black Population in the United States: March 2002. http://www.census.gov/population/www/socdemo/race/black.html. Accessed February 2008

55. U.S. Department of Commerce, Economics and Statistics Administration. U.S. Census Bureau. The Hispanic Population in the United States: March 2002. http://www.census.gov/population/www/socdemo/hispanic/ho02.html. Accessed February 2008

56. Rawlings, MK. "Are There Adequate Clinicians Experienced in HIV Care to Meet the Current Demand in the United States?" Poster MoPe0643, XV International AIDS Conference, Toronto, Canada, August 2006

57. Landon BE, Wilson IB, Wenger NS, et al. Specialty training and specialization among physicians who treat HIV/AIDS in the United States. J Gen Intern Med. 2002; 17(1): 12–22

Moving Toward a Unified Global HIV/AIDS Agenda: Communities of Color in Crisis

Bisola Ojikutu and Jamal Harris

Introduction

At the conclusion of 2007, UNAIDS and the World Health Organization (WHO) estimated that there were 33.2 million people living with HIV (PLWHA) worldwide.[1] Since the first cases were identified more than 25 years ago, HIV infection has been reported in every region of the world. However, the most dire consequences of this disease have been manifested in resource-poor settings where health care infrastructure is suboptimal, access to education is minimal, and poverty is rampant. Over the course of the last 5 years, efforts have been initiated to mitigate the disparate impact that HIV has in these settings. Though universal access to treatment is an unmet and distant goal, antiretroviral therapy is now more widely available. In addition, there has been a decrease in the number of new HIV infections, primarily due to strides made in both prevention and access to effective care and treatment.[1]

This chapter will focus on the HIV epidemic in three of the most resource-limited regions of the world: sub-Saharan Africa, the Caribbean, and Latin America. Each of these regions has been impacted by varying degrees by HIV/AIDS. Each faces ongoing challenges while combating the spread of infection and struggling to treat those who are already infected. However, progress has been made. Lessons that can be derived from the development of successful prevention interventions and from scale-up of treatment programs in these regions will be highlighted.

Equally important is the recognition that this epidemic is borderless. Immigration from the three selected regions to other parts of the world, including the U.S., is constant. Providers in the U.S. are caring for and treating culturally diverse populations, including immigrants from all corners of the globe, particularly in minority communities. Therefore, it is important for health care providers to have an understanding of the international HIV epidemic. Moreover, some of the lessons learned from

B. Ojikutu (✉)
Massachusetts General Hospital, Office of International Programs, Division of AIDS, Harvard Medical School, Boston, MA
E-mail: bojikutu@partners.org

V. Stone et al. (eds.), *HIV/AIDS in U.S. Communities of Color*.
DOI: 10.1007/978-0-387-98152-9_15, © Springer Science + Business Media, LLC 2009

experiences internationally may be extrapolated to vulnerable, relatively resource-constrained populations here in the U.S. Suggestions for the potential integration of international and domestic strategies will be discussed.

Sub-Saharan Africa

Though the HIV epidemic has adversely affected inhabitants of every corner of the globe, sub-Saharan Africa has suffered the most widespread and catastrophic blow from this disease. Home to only 10% of the world's population, this region shoulders the burden of approximately 75% of all HIV cases. Nearly 7 out of 10 HIV-infected adults and 9 out of 10 HIV-infected children live in sub-Saharan Africa.[1] Furthermore, biological factors, economic inequality, violence against women, and cultural practices, including early marriage, have led to gender-based disparities in HIV prevalence.[2–6] Today, 61% of those living with HIV in the region are women and adolescent females. Because of the high prevalence of infection, poor health care infrastructure, and limited access to care and treatment, HIV-related mortality has been devastating. In 2006, 76% of AIDS deaths worldwide occurred in sub-Saharan Africa.[1]

Sub-Saharan Africa's 47 countries can be divided into southern, eastern, western, and central regions. Each is distinct in its geography, its history, and the characteristics of its HIV epidemic. The southernmost nations have the highest rate of HIV infection on the continent. Eight countries in southern Africa reported an HIV prevalence greater than 15% in 2007 (Table 1). With 5.5 million PLWHA, South Africa has the largest population of HIV-infected adults and children in the world. Kwa Zulu Natal, one of South Africa's nine provinces, has the highest HIV prevalence rate based on seroprevalence surveys of antenatal clinic attendees (39.1%) in the country. Nationwide, 29% of pregnant woman were estimated to be HIV-positive in 2006. However, there is new evidence that the rate of new infections throughout the country has leveled off.[7]

Though rates of HIV throughout southern Africa are exceptionally high, Zimbabwe has noted a recent decline in prevalence. Rates dropped from 22.1% in 2003 to 20.1% in 2005.[8] Amongst Zimbabwean women, a considerable decline in HIV prevalence has been observed. For example, in the capital city of Harare, HIV prevalence in women attending antenatal or postnatal clinics fell from 35% in 1999 to 21% in 2004.[9] Similarly, Botswana has noted a decline in HIV prevalence rates among young, pregnant women, from 39 to 29% in 20–24-year-old antenatal clinic attendees nationwide. However, nationwide prevalence estimates in that country remain high, approximately 24% in 2005.[1,8]

Throughout much of eastern Africa, HIV prevalence has remained lower than that noted in its neighbors to the south. Over time, the difference between the two regions has widened as several countries in eastern Africa have reported remarkable declines in HIV prevalence. The most notable are Uganda and Kenya where the proportion of adults living with HIV dropped from 15% and 14% in the early 1990s

Table 1 Adult[15–49] HIV prevalence in selected Sub-Saharan Africa, Caribbean, and Latin American countries, 2005

Sub-Saharan Africa	(%)
Swaziland	33.4
Botswana	24.1
Lesotho	23.2
Zimbabwe	20.1
Namibia	19.6
South Africa	18.8
Zambia	17.0
Mozambique	16.1
Cote d'Ivoire	7.1
Uganda	6.7
Kenya	6.1
Cameroon	5.4
Nigeria	3.9
Chad	3.5
The Caribbean	
Haiti	3.8
Trinidad and Tobago	2.6
Jamaica	1.5
Dominican Republic	1.1
Cuba	0.1
Latin America	
Belize	2.5
Guyana	2.4
Honduras	1.5
Brazil	0.5
Mexico	0.3

to 6% and 5.1%, respectively, by the end of 2006.[1] HIV prevalence in the remaining east African nations has either decreased or remained relatively stable (Table 1).

Significantly lower HIV infection rates have been observed in western and central Africa. The majority of the countries in these two regions have a national prevalence less than 2% (Table 1). HIV infection rates are somewhat higher in the central nation of Cameroon and the western nations of Chad, Cote d'Ivoire, and Nigeria (Table 1). Though Nigeria's HIV prevalence is currently estimated to be less than 4%, more than three million HIV-infected individuals live in this heavily populated nation. Wide variations in HIV prevalence have been noted across the country, from 1.6% in the western states to 12% further east.[10]

A combination of several factors helps explain the pervasive discrepancy in HIV epidemiology between the regions in sub-Saharan Africa. Male circumcision has been identified as a significant factor mediating HIV transmission in Africa. Circumcised males have a 50–60% decreased risk of contracting HIV from their female partners.[11–13] The prevalence of male circumcision differs widely across the continent. Higher rates have been noted in western Africa, particularly amongst Muslim populations where HIV prevalence is low. Male circumcision is much less common

in southern Africa where HIV prevalence is significantly higher. The WHO estimates the prevalence of circumcision in Botswana and Zimbabwe, both with raging
HIV epidemics, to be less than 20% countrywide.[14]

But low circumcision rates alone do not explain the enormously high HIV prevalence rates in southern Africa. A second contributing factor is genital herpes simplex
virus infection-2 (HSV). Numerous epidemiologic studies have identified HSV-2
as a biological cofactor in transmission and acquisition of HIV infection in both
males and females.[15–17] HSV-2 seroprevalence in sub-Saharan Africa ranges from
less than 10% amongst males in the western African country of Benin, which has
an HIV prevalence of 2%, to over 50% amongst males in Zimbabwe, which has
an HIV prevalence of 27%.[18] Recent studies have explored the use of antivirals,
such as acyclovir, to reduce HSV-2 replication, and therefore inhibit HIV transmission and acquisition. Though epidemiologic data validate this intervention as a
reasonable approach to HIV prevention, two recent large-scale trials employing this
strategy have failed to show any efficacy of HSV-2 suppressive therapy. Studies are
underway to determine why no effect was noted.[19, 20]

Behavioral factors also help explain variation in HIV prevalence across Africa.
Though HIV transmission via intravenous drug use (IDU) and men having sex with
men (MSM) have been reported in Africa (most notably in Kenya, Tanzania, South
Africa, and Mauritius), heterosexual sex is the predominant mode of transmission
across the continent. Numerous lifetime sexual partners, young age at sexual debut,
and low condom use contribute to increased risk of HIV acquisition. But a key
feature that may differentiate high-prevalence regions from those that have lower
prevalence is the rate of multiple *concurrent* sexual partnerships. The per act risk
of heterosexual transmission of HIV is low.[21] However, engaging in multiple concurrent partnerships over an extended period of time increases one's risk of HIV
acquisition because of exposure to a higher number of cumulative sexual acts. A
recent study revealed that 22% of men in Zambia and 55% of men in Lesotho (both
high HIV prevalence countries) reported engaging in two or more concurrent sexual partnerships lasting at least a year within the previous year.[22] This pattern of
concurrent partnerships is less common in western African nations where, as aforementioned, HIV prevalence is lower. Though polygamy, a type of concurrency, is
common in north and western Africa, other factors, such as the higher prevalence
of circumcision and the lower likelihood that women in polygamous relationships
in those regions are also engaging in multiple partnerships, most likely diminish the
risk of HIV transmission.

The Caribbean

Though the Caribbean is small in both land mass and population, its HIV prevalence
is second only to that observed in sub-Saharan Africa. The first case in the region
was noted in Jamaica in 1982.[23] By the end of 2007, a total of 230,000 people were
living with HIV in the Caribbean Islands.[1] Approximately 50% of infections have

been noted in women. Most recent data indicate that HIV prevalence has ranged from a high of 3.8% in Haiti to a low of 0.1% in Cuba (Table 1). As in sub-Saharan Africa, the spread of the epidemic has been fueled by poor health care, poverty, and behavioral factors, such as young age at sexual debut. Commercial sex work has also significantly contributed to HIV spread in most of the Caribbean nations. More than 31% of female sex workers in Guyana have been noted to be HIV positive.[24] In addition, 12% of the HIV cases that were reported in 2007 were secondary to MSM. High levels of stigma and discrimination toward MSM have been documented; therefore, the percent attributed to this transmission mode may be underreported and thus deceptively low.[24] Injection drug use has rarely been reported as a risk factor for infection in this region.

Haiti, the poorest country in the Western Hemisphere and the country with the largest epidemic in the Caribbean, deserves special consideration. More than one-half of those living with HIV in the Caribbean (or 190,000 people) are Haitians. At the height of the epidemic in that country Haiti's HIV prevalence was esti-mated to be 6%. Among women aged 15–49, AIDS continues to be the leading cause of death.[1] Though HIV has impacted other countries throughout the region, several factors have made Haiti's epidemic particularly severe and in many ways similar to epidemics in sub-Saharan Africa. Throughout the epidemic, Haiti has been embroiled in political upheaval. The lack of an effective government has led to disruption of economic activity and limited development and upkeep of public services, including health care facilities. Therefore, most Haitians have had lim-ited access to health care and accurate education regarding prevention strategies. In addition, most Haitians live on less than 1 U.S. $ per day; therefore, extreme poverty has contributed to severe deficits in health care access. Extensive internal (rural to urban) and external migration has also limited the ability to trace exposed individu-als, establish accurate epidemiologic data, and treat known cases.[26] Immigration has led to a higher HIV prevalence rate in some areas of neighboring Dominican Repub-lic, particularly in camps housing sugar cane plantation workers, many of whom are Haitians.[27]

In spite of severe economic and political strife throughout the 25 years of the AIDS epidemic, Haiti has made significant progress in addressing the epidemic. Though 6% of women tested in antenatal clinics were found to be HIV infected in 1996, 3.1% were HIV positive in 2004.[28]

National HIV prevalence is also relatively high in the Bahamas (3.3%). Trinidad and Tobago and Guyana are also combating significant epidemics; countrywide prevalence rates are 2.6% and 2.4%, respectively (Table 1).

As mentioned previously, Cuba has maintained an extremely low HIV preva-lence throughout the epidemic (0.1% in 2005). More than 80% of cases are amongst MSM. Several factors have contributed to this country's low infection rate. Cuba established its National Programme on HIV/AIDS in 1983 soon after the first cases of HIV were noted in the region. This program has been simultaneously lauded and critiqued for its proactive and aggressive approach. Integral to the pro-gram was mandatory confinement of known HIV-positive individuals in sanatoriums until 1994, after which confinement became voluntary. Confinement limited sexual contacts and allowed for close follow-up of patients. Though controversial, this practice helped contain the epidemic. In addition, Cuba implemented an HIV testing policy, which included partner tracing and notification, testing of pregnant women, and extensive follow-up of HIV-positive persons.[29] Antiretroviral therapy became available through Cuban drug manufacturers in 2000, prior to availability of treatment in other countries within the region. According to the Cuban government, all patients who qualify receive treatment free of charge.[30] Regarding prevention, the Cuban government recently announced a national prevention initiative that will specifically target the largest population affected by the epidemic, MSM.[31]

Unlike other countries in the Caribbean, Puerto Rico's HIV epidemic has been driven by IDU. Although national HIV prevalence is estimated to be less than 1% (Table 1), HIV prevalence amongst IDU(s) ranges from 42.4 to 55.2%.[32] According to the Puerto Rican Department of Public Health, 50% of AIDS cases in the country are amongst heterosexual IDU(s) and another 7% are in intravenous drug using MSM. Intravenous heroin and cocaine use has been difficult to combat because Puerto Rico serves as an efficient drug trafficking route from South America to the U.S. and Canada. Further compounding the problem is the lack of methadone and needle exchange programs on the island.[33]

Latin America

HIV prevalence in Central and South America ranges from 0.1% in Bolivia to 2.5% in Belize (Table 1). Throughout Latin America, HIV has remained concentrated in high-risk groups: IDU(s), MSM, and commercial sex workers and their clients. However, several nations are experiencing generalized epidemics.[1]

Brazil, the most populous country in South America, has the largest number of PLWHA in South America and accounts for approximately one-third of the HIV cases in the region. As is the case in most Western nations, HIV was first noted in Brazil among MSM in the mid-1980s. By the early 1990s, cases had been reported in heterosexual men, women, and IDU(s). Though a rise in cases has been observed over time, AIDS experts and advocates praise Brazil for limiting an epidemic predicted to spread much farther than the estimated 620,000 infected adults.[34, 35] HIV prevalence within the country has remained stable at 0.5% (Table 1). This is largely due to an early, aggressive HIV program, which included simultaneous prevention programming and universal access to antiretroviral treatment.[36]

In most South American countries MSM is the most commonly reported risk factor for HIV.[1] The exceptions are Argentina and Uruguay, where heterosexual transmission has caused the majority of new cases in recent years. Transmission due to IDU is significant in many South American countries as well as in Mexico.[37]

In Central America, migrant life styles and the frequenting of commercial sex workers has driven the spread of HIV. As mentioned, Belize has the highest rate in the region. Factors contributing to Belize's high HIV-prevalence rate include multiple sexual partners, young age at sexual debut, and low condom usage. In addition, high HIV prevalence has been noted amongst commercial sex workers. Significant epidemics also exist in Honduras, Guatemala, El Salvador, Costa Rica, Nicaragua, and Panama.[1]

Mexico has maintained an HIV infection prevalence of 0.3%, lower than the 0.6% in the U.S. to its north and lower than the HIV prevalence rates of its Central American neighbors (Table 1). There continues to be significant HIV rates among MSM. Unprotected sex between MSM contributes to more than half of new infections per year.[1] Because of migration, HIV infection rates have also increased in border communities, including rural areas around the southern and northern borders of the country.[38, 39]

Treatment

Though highly active antiretroviral drug therapy (HAART) for HIV was widely available in high-income nations by the mid-1990s, treatment was largely unavailable in most low- to middle-income countries until recently. Drug prices, concern that poverty-stricken patients in resource-poor settings would not be able to manage complicated drug regimens, and the lack of trained human resources to provide the drugs inhibited widespread access. In response to this glaring inequity and increasing AIDS-related mortality, several critical funding initiatives were implemented, which have improved the availability of HIV treatment and prevention around the world. In 2001, the Global Fund to Fight AIDS, Malaria, and Tuberculosis, a multilateral partnership of governments, civil society, the private sector, and affected communities was created to collect and disburse financing for international health projects. Securing and distributing funds for HIV treatment integrated with prevention services is a major function of this organization. During its first two rounds of grant making, the Global Fund committed U.S. $1.5 billion in funding to support 154 programs in 93 countries worldwide.[40]

In 2003, the WHO and the United Nations Program on HIV/AIDS launched the 3×5 initiative with the goal of having three million people living with HIV/AIDS in low- to middle-income countries on HAART by the end of 2005. By the end of 2005, 1.3 million people were receiving HAART, tripling the total number of people on these lifesaving medicines in a 2-year period.[41] The estimated number of people on treatment jumped to nearly three million by the end of 2007.[42] A significant amount of money to support treatment has come from the U.S. through the President's Emergency Plan for AIDS Relief (PEPFAR), which committed 15 billion U.S. $ to support HIV care, treatment, and prevention initiatives in 15 focus countries in Africa, the Caribbean, and Asia. This unparalleled funding initiative supported treatment for more than 1.6 million HIV-infected adults and children by March 2008.[43] National governments of some of the most highly impacted countries in the developing world have also contributed resources. Further contributing to the ability to increase access to treatment is the drop in the yearly cost of annual antiretroviral treatment. The prices of antiretroviral drugs in the developing world

Table 2 Estimated number of people needing and receiving antiretroviral therapy in Sub-Saharan Africa, the Caribbean, and Latin America, 2007

Region	Number needing ART	Number receiving ART	Coverage (%)
Sub-Saharan Africa	7,000,000	2,120,000	30
Eastern and Southern	5,300,000	1,690,000	32
Western and Central	1,700,000	430,000	25
Latin America	630,000	390,000	62
Caribbean	70,000	30,000	43

declined from $10,000–$15,000 per patient per year to as little as $140 per patient per year for a first-line WHO combination antiretroviral treatment regimen largely due to advocacy efforts.[44,45]

The influx of new funding changed the landscape of HIV treatment throughout the developing world. In 2003, approximately 100,000 people were receiving antiretroviral therapy in sub-Saharan Africa. By the end of 2007, over two million people were on therapy. Unfortunately, this is only 30% of those who require treatment in the region (Table 2). In addition, wide disparity in access has been evident between countries. Botswana reported that 79% of those who qualified were receiving treatment by the end of 2007, while other countries, such as Ghana, struggled to provide access to a mere 15% of patients.[42] With 5.5 million people infected countrywide, South Africa has the greatest need, yet scale-up has been criticized for its slow pace.[46] By the end of 2007, approximately 300,000 people had initiated treatment.[42]

The scale-up of antiretroviral therapy in both Latin America and the Caribbean has occurred more quickly than in Africa with an estimated 64% and 43% of those needing treatment receiving it by December 2007 (Table 2). Within the region there is also great variation in coverage. Countries such as Brazil, Argentina, Cuba, Costa Rica, and Chile have covered more than 70% of those needing treatment, while in the Dominican Republic and Haiti the coverage is much less widespread.[42]

The challenges facing those working to expand effective treatment programs for both adults and children in resource-poor settings have been substantial. Skilled human resources, including doctors, nurses, pharmacists, and laboratory technicians are severely lacking in most developing countries because of early death due to HIV and brain drain. With 1 doctor for every 60,000 patients, Malawi, a country with an HIV prevalence of 14%, is facing a grave plight.[47] In addition to human resources, general health care infrastructure is sorely lacking. Combating coinfection with tuberculosis (TB) is also a major concern. In many developing countries, the TB case rate has increased fivefold to tenfold since the identification of HIV, and the prevalence of HIV infection among individuals with newly diagnosed TB exceeds 80%.[48] Furthermore, even though drug prices continue to decline, medication stock-outs (both of antiretrovirals and drugs for the prophylaxis and treatment of opportunistic infections such as TB) continue to occur. These deficits place patients at risk for antiretroviral therapy resistance due to nonadherence to first-line regimens. Currently, second-line treatment, which usually includes a protease inhibitor, is costly and less available at treatment sites.

Although these challenges exist, availability of antiretroviral therapy for the prevention of mother-to-child transmission has increased. From 2004 to 2007, access to PMTCT increased from 10 to 33% in all low- and middle-income countries. Undoubtedly, room for improvement in access remains; 420,000 children were newly infected in 2007.[42] Once infected, outcomes are often poor for children. The lack of clinical and laboratory facilities for diagnosing HIV infection, lack of human resource capacity skilled in treating children, and lack of appropriate liquid drug formulations have contributed to a severe deficit in access. Moreover, some have sited lack of political and social will to treat children for HIV as a major barrier that must be overcome if progress is to be made.[49]

Outcomes in Resource-Limited Settings

For those patients in resource-poor settings who have been able to access treatment for HIV, HAART has proven to be very effective. Mortality and morbidity for HIV-infected patients in resource-limited settings have declined markedly with increased access to combination antiretroviral therapy. Short-term follow-up studies from numerous low-income countries in sub-Saharan Africa, the Caribbean, and Latin America have observed sustained immunologic benefit and virologic suppression.[50–52]

Although outcomes have been positive, studies have noted increased mortality secondary to late presentation and lost to follow-up. Braitstein et al. compared outcomes from 18 treatment programs through out Africa, Latin America, and Asia to results from the U.S. and Europe. Immunologic and virologic response to therapy was similar after 6 months in both settings. However, mortality in the lower income countries was higher secondary to more severe disease at the initiation of treatment.[53] Dalal et al. observed high rates of lost to follow-up in South Africa. Nearly 1 in 6 patients were lost to follow-up in a 15-month period.[54]

Success Stories

Antiretroviral Therapy Adherence

Prior to the more widespread availability of antiretroviral therapy in the developing world many questioned the ability of HIV-positive patients in resource-limited settings to adhere to complicated drug regimens. In actuality, higher rates of adherence to HAART have been noted in sub-Sahara Africa than in North America. Millis et al. compared data from 31 adherence studies in North America and 27 studies from Africa. In the North American studies 55% of patients demonstrated adequate adherence compared with 77% of the African participants.[55] High rates of adherence in both adults and children at individual sites throughout the developing world have also been widely reported.[56–58] Several reasons for this finding have been proposed: intense, mandatory adherence training and patient education prior to HAART start, compulsory adherence tools and monitoring, treatment supporters, and the sense of overall emergency in regard to the epidemic. Models of adherence that emphasize communal relationships and social capital have also been employed and may be another factor for the high adherence rates.[59] Though adherence is high, Hardon et al. noted that transportation costs, excessive waiting times at health care facilities, and hunger may threaten long-term adherence to first-line regimens in low-income settings.[60]

National Prevention Strategy

Few countries have experienced a decline in HIV prevalence as significant as that noted in Uganda. The first African nation to successfully reverse the course of its HIV epidemic, Uganda was noted to have a nationwide adult prevalence of 15% in the early 1990s, which fell to approximately 4% by 2003.[1] Evidence of a decline in HIV incidence has also been documented.[61] Some debate has surrounded the reasons for this large-scale decline. However, several facts are incontrovertible. Uganda's National AIDS Control Program began very early in the epidemic and included strong political leadership as well as a significant amount of funding. The centerpiece of Uganda's campaign was health education and widespread communication of messages like "zero grazing," which promotes monogamy as opposed to abstinence. Incorporation of recognized church leadership and PLWHA was also critical to Uganda's multisectoral response. In addition, early efforts to secure the blood supply and develop a comprehensive countrywide surveillance system were key. Efforts also focused on empowering girls and women and targeted young people. Interestingly, the promotion of condom usage was not a program element until the late 1990s.[62,63]

The major effect of these efforts was the alteration of cultural and sexual behavioral norms.[63] Delay in sexual debut, decreased frequency of multiple sexual partners, and narrowing in the age gap between women and men have been documented in numerous studies. Increases in condom usage and voluntary counseling and testing also occurred in the mid to late 1990s.[64,65]

In recent years, there is evidence of stabilization and possibly a slight increase in the prevalence of HIV in Uganda. This trend coincides with a dramatic increase in the availability of HAART and further uptake of condoms and voluntary counseling and testing. Evidence suggests that more young people are having sex with multiple partners, although the age of sexual initiation continues to rise.[62] Understanding the interplay of these factors and developing interventions that will be effective in reversing this rise in HIV prevalence is Uganda's new challenge.

Evidence for population level decline in adult HIV prevalence has also been noted in Kenya and Zimbabwe. In both cases, similar alterations in sexual behavior with decreases in multiple partnerships and delayed age at sexual debut have been cited as causal factors.[66,67]

Circumcision

As mentioned previously, studies have determined that male circumcision decreases HIV transmission from female to male upward of 60%. Though these studies did not demonstrate a direct benefit to the female partners of circumcised men, this discovery has been heralded as the most significant finding since the development of HAART or triple drug regimens.[68] Modeling estimates indicate that male circumcision could avert two million new HIV infections and 0.3 million deaths in sub-Saharan Africa in the next 10 years.[69] However, challenges to widespread dissemination of this intervention remain. Safety in settings where health care infrastructure is suboptimal is a concern.[70] In addition, there is evidence to suggest that transmission risk is increased during the healing period postprocedure.[71] Attention must also be directed toward the implications for not only the patient, but toward his sexual partner(s). Though these challenges exist, the benefit of this procedure outweighs current known risks. Therefore, the WHO recommends rapid establishment of circumcision services to optimize HIV prevention in countries with the highest prevalence.

Condom Use and HIV Prevention

According to estimates made by UNAIDS, the HIV epidemic in Brazil appears to be stabilizing.[1] The simultaneous institution of early treatment access and a vigorous prevention campaign have contributed significantly to this stabilization. Condom use has been central to Brazil's national prevention campaign. The country's aggressive promotion of condoms amongst the general population and within high-risk groups has successfully contributed to sustained control of the epidemic. While in other countries condom ads, if broadcast, have been shaded in nuance, Brazil's media campaign has been glaringly overt. For example, a new line of condoms depicting the logos of the most popular Brazilian soccer teams was promoted using nationwide television ads featuring supporters wearing condom-shaped caps in their team's colors. The condoms broke sales records. Contrary to findings from other countries, the acceptability of the female condom has been high in some studies; therefore, both male and female condoms have been promoted and distributed widely.[72]

Opt-Out Testing

The WHO currently recommends opt-out HIV testing and counseling for all individuals attending healthcare facilities, irrespective of the presence of symptoms or the patient's reasons for accessing healthcare. In the developing world, Botswana was a forerunner in the implementation of opt-out testing in medical settings. Prior to 2003, HIV testing was performed after individuals were counseled with patients actively choosing whether or not they agreed to be tested. Though antiretroviral therapy was available for PMTCT since 2001, very few women who received care at antenatal clinics opted to be tested for HIV. To increase the percentage of women who benefited from HIV testing and subsequent PMTCT, Botswana initiated a nationwide opt-out testing program in 2004. Testing remained confidential and noncompulsory.[73] Creek et al. assessed the efficacy of Botswana's approach and found that the percentage of women receiving PMTCT interventions increased from 29 to 56%.[74] According to the 2007 UNAIDS report, 77% of all pregnant women were tested for HIV in 2007 and more than 95% received antiretroviral therapy for PMTCT. Kenya, Malawi, Uganda, and Zambia have implemented similar programs.[1]

Applying Lessons Learned Internationally to the U.S.

The U.S. has suffered from a concentrated epidemic since the first cases were noted in the early 1980s. MSM, minority populations, particularly African Americans and Latinos, and injection drug users have been disproportionately affected. As of 2007, 1.2 million people were estimated to be living with HIV nationally. Annual incidence is down from its peak in the 1980s. However, a potential rise in new cases amongst the most highly impacted populations has been noted.[75] In Washington, DC, the nation's capitol, HIV prevalence within certain populations has been found to be similar to that noted in resource-limited regions of the world.[76]

As scale-up of international treatment programs has progressed, expertise from the U.S. and other western nations where HAART has been available since the mid-1990s has been instrumental. Can any lessons learned through rapid scale-up in the developing world be utilized in the U.S.? As discussed earlier, one of the primary reasons that several countries have noted for a decline in HIV prevalence is the presence of a national strategic plan that incorporates both comprehensive prevention programming and universal access to treatment. Some progress has been made in the development of a national strategy that will specifically target the most vulnerable, disproportionately impacted populations in the U.S. In June 2008, the U.S. House of Representatives Financial Services Appropriations Subcommittee approved a bill that includes $1.4 million to the White House Office of National AIDS Policy for the development of a National AIDS Strategy.

Opt-out testing has a proven benefit in increasing the acceptability of HIV testing and in normalizing the process of obtaining an HIV test. Opt-out testing has been implemented successfully in resource-limited settings. In the U.S. one in four people who are estimated to be HIV positive are unaware of their status. Those who are unaware of their status are more likely to engage in risky behaviors and therefore have a higher likelihood of transmitting HIV. In 2006, the Centers for Disease Control and Prevention (CDC) recommended that opt-out HIV screening be a part of routine clinical care in all health-care settings for patients of age 13–64.[77] Though opt-out testing has been recommended, few programs have been implemented. Many challenges exist for widespread opt-out testing strategies to be successfully implemented. These include limits on funding for treatment, human resource shortages, and time constraints.[78] However, most agree that opt-out testing is an appropriate and long overdue intervention that must be undertaken in order to reach those who are unaware of infection and ultimately lower the rate of new HIV infections.

Lastly, although studies have shown that adherence to HAART is higher in many resource-limited settings than it is in settings such as the U.S., little is known about whether or not models that promote adherence in the developing world can be transferred to domestic health care settings. As mentioned, many national treatment plans in the developing world have mandated adherence training prior to starting HAART. Intensive adherence training is not standard in health care settings where HIV-infected patients are treated in the U.S. In addition, treatment supporters who assist patients to remain adherent to HAART are a frequent component of programs in resource-limited settings. This model has been implemented in a few locations in the U.S. with some success.[79] Further research should be undertaken to identify the factors that promote adherence in the developing world and to determine their applicability to the U.S. setting.

Remaining Challenges and Conclusions

Over the last few years significant strides have been made that have decreased morbidity and mortality secondary to HIV/AIDS. However, many challenges remain if the rate of new infections is to be further slowed and the goal of universal access to care and treatment is to be reached worldwide. There have been notable failures in critical areas. For example, minimal progress has been made in vaccine development. The most recent vaccine trial sponsored by Merck Pharmaceuticals yielded negative trial results and in post hoc analysis actually increased the risk of HIV transmission.[80] In addition, though studies are ongoing, researchers have thus far been unable to identify an effective microbicide that would decrease the vaginal or rectal transmission of HIV.[81] Both of these factors have led to a reaffirmation of the need to emphasize known prevention strategies and treatment.

Although these and other challenges that have been discussed do exist, efforts to end this epidemic must intensify. Continued focus must be directed toward those populations who are most highly impacted by this disease both domestically and internationally. Failure to do so will lead to increased inequality within populations already suffering from extreme health care disparities.

References

1. UNAIDS. 2007 AIDS Epidemic Update. Available at: http://www.unaids.org/en/ KnowledgeCentre/HIVData/EpiUpdate/EpiUpdArchive/2007/. Accessed on June 30, 2008.
2. European Study Group on Heterosexual Transmission of HIV. Comparison of female to male and male to female transmission of HIV in 563 stable couples. BMJ. 1992;304:809–13.
3. Mastro TD, de Vincezzi I. Probabilities of sexual HIV transmission. AIDS. 1996;10 Suppl A:S75–82.
4. Vittinghoff E, Douglas J, Judson F, et al. Per-contact risk of human immunodeficiency virus transmission between male sexual partners. Am J Epidemiol. 1999;150:306–11.
5. Sa Z, Larsen U. Gender inequality increases women's risk of hiv infection in Moshi, Tanzania. J Biosoc Sci. 2008;40:505–25. Epub 2007 Dec 19.
6. Clark S. Early marriage and HIV risks in sub-Saharan Africa. Stud Fam Plann. 2004;35: 149–60.
7. Report National HIV and Syphilis Prevalence Survey South Africa 2006 Department of Health South Africa, 2007. Available at: http://www.doh.gov.za/docs/reports/2007/hiv/part1. pdf. Accessed on June 30, 2008.
8. UNAIDS Fact Sheet: Sub-Saharan Africa. 2006. Available at: http://data.unaids.org/pub/ GlobalReport/2006/200605-FS_SubSaharanAfrica_en.pdf. Accessed on June 30, 2008.
9. Mahomva A, Greby S, Dube, S, et al. Sexually transmitted infections HIV prevalence and trends from data in Zimbabwe, 1997–2004. Sex Transm Infect. 2006;82 Suppl 1:i42–7.
10. Federal Ministry of Health Nigeria, 2005 Sentinel Survey. Available at: http://www. nigeria-aids.org/pdf/2005SentinelSurvey.pdf. Accessed on: June 30, 2008.
11. Auvert B, Taljaard D, Lagarde E, et al. Randomized, controlled intervention trial of male circumcision for reduction of HIV infection risk: the ANRS 1265 Trial. PLoS Med. 2005;2:e298.
12. Bailey RC, Moses S, Parker CB, et al. Male circumcision for HIV prevention in young men in Kisumu, Kenya: a randomized controlled trial. Lancet. 2007;369:643–56.
13. Gray RH, Kigozi G, Sirwadda D et al. Male circumcision for HIV prevention in men in Rakai, Uganda: a randomized trial. Lancet. 2007;369:657–66.
14. World Health Organization. Male circumcision for HIV prevention. Available at: http://www.who.int/entity/hiv/topics/malecircumcision/JC1320_MaleCircumcision_Final\ _UNAIDS.pdf. Accessed on June 30, 2008.
15. Freeman EE, Weiss HA, Glynn JR, et al. Herpes simplex virus 2 infection increases HIV acquisition in men and women: systematic review and meta-analysis of longitudinal studies. AIDS. 2006;20:73–83.
16. Wald A, Link K. Risk of human immunodeficiency virus infection in herpes simplex virus type 2-seropositive persons: a meta-analysis. J Infect Dis. 2002;185:45–52.
17. Celum CL. The interaction between herpes simplex virus and human immunodeficiency virus. Herpes. 2004;11 Suppl 1:36A–45A.
18. Weiss H. Epidemiology of herpes simplex virus type 2 infection in the developing world. Herpes. 2004;11 Suppl 1:24A–35A. Review.
19. Celum C, Wald A, Hughes J, et al. HSV-2 suppressive therapy for prevention of HIV acquisition: results of HPTN 039. 2008. Fifteenth Conference on Retroviruses and Opportunistic Infections, Boston, abstract 32LB.69.
20. Watson-Jones D, Rusizoka M, Weiss H, et al. Impact of HSV-2 suppressive therapy on HIV incidence in HSV-2 seropositive women: a randomised controlled trial in Tanzania. 2007. Abstract MOAC104. Fourth IAS Conference on HIV pathogensis, treatment and prevention 2007, Sydney, Australia.

21. Mastro TD, Satten GA, Nopkesorn T et al. Probability of female-to-male transmission of HIV-1 in Thailand. Lancet.1994;343:204–7.
22. Halperin DT, Epstein H. Concurrent sexual partnerships help to explain Africa's high HIV prevalence: implications for prevention. Lancet. 2004 Jul 3–9;364:4–6.
23. CAREC. CAREC Surveillance Report Supplement, Vol. 23, Supplement 1; October 2003.
24. Allen CF, Edwards M, Williamson LM et al. Sexually transmitted infection service use and risk factors for HIV infection among female sex workers in Georgetown, Guyana. J Acquir Immune Defic Syndr. 2006;43:96–101.
25. UNAIDS Epidemic Update, December 2005. Available at: http://www.who.int/hiv/epi-update2005_en.pdf. Accessed on June 30, 2008.
26. Caistor N, Henrys JH, Street A. HIV and AIDS in Haiti. Catholic Institute for International Relations, UK; 2008:6–17.
27. Cohen J. HIV/AIDS: Latin America & Caribbean. HAITI: making headway under hellacious circumstances. Science. 2006;313:470–3.
28. Gaillard EM, Boulos LM, Andre Cayemettes MP, et al. Understanding the reasons for decline of HIV prevalence in Haiti. Sex Transm Inf. 2006;82 Suppl 1:i14–20.
29. Hsieh YH, Arazoza H, Lee SM, et al. Estimating the number of Cubans infected sexually by human immunodeficiency virus using contact tracing data. Int J Epi. 2002;31:679–683.
30. Arazoza H, Joanes J, Lounes R, et al. The HIV/AIDS epidemic in Cuba: description and tentative explanation of its low HIV prevalence. BMC Infect Dis. 2007;7:130.
31. Cohen J. Cuba Increasing HIV Prevention Efforts Targeted at MSM, Health Officials Says. Available at: www.medicalnewstoday.com/articles/107389.php. Accessed on June 30, 2008.
32. Aceijas C, Stimson GV, Hickman M, et al. Global overview of injecting drug use and HIV infection among injecting drug users. AIDS. 2004;18:2295–303.
33. Cohen J. HIV/AIDS: Latin America & Caribbean. Puerto Rico: rich port, poor port. Science. 2006;313:475–6.
34. Berkman A, Garcia J, Munoz-Laboy M, et al. A critical analysis of the Brazilian response to HIV/AIDS: lessons learned for controlling and mitigating the epidemic in developing countries. Am J Public Health. 2005;95:1162–72.
35. Levi GC, Vitoria MA. Fighting against AIDS: the Brazilian experience. AIDS. 2002;16:2373–83.
36. Okie S. Fighting HIV-Lessons from Brazil. NEJM. 2006;354:1977–81.
37. Cohen J. HIV/AIDS: Latin America & Caribbean. Overview: the overlooked epidemic. Science. 2006;313:468–9.
38. Bronfman MN, Leyva R, Negroni MJ, et al. Mobile populations and HIV/AIDS in Central America and Mexico: research for action. AIDS 2002;16 Suppl 3:S42–S49.
39. Magis-Rodriguez C, Gayet C, Negroni M, et al. Migration and AIDS in Mexico: an overview based on recent evidence. J Acquir Immune Defic Syndr. 2004;37 Suppl 4:S215–S226.
40. The Global Fund to Fight HIV, TB and Malaria. Available at: http://www.theglobalfund.org/en/about/how/. Accessed on June 30, 2008.
41. World Health Organization. Progress on Global Access to HIV Antiretroviral Therapy: A Report on "3 by 5" and Beyond, March 2006. Available at: www.who.int/hiv/fullreport_en_highres.pdf. Accessed on July 20, 2008.
42. UNAIDS. Towards Universal Access: Scaling Up Priority HIV/AIDS Interventions in the Health Sector. 2008. Available at: www.who.int/hiv/mediacentre/2008progressreport/en/index.html Accessed on June 30, 2008.
43. President's Emergency Plan for AIDS Relief. Available at: http://www.pepfar.gov/. Accessed on June 30, 2008.
44. Steinbrook R. Providing antiretroviral therapy for HIV infection. NEJM. 2001;344:844–6.
45. Drug Access: Clinton Foundation, Global Fund, World Bank, UNICEF Extend Low-Cost Generic AIDS Drug Prices to More Than 100 Countries. Available at: http://www.kaisernetwork.org/daily_reports/rep_index.cfm?DR_ID=23059. Accessed on July 4, 2008.
46. Ojikutu B, Jack C, Ramjee G, et al. Provision of antiretroviral therapy in South Africa: unique challenges and remaining obstacles. J Infect Dis. 2007;196 Suppl 3:S523–27.

47. Malawi: Health Worker Shortage a Challenge to AIDS Treatment. http://www.irinnews.org/report.aspx?reportid=61598. Accessed on: June 30, 2008.
48. Corbett EL, Marston B, Churchyard GJ, et al. Tuberculosis in sub-Saharan Africa: opportunities, challenges, and change in the era of antiretroviral treatment. Lancet 2006;367:926–37.
49. Kline M. Perspectives on the pediatric HIV/AIDS pandemic: catalyzing access of children to care and treatment. Pediatrics. 2006;117:1388–93.
50. Ferrandini L, Jeannin A, Pinoges L, et al. Scaling up of highly active antiretroviral therapy in a rural district of Malawi: an effectiveness assessment. Lancet. 2006;367:1335–42.
51. Brigido L, Rodrigues R, Vasseb J, et al. CD4+ T-cell recovery and clinical outcome in HIV-1-infected patients exposed to multiple antiretroviral regimens: partial control of viremia is associated with favorable outcome. AIDS Patient Care STDS. 2004;18:189–98.
52. Kilaru KR, Kumar A, Sippy N, et al. Immunological and virological responses to highly active antiretroviral therapy in a non-clinical trial setting in a developing Caribbean country. HIV Med. 2006;7:99–104.
53. Braitstein P, Brinkhof MW, Dabis F, et al. Mortality of HIV-1-infected patients in the first year of antiretroviral therapy: comparison between low-income and high-income countries. Lancet 2006;367:817–24.
54. Dalal RP, Macphail C, Mqhayi M, et al. Characteristics and outcomes of adult patients lost to follow-up at an antiretroviral treatment clinic in johannesburg, South Africa. J Acquir Immune Defic Syndr. 2008;47:101–7.
55. Mills EJ, Nachega JB, Buchan I, et al. Adherence to antiretroviral therapy in sub-Saharan Africa and North America: a meta-analysis. JAMA. 2006;296:679–90.
56. Remien RH, Bastos FI, Jnr VT, et al. Adherence to antiretroviral therapy in a context of universal access, in Rio de Janeiro, Brazil. AIDS Care. 2007;19:740–8.
57. Etard JF, Lanièce I, Fall MB, et al. A 84-month follow up of adherence to HAART in a cohort of adult Senegalese patients. Trop Med Int Health. 2007;12:1191–8.
58. Reddi A, Leeper SC. Antiretroviral therapy adherence in children: outcomes from Africa. AIDS. 2008;22:906–7.
59. Ware NC, Wyatt MA, Bangsberg D. Examining theoretic models of adherence for validity in resource-limited settings. A heuristic approach. J Acquir Immune Defic Syndr. 2006;43 Suppl 1:S18–22.
60. Hardon AP, Aukurt D, Comoro C, et al. Hunger, waiting time and transport costs: time to confront challenges to ART adherence in Africa. AIDS Care. 2007;19:658–65.
61. Mbulaiteye SM, Mahe C, Whitworth JA, et al. Declining HIV-1 incidence and associated prevalence over 10 years in a rural population in south-west Uganda: a cohort study. Lancet. 2002;360:41–6.
62. Green EC, Halperin DT, Nantulya V, et al. Uganda's HIV prevention success: the role of sexual behavior change and the national response. AIDS Behav. 2006;10:335–46.
63. Slutkin G, Okware S, Naamara W, et al. How Uganda reversed its HIV epidemic. AIDS Beh. 2006;10:351–60.
64. Ukwuani FA, Tsui AO, Suchindran CM, et al. Condom use for preventing HIV infection/AIDS in sub-Saharan Africa: a comparative multilevel analysis of Uganda and Tanzania. J Acquir Immune Defic Syndr. 2003;34:203–13.
65. Wakabi W. Condoms still contentious in Uganda's struggle over AIDS. Lancet 2006;367:1387–8.
66. Cheluget B, Baltazar G, Orege P, et al. Evidence for population level declines in adult HIV prevalence in Kenya. Sex Transm Inf. 2006;82:i21–i26.
67. Gregson S, Garnett GP, Nyamukapa C, et al. HIV decline associated with behavior change in eastern Zimbabwe. Science. 2006;311:664–66.
68. Turner AN, Morrison CS, Padian NS, et al. Men's circumcision status and women's risk of HIV acquisition in Zimbabwe and Uganda. AIDS. 2007;21:1779–89.
69. Williams B, Lloyd-Smith J, Hankins C, et al. The potential impact of male circumcision on HIV in Sub-Saharan Africa. PLoS Med. 2006;3:e262.
70. Johnson KE, Quinn TC. Update on male circumcision: prevention success and challenges ahead. Cur Inf Dis Rep. 2008;10:243–51.

71. Kigozi G, Gray RH, Wawer MJ, et al. The safety of adult male circumcision in HIV-infected and uninfected men in Rakai, Uganda. PLoS Med. 2008;5:e116.
72. Barbosa RM, Kalckman S, Berquo E, et al. Notes on the female condom: experiences in Brazil. Int J STD AIDS. 2007;18:261–6.
73. Centers for Disease Control and Prevention. Introduction of routine HIV testing in prenatal care–Botswana, 2004. MMWR Mord Mort Weekly Rep. 2004;53:1083–86.
74. Creek TL, Ntumy R, Seipone K, et al. Successful introduction of routine opt-out HIV testing in antenatal care in Botswana. J Acquir Immune Defic Syndr. 2007;45:102–7.
75. Centers for Disease Control and Prevention (CDC) Increases in HIV diagnoses–29 States, 1999–2002. MMWR Morb Mortal Wkly Rep. 2003;52:1145–8.
76. Government of the District of Columbia DoHHAABoSaE. The District of Columbia HIV/AIDS Epidemiology Annual Report 2007.
77. Branson BM, Hansfield HH, Lampe MA, et al. Revised recommendations for HIV testing of adults, adolescents, and pregnant women in health-care settings. MMWR Recomm Rep. 2006;55:1–17.
78. Saag M. Opt-out testing: who can afford to take care of patients with newly diagnosed HIV infection? Clin Inf Dis. 2007;45 Suppl 4:S261–5.
79. Behforouz H, Farmer P, Mukherjee J. From directly observed therapy to accompagnateurs: enhancing AIDS treatment outcomes in Haiti and in Boston. Clin Infect Dis. 2004;38 Suppl 5:S429–36.
80. HIV vaccine failure prompts Merck to halt trial. Nature. 2007;449:390.
81. Padma TV. After microbicide failures, hope that antiviral approach will gel. Nat Med. 2008;14:354.

Index